The
Opposite
of
Butterfly
Hunting

The Opposite of Butterfly Hunting

The Tragedy and The Glory of Growing Up

A Memoir

Evanna Lynch

Ballantine Books

New York

Published in the United States by Ballantine Books,
an imprint of Random House, a division of
Penguin Random House LLC, New York.

Ballantine and the House colophon are registered trademarks of
Penguin Random House LLC.

Published in the United Kingdom by Headline Publishing Group,
a Hachette UK Company, in 2021.

Trade paperback ISBN 978-0-593-35841-2
Ebook ISBN 978-0-593-35840-5

Printed in the United States of America on acid-free paper

randomhousebooks.com

2nd Printing

For Simon –
a fearless writer, passionate storyteller
and an irreplaceable friend

Man builds on what he has known in the course of the first months of his life: if he has not felt hungry, he will be one of those strange elect, or those strange damned souls who refuse to build their lives around a lack.

— Amélie Nothomb, *The Life of Hunger*

Foreword

'Is this perhaps a bit cruel?'

This was the note that repeatedly cropped up in the margins from everyone who read or worked on the early drafts of this book – from my friends, family, editor, copy-editor, lawyer, doctor and also, very often, from myself. The cruelty of the words I'd written unsettled me but did not surprise me. And despite my own and my editor's most mindful and considered efforts, this book remains, at times, kind of mean. So, I wanted to prepare you for that.

I knew it would be impossible to write a memoir about my journey towards self-love and acceptance without also writing an in-depth exploration of my self-hate. Too often in life – and in stories – we rush to find the happy ending, even if that ending is an artifice. We have this compulsion to turn every story into a fairy tale. People want to believe in fairy tales, I get that, and that childlike insistence on believing good things will happen is beautiful, and the ability to find the light in the midst of darkness is the mark of a truly resilient spirit. Absolutely, there is something admirable about our capacity to smile and present a brave face even when we are hurting. But I think there is also something else going on here, something a little bit sinister and concerning about our refusal to admit to anything other than perfect happiness, and I think it's because we're afraid of our own darkness. We're afraid that if we fully surrender to our darkness, we'll never come back from it. We're afraid our darkness will go on and on and on, that there *is* no end to it and that we will get lost in it. We're afraid that if we show these ugly, unpalatable parts of ourselves, it will be too much for others; that nobody will love and accept us, and we'll be left alone with only the worst parts of ourselves for company. So, we don't let ourselves get too deep into self-hate – at least, not in public. We hurry to slap on the happy ending and construct a heroic tale before the healing has even begun.

The thing is, I don't believe this coping mechanism is the healthiest way of dealing with darkness. I've read articles depicting my life as a fairy tale even as I sat at home consumed by darkness, and those stories only compounded my feelings of isolation and disillusionment. And what I've found out is that darkness is not infinite, that you *do* actually get to the other side of it, but first you have to submerge yourself in it. You have to stop skating above the surface of your depths. You have to confront and accept this darkness in order to heal from it. This is why there are parts of this book where I had to submerge myself and the reader in moments of utter desolation. Why I had to be honest about the moments where it felt like every light had gone out.

I know that stories of eating disorders – such as the one I'm sharing in this book – can seem unendingly bleak, and therein lies our frenzied need to truncate the long road to recovery and rush to a place of positivity, a hearty commitment to self-love, but I think in doing so we gloss over the intense cruelty inherent within them; after all, the cruelty of eating disorders can literally starve a person to death. I've found, when reading other stories similar to mine, that the book often ends at the point where the person dissociates themselves from their disorder. They create a distance and step back, attributing all those dark, hateful thoughts neatly to this thing that's been identified as a sickness. But personally, I found that even after my fixation on food and controlling my body had gone away, that darkness was still present – and, indeed, it had been there long before the eating disorder ever took residence in my mind. In so many ways, the anorexia was just a distraction. And – both in my healing journey and in writing this book – I wanted to get to the bottom of that darkness. I wanted to unpack it and understand what really was beneath this compelling distraction: an addiction not to thinness, but to negative thinking, to safety, to staying small in all ways so that I wouldn't have to deal with the terrifying reality of fully living life. I wanted to submerge myself in this darkness for this book and find my way through it, because, ultimately, I do actually believe in fairy tales. Not the shallow, saccharine sort peddled by tabloids and short-lived self-help manifestos. I believe in the kind of fairy tales that have depth, complexity, profundity and moments of darkness that birth a fiercer belief in light; the kind where the endings are not endings but breakthroughs that lead to the next adventure. And my intention with this book was to shed light on a darkness that is most often obscured by myths, misunderstanding and sensationalism.

In order to tell the story with integrity, I had to discuss moments and thoughts that provide insights into the mind of someone with an eating disorder, and, certainly, many of these parts could be triggering to readers. That's why, before you read any further, I need to highlight that this book explores a variety of sensitive topics, including eating disorders, self-harm, suicide, fat-phobia and self-hate in various other guises. I would advise any reader to use their personal discretion when reading this book, and to step away from it if it triggers unhealthy thoughts. I'm of the belief that when struggling with mental-health issues or the early stages of recovery, virtually everything is triggering, and the onus is on the individual and on their support system to identify the things that are disproportionately triggering, and to take precautions to avoid being bombarded by these things. I would advise you to do whatever feels best to you, and to keep reading only as long as this book feels eye-opening, inspiring or comforting, which I hope it is.

I was determined from the start that this book would not become a 'how-to' manual for eating disorders. For this reason, I've decided to omit any specific details of weight, calorie counting, and health statistics. I don't feel they are relevant or necessary to tell this story, and any urge to include these details in any conversation around eating disorders is actually the voice of the eating disorder, which wants to provoke horror and awe, to be identified by a series of numbers and statistics, and to distract its audience from the deeper issues. I would go further and say that any publication or book that reveals the weight and calorie count of a person with an eating disorder does not serve the reader's best interests, and personally I would avoid them. We need to stop playing so neatly into the hands of eating disorders by measuring people's sickness and health by the numbers on the scale. That's a belief I stand by. There is mention of specific foods, the concept of 'safe foods' and 'fear foods', and descriptions of eating, but I have tried to keep these vague and have only included these details where they were relevant to telling the story. Once again, I hope you will use your discretion and skip any part that is triggering to read.

On a separate note, I'd like to mention that all names and identifying characteristics of doctors, nurses, hospital staff and of other young people I encountered in hospitals and clinics have been changed to protect their privacy. The hospital and clinic I attended have been given pseudonyms. All of the stories recounted are true, but a few times I have deliberately given a certain anecdote or moment to a different person in the story. This was done to further protect privacy. I've endeavoured to tell the story chronologically but, as you will see, the road to recovery is a difficult one to track, and there were a few times where it made narrative sense to alter the timeline of the actual events, though this was only done in a couple places.

Ultimately, this is a story of choosing creativity, love and a positive outlook on life, so I promise, however dark it gets at points, not to leave you in that place. I hope that by submerging readers in my darkness at times when it really felt like my situation was hopeless, this story will inspire in you the courage, vision and determination to confront your demons. More than anything else, I hope this story helps you find the lighted path out of your own darkness.

1

'What's rape?' I pipe up from my spot on the floor, craning my neck around to peer at my mother. It feels like the kind of subject that warrants eye contact and careful scrutiny of her micro-expressions.

'Hmm?' she asks. Her expression is frozen, her widened eyes fixated on the TV screen as her hands pass absent-mindedly over a pillow slip on the ironing board.

'Rape,' I enunciate clearly, as the newsreader continues on in a sombre monotone in the background. 'What does he mean by that, exactly?'

I see her eyes dart to my dad in his armchair, but his gaze is fixed determinedly on the TV, his mouth pressed into a stern line. She is going to have to take this one.

'Ahhhhm . . .' She deliberates, returning to her ironing, but then answers plainly: 'It's when a man forces a woman to have sex with him.'

My hands freeze in mid-air, and a few of the beads I am stringing together drop to the floor in front of me. There's no denying that my mother has just uttered a rare and spicy word, one uncommonly breathed within the four walls of our living room. Its sudden, shocking presence is felt in the silence of my parents, a silence that is bursting with the tension of things held back. The iron releases a sensual, throaty exhale. I see Mum is steadily avoiding my gaze, but the 'sex' word has ignited a spark in the room, and I know I must pounce before it goes out and we all fall back into a comfortable inertia.

'Why would he want to do that?' I ask, not managing to mask the excitement in my voice. My dad's frown flickers over to me from beneath bushy eyebrows and then back to the telly. He will probably work on feigning sleep in a moment. Mum looks anxious and deeply uncomfortable as she strains to articulate the inner motives of your average rapist to a ten-year-old.

'Well, it's because . . . I suppose . . . he wants the woman so much that he decides to just . . . take her.' She grimaces as she props the iron upright and starts to fold the pillow slip.

'And the woman doesn't want it?' I press her, the string of beads stretched taut between my hands, my attention rapt with my mother's discomfort.

'Well, no, she doesn't . . . that's what rape is. The woman doesn't want it.' She wrinkles her nose as she spreads the folded pillow slip on top of her pile of ironing and pats it. 'Not very nice,' she summarises, and then plucks a school shirt from the pile of laundry, starting on the sleeves.

'THE TAOISEACH HAS ANNOUNCED A REFERENDUM WILL BE HELD—' the newsreader blares, rudely interrupting my thought spiral, and I see my dad pressing down hard on the remote control volume button.

'*Whissht!!*' he says to the room, his glasses glinting. 'I want to hear this.'

I steal another glance at Mum, who is serenely working on the collar now, all trace of sordid sex words wiped from her face. Ostensibly, I return to my beadwork, where a neat little fairy is taking shape, but my mind lingers stubbornly on rape. *Not very nice*, I think, puzzled. I snip a fresh length of wire and start on a wing, threading three iridescent seed beads and weaving them into a point. Her assessment of rape is at odds with my understanding of the mechanics of sexual intercourse. Everything about the context of this conversation suggests rape is something not to be coveted: something dark, unspeakable, serious. Something thematically similar to sex, but worse. I turn the words and images of unsolicited sex over in my mind as I weave another row of beads that shimmer with rainbow reflections. *Wants the woman . . . so much . . . he just takes her. Wow!* I think. *How flattering!* Imagine being so beautiful, so attractive, so irresistibly desirable that someone can't help themselves from having you! *Fabulous*, I think enviously, trying to picture these mythically intoxicating women whose bodies turn men into slavering sex-thieves. I couldn't understand the reactions of my parents to the mention of rape – the look of disturbed anguish that crossed Mum's face, along with an unmistakable hint of reproval, as if the newsreader had thoughtlessly implicated her in this all-too-sordid affair; the sudden stiffness in my dad's crossed arms as he stared owlishly at the TV screen, his chin seeming to retreat into his collar in distaste – but their body language, and the fact that this was on the national news, told me that rape was serious. The police were looking for a man of about twenty-five, the newsreader had said, who'd raped an unnamed schoolteacher at her home one evening. He'd described it with the same sober tones applied to other violent crimes, making it clear that rape was illegal. I could imagine how it would be a bother to be put upon, when one wasn't expecting it, quietly making beans on toast on a school night. I could see that it might even be unpleasant. But sinful? Illegal? My understanding of the finer logistical details of sex was limited, certainly – I'd had no desire to sink my mind into the wormholes of humanity's lowest, most perverse instincts, and my curiosity had been satisfied by an understanding of the absolute basics – but even I had heard tell that sex was something every adult wanted and sought, something natural, something inevitable, something that was possibly – allegedly – even pleasurable. Hadn't we all got here, many of us accidentally so, by an act of sex? But, playing devil's advocate, my mind flicked through a series of men I wouldn't like to be put upon by. The dopey-eyed boy who sat beside me in class, who always had a stream of toxic-green snot dripping from the nostril I sat nearest to. The freckly farm boy who would hiss graphically violent threats from behind his pile of books, detailing how he was going to run down my cats with his dad's combine harvester. *No, thank you.* The tendrils of my mind even snaked their way to the image of a sharp-nosed, elderly neighbour, who I imagined had a sort of dense, moss-covered mass rather than a naked body beneath those sleeveless wool jumpers and pressed slacks. I suppressed a shiver. I'd most definitely prefer to be left to my own devices. But even with the bad breath, musky man-stink and suffocating bulk, I couldn't help but feel a wave of magnanimous sympathy towards these poor, pathetic male speci-mens, mollified as I was by the overriding sentiment of being, above all things, flattered by their hypothetical feverish desire. The idea that someone could crave and admire your very flesh so much that they would commit a criminal act was impossible to grasp, and I wondered how special you had to be to be so desired. And, after all, wasn't sex otherwise commonly known as 'love-making'? Nobody really got hurt, did they? No harm, no foul. Wasn't the simplest solution to just lie back and accept the love? Shake it off and take the compliment? There was something else intriguing lingering within this interesting new concept of rape and uncontrollable sexual urges: something the woman in this news story seemed to possess that the man clearly didn't. Something the female body had that drove men into a wild, primitive frenzy; something so precious and rare that, with it, womankind had an aura of something greater than her sex or her flesh or her beauty: she had power.

Later that evening, I sit in my piano teacher's hallway, my religion homework open on my lap, my mind absolutely teeming with scandalous visions of rape. My older sister is dutifully plunking her way through her Grade 6 sonatas in the next room. She is a grade ahead of me, playing dizzyingly complex pieces with inscrutable time codes and an unfathomable number of extra notes crammed into the bars. I always catch up a year later, her passing me the now slightly yellowed and creased songbook, and learn the very same pieces she'd mastered – but, somehow, by the time I learn them, they don't sound impressive anymore, or even difficult. She falters and slips up far less than I did half an hour previously, and now I hear her finish the piece to the end of the phrase, and the muffled trill of praise my teacher gives her. My sister practises more often than I do, but she is also more naturally talented, which makes her inclined to practise more, and me less. I sigh, frustrated, and strain my mind to focus only on my religion homework, my religion homework, my religion homework, but all I can think about is rape, rape, rape. If, as legend had it, every man who gets married has sex, and if, as my teacher explained it, they're not having sex *until* they get married . . . do they all want to rape the rest of the time? Are all unmarried men . . . rapists? Are they all gasping thirstily in secret at the unbearable, tantalising sensuality of womankind?

In the Gospel of Matthew, my textbook enquires, *why would nobody approach the leper?*

Possibly because he was a rapist? my mind provides. Being a single man with a flesh-eating disease who nobody would touch, let alone sleep with, it seems inevitable he would also become a rapist – and, based on my studies in Catholicism so far, that would be even worse than the leprosy. *Was Jesus . . . a rapist?* my mind dares. Images of the Stations of the Cross at our local church, where mournful, hooded women draped themselves sorrowfully at the foot of a scantily clad Jesus swim to mind. Heaven knew he had his pick of fawning groupies. But then I think of how much my dad reveres Jesus, and how he cringes at the very mention of sex, and the incongruous nature of a sex-having Jesus. *No,* I think, *impossible, that's why he's Jesus.*

My mind is working overtime, rapidly attributing the sins of mankind to this vital, previously unknown piece of the puzzle of life. It suddenly seems an impossible task to complete my religion homework without the mention of rape.

At that moment, as though overhearing my train of thought, the TV in the kitchen pipes up with the same fateful story. It's just after 9pm (early bedtimes are not a concept my family understands so yes, absolutely, piano lessons 'til 9pm on a school night), so of course RTE news is on again. This is one thing you must understand about

Irish culture: RTE news is always on. Daily life is *built* around RTE news. Dinner is served *after* the 6pm news, and homework is done *before* the 9pm news. 'That's *desperate*,' my mother would say almost daily while watching the 6pm news, her right hand paused in the action of chopping carrots, her left hand clutching absent-mindedly at her chest. 'Terrible. Yeah. Yeah,' my dad would agree, nodding solemnly in perfect chorus with dads across the country at the story of a middle-aged woman who's burned down her family home with her three sleeping children inside. And though they may appear increasingly distressed and horrified at each grim news story, though they watched the same depressing stories three hours ago and nothing has improved since, let me assure you, they fucking *love* the news. It makes them feel simultaneously grateful for and ashamed of their own humble, comfortable lives. I think it even makes them feel like they're *doing* good – that virtuous, charitable, kind people sit down at the end of a long working day and stoically subject themselves to all manner of real-life horrors that are occurring in the lives of strangers, rather than relaxing and enjoying their own evenings too much, like godless hedonists. In Ireland, you can always rest assured that when you're going through a painful period in your life, there is, at any moment, a sea of people in armchairs all across the nation who are so racked with guilt and embarrassment at their own nice lives that they will attempt to psychically shoulder the burden of your personal trauma. Your suffering is never in vain in Ireland; it's almost like you're providing a service.

I am sitting very still, barely breathing, trying to glean any further texture on the rape story that the 6pm news may have glossed over, when the kitchen door snaps open. A plate of biscuits emerges, followed by Sheila, my piano teacher's mother.

'Hello, love,' Sheila coos as I quickly scan the biscuit selection, mentally planning which one I'll have: custard creams, bourbons and plain digestives, a standard but satisfactory working-class array. Sheila often visits me on my stool in the hallway between lessons for a chat, asking about school and piano exams, though the biscuits are a rare perk. 'Will ya have a biscuit?' She proffers the plate and I try my luck, clumsily grasping a bourbon and custard cream together in the one fist. I think I have done so covertly until Sheila chuckles in amusement.

'How's school, love?' she asks kindly.

'Yeah, fine.'

'And how was your lesson?'

'Yeah, it was good,' I reply, hoping she hadn't overheard me playing while passing through the hallway.

'And you're doing your homework, good girl.' Her eyes light up as they fall on my religion copybook. 'Did you do these?' she says, picking up the copybook and gesturing to the coloured-pencil drawings of Jesus and his disciples.

'Yes.' I shrug, quietly pleased by her tone of exaggerated awe. I've worked particularly carefully to give each of Jesus's twelve disciples a differently patterned robe, accentuating their individuality. They are a stunningly characterful bunch, who I hope will earn me a gold star the next day at school. Sheila flicks through the pages of my copybook, 'ooh'-ing and 'aah'-ing at my artistic interpretations of the New Testament, and it gives me a chance to contemplate her, with her cream-coloured, candy floss hair and knee-length wool cardigans. She is approximately seventy-five, maybe a fit-looking eighty. In the kitchen, Sheila's shy husband Jack is glued to the news, the yellow glare of the overhead strip light glancing off his shiny pate. I stare at the back of his head and wonder if his mind is also pulsing with the scandalous news story. I look back at Sheila, my mind whirring as I contemplate this sweet, wholesome couple. If they had sex, at some point or another had he only wanted sex a sensible amount, a procreative amount? Sheila hands me back my copybook, calling me a good girl once again. I smile back, warily though, as she returns to the kitchen, shutting the door behind her, and I feel more confused than ever by these sordid adult secrets wriggling their way into my daily life like worms from damp earth.

And then – I can't help it – later that evening, I ponder my parents' relationship in the kitchen as I chew on some leftover pasta bake. I size up my dad as he reads the paper and munches a large handful of almonds. No – I strike him off easily. There just isn't enough passion there for any swell of sexual fervour – it's all siphoned into his hurling team. Jesus and my dad are both characteristically unsuited towards those carnal proclivities. But everyone else . . . I wonder at them all.

What would it take to be so wanted that someone couldn't help but have you? That night before bed, I scrutinise my flesh in the bathroom mirror, this mirror that has seen far too much of me and my family, all these private, unpleasant moments, witnessed and reflected back. But now I'm ten years old, and for the first time I'm looking beyond the glitter-spangled jeans that I begged Mum to buy, or the candy-coloured clunky friendship bracelets crowding my wrists. I am pink and blotchy, not white, not all that unlike a pig. There are compression marks from the waistband of my jeans, which remind me of the lines on a boiled ham when it's been wrapped in string. I am sort of shapeless, nothing remarkable, but overall I am functional, sufficient. My body has never stopped me from doing anything I've set my mind to. But to be *wanted*? I think of the women whose flesh is so desirable that rather than having to put on an attractive and showy display of their best assets, they have to fight off the attentions of men, who want them so much it is actually an inconvenience, an encumbrance to their lives. *Maybe someday, someone will desire me that fiercely,* I think dreamily, spinning and posing like a model. But then I stop, and fixate on an angry-looking allergic rash covering my upper arms, and it seems absurd, absurd to imagine that anyone could ever want me, even a little bit, even a legal amount. Looking back at my nondescript form, I'm not sure *I* would even want me – but then I've never had to. My body has always just been there. I have used, inhabited, and sprung about in my body my whole life, seemingly unconsciously, because at the end of the day, it's just . . . me. Up until this moment I hadn't realised I could view it objectively as a separate entity, one that I can choose to love or hate, decline or accept. And though, in this moment, I don't love or hate it, because it just is what it is, the more I look, the more ridiculous it seems that anyone else would ever admire and want this flesh vehicle. *So silly*, I think, deflating from my poses, giving my body one last cursory scan. Mine just isn't the kind of body people want. *But no matter*, I think, easily shrugging it off and flicking off the bathroom light. It doesn't matter that I'm not beautiful, that nobody will ever want to take or have or even borrow my body. I don't need to be desired! I certainly don't need a man! I have far bigger and more beautiful dreams for me and this perfectly average body that has, I now realise, been foisted upon me.

It didn't matter that I didn't possess any beauty of my own, because my body was a conduit for beauty! Beauty and creativity. Its energy flowed through me and off my fingertips like rainwater. I was, as the rest of my family referred to me, when casting around for that indistinct defining trait of the third daughter, 'the artistic child'. I had eyes that roved hungrily for beautiful, sparkly, intricate details, and hands that grasped for crayons, markers, pencils, flowers, ribbons, printed fabrics, beads and blank white pages on to which I could pour the images that crowded my mind. Whatever it was that caught my imagination – the princesses in fairy tales, the glittery eyeshadow my teenage cousins wore, or an impossibly intricate origami rose in an arts and craft book – I had a need to touch it, gaze at it, feel it, capture it. And I was content as long as I was drawing pictures, or dressing up dolls, or crafting tiny, delicate things out of paper and beads. It was a restless, curious energy, a near compulsive need to create and beautify my surroundings, and I wasn't too concerned with whether the product of these explorations was good or not; it was just the way I showed up in the world each day: the way I existed. It kept me *busy*, too. I was always hunting for precious and unlikely new materials to help realise my latest art project. Pipe cleaners. Tights. Jeans. Jewels. The slippery reel from the inside of a cassette tape. *Many* shoeboxes. Empty toilet rolls were a particularly precious entity in our household. A devotee of *Art Attack*, an *iconic* publication for artistic children of the nineties, I would tot up the number of empty loo rolls required for my chosen works in my journal, and then announce over dinner that everyone must please use toilet roll very liberally this month, and that we should also exercise our most comely charms on our teachers in exchange for the classroom's empty toilet rolls – if, that was, we were to have the new papier-mâché Spooky Dolls Haunted House project in time for Halloween. I would loiter in the shadows of our hallway when anyone made a bathroom visit and elfishly scamper in after them to monitor the loo roll status. It boded well for my aspirations when I saw my dad enter the bathroom with a newspaper. At times, I would have sold my own hair for toilet rolls, there were simply never enough. *Fuck's sake*, I would think a few weeks later when Mum brought home the newest issue of *Art Attack* and I realised I would need another *thirteen* loo rolls to construct my towering and majestic new jewellery holder. Who *was* this Neil Buchanan character with his bottomless supply of toilet-roll-less tubes? It was clear a career in the arts was for the affluent.

But toilet roll poverty aside, life was good as long as I could spend my time making beautiful things with my mind and hands and words. Making things was how I communicated with the world around me. Though I was shy around strangers, reserved even, I forgot myself when I had *a project*, becoming bossy and ultra-focused, seeing myself as some kind of child-auteur who had a culturally important and extremely significant story to direct/paint/light/write/act. At Christmas, everyone received a handmade card. Then there were birthday cards, Easter cards, cards when there was no occasion – just for something to do with my hands. Everything was an opportunity for creativity. Nothing was left in its original state: it could always be enhanced, brought out and made shine. Jeans were turned into shoulder bags, flesh-coloured tights into dolls, newspapers into papier-mâché fruit bowls and, each Christmas, still more toilet rolls were painted to become Jesus, Mary and Joseph in their shoebox manger.

There was also the feeling of how, after spending three hours on my bed, head bent over my box of beads, a strange, gangly little creature would take shape and be realised limb by limb, a spindly leg, a rainbow wing, then another, and two bright little beady eyes, until, finally, it was a magnificent bird! How it felt to race down the stairs to Mum in her usual spot by the cooker, elbows raised in chaotic direction of a choir of mismatched steaming saucepans, and plant the spangled creature, already starting to sag and droop sadly in places – not like the pictures in the book – in the centre of the palm of her hand. How my little gift would light up her whole face.

'Beautiful, pet! Did you make this all by yourself? That's *amazing*! I think it's even nicer than the one you made last week!'

She would perch it on the dresser, be it a beaded bird, a card, a doll, a fairy, and there it would sit, clumsily made, curling and crumpling awkwardly, but still beautiful. More beauty I'd brought into the world. The beauty I made filled our kitchen walls and mantelpieces and dressers, and it made Mum beam.

I remember a lot of my childhood from the vantage point of corners. Wherever there was a quiet corner of the living room, the kitchen, the bedrooms, I would claim it, stationing myself at a small craft table or pouffe and unhurriedly unpacking my shoebox of beads, paints, glitter and glue, piece by piece. There, where I would spend the rest of the evening bent over patterns, notebooks or a tottering papier-mâché castle. It was absorbing, intricate work, drowning out my surroundings, my eldest sister's screechy violin practice or my second sister and younger brother tearing about the house with hurley sticks and ping-pong balls. I never really thought beyond my current project; my creations demanded my full attention and anchored me to the present moment. It was an idyllic way to spend a childhood, my inner muse free, as soon as homework was done, to run riot across the endless reams of blank paper supplied by my very loyal, long-suffering patron: Mum. As long as she kept me in string, beads, paints, and yes, of course, toilet rolls – which she always did – I didn't care about tomorrow or the next day or the next. I didn't know who or what or why I was, but that was always the furthest thing from my mind when I was working on a project. If only the world had just let me be, weaving and scribbling and stitching in my crafts corner. But gradually, I noticed that people wanted to know who I was, the enigmatic artist behind the Christmas cards and beaded birds. That was the thing, though. She wasn't enigmatic. Or interesting, or memorable, or particularly charming. She certainly wasn't a conversationalist. But they persisted. *Who are you? What do you like? What are you going to do with your life?* they demanded. They looked at me expectantly, as though I had the answers.

'And what do you want to be when you grow up?' a friend of Mum asked one day in my early childhood, bending down at my crafts table, where I was energetically scribbling my way through a Disney colouring book. I looked up at this enquiring face, curling a protective arm around a picture of one of the seven dwarfs. Clíodhna, Mum's best friend, had transparent eyelashes and invisible eyebrows. She never let her three children have sugar, not even the odd Penguin bar, and her household's bedtime was at the unthinkably early time of 8.30pm sharp, an hour when the younger generation of *our* household was usually still noisily mucking about in the back garden. I saw her rosy complexion and preternaturally pale eyebrows as evidence of her peerless virtuosity.

'Hmm?' she probed gently, as I continued to stare at her eyebrows.

This was an easy question when people had first started asking it. What *didn't* I want to be! I had an inexhaustible list, one that lengthened every time I read a new fairy tale. But for the purpose of brevity in social situations, I had narrowed it down to my three most profound callings in life.

'I'm going to be a blue butterfly with patterns, or a pink stripy cat or a white pony with purple hair,' I told Clíodhna with complete sincerity, carrying on with my colouring.

Mum laughed lightly from the couch and, after a moment of puzzlement, Clíodhna joined in, chuckling uncertainly. 'Ohhhh,' she said. 'Fabulous! Aren't you going to be very busy!'

Yes, I thought, *I am.* I was glad somebody could empathise with the sheer enormity of my dreams. *But I can handle it,* I thought, smiling as I imagined my purple pony hair unfurling behind me and rippling in the wind as I cantered joyfully in the wilderness, my powerful flanks propelling me across a dazzling meadow of wild forget-me-nots.

Clíodhna and Mum continued chuckling light-heartedly on the couch with their cups of tea and biscuits. This was the usual reaction when I shared my lofty life plans, and I couldn't really work it out. Jealousy, presumably. They'd not meticulously planned out or thought through their own metamorphoses and had ended up as mere ladies on couches drinking a murky, flavourless beverage rather than dancing – childless, jobless, carefree – amid flowers and over cabbage patches: a gorgeous, periwinkle-blue winged flake, being carried where the wind takes her. They had hair that ranged only within the colour spectrum of mushy piles of autumn leaves, from dull brown to russet red, and sometimes, for a brief hot fortnight of summer, to a pale blonde – but never candy-pink or violet-purple. They had not thought creatively enough about their potential and now they were trapped in their lady-bodies. I pitied them deeply.

But as I got older, people didn't laugh so merrily at my dreams.

One day, sometime later, my relatives came to visit and I obliged everyone once again by reciting my future feline ambitions for an audience. My mum smiled fondly as my cousins giggled in the background, but a small frown creased her forehead as she explained to me that I couldn't actually be a cat or a pony or a butterfly. I was a girl, and that meant that I'd grow up to be a woman. Woman. I let the word pass quickly and inconsequentially over me like a bad smell. Caterpillars grow into butterflies, she explained. Foals grow into ponies, kittens grow into cats – and none of those cats, regrettably, had ever been pink.

'But why?' I still couldn't really see the issue. *Who's to say one of them couldn't just turn into something else if they* really *felt like it?* I reasoned. What daft law of nature insisted we must all live such dull, segregated lives?

'That's just science,' Mum answered. 'That's just our biology; it's not something we get to choose.'

I decided, in that moment, that I didn't like science. It forced brutal, uncompromising restraints on my imagination that there was no coming back from. I held fast to my dreams for a while, becoming more defensive of them the more adults insisted on *science*, but slowly I started to worry that given that every human girl on the planet and in the history of human evolution had never matured into anything beyond the scope of Homo sapiens, it was unlikely that I was going to be the first. Apparently, out of the 8.7 million forms of life on earth, I'd been born into the most mundane of them all. Eventually, reality set in and I stopped answering their questions, annoyed at their insistence and heartbroken by the dullness of my furless, magic-less, flightless future. *What are you going to be?* all manner of strangers probed. *I don't know.* I would shrug evasively, uncomfortable. They wanted to know what kind of woman I'd be: a teacher-woman, a singer-woman, a lawyer-woman, a spacewoman? *You can be any of those things!* They beamed, wearing expressions of bountiful enthusiasm that suggested they thought themselves very generous. Sometimes I would mumble that I was going to be 'an actress' to shut them up, because it was perhaps the least tragic alternative to my previously fixed plans. Actresses could be trees, cats, teapots, princesses. But not really . . . It didn't matter what kind of guise she came in, and that was where everyone misunderstood me: I didn't want to be any kind of woman. I wanted to be a mermaid. I wanted to be a Jigglypuff. I wanted to be a hand-drawn cartoon fairy. I wanted to be a singing pony with magic rainbow hair. I even wanted to be a girl in glittery jeans and a butterfly top. I just could not see myself becoming a woman.

Women. I didn't hate them yet. I admired them. I was in awe of them. Women made a room safe. They had long sweeping skirts behind which I could hide from strangers, and warm, perfumed necks I could nestle into. They had pockets that jangled with the promise of warm car interiors and kitchens filled with the familiar aroma of shepherd's pie. They had tidy ponytails and conical heels that *clicked* elegantly in their wake. They were the unassuming gatekeepers of beauty and colour – hidden rose gardens, face-painting studios, delicatessen cake shops – and they possessed an internal radar that guided them to these treasure-laden enclaves. Wherever women were, men loitered greyly, blurrily in the background, in shapeless, heavy flaps of material that folded their blocky bodies into plain, unexciting right angles. And everywhere they went, women left traces. Blurry little lip prints on wine glasses, stained faintly in rose hues of red or pink. Citrus-scented silk neck scarves hanging over the backs of chairs.

Delicious brown paper packages of food they'd made with their hands. Mysterious yellow wrappers discreetly tucked into the corners of bathroom bins. Handwritten notes in curly, cursive script, with clear instructions, and kisses. Everywhere they went, they made their presence seen and felt. Women were not inclined to sit in corners monosyllabically deflecting questions from passers-by, and watching life flicker past, hoping no one would notice them. Women were front and centre, running the show, feeding everyone, doing several things at once. Women had opinions, and large bosoms, and they took up plenty of space with both. But even though everyone told me I'd grow into one, inevitably, soon, I didn't believe them, feeling that I had much more in common with the inanimate dolls I filled my bed with at night, or the tabby cat sleeping peaceably, passively at the end of it. But I studied women from my corner, fascinated, finding them interesting, powerful, large. Remote.

Elsewhere, the question of who I was persisted, and I'd begun to ask it myself. Who was I when I left my crafts corner? What could I say? What could I offer? I was drawn to loud girls, confident girls. They knew exactly who they were and they filled all the silence with it, while I sat there feeling paralysed, empty, wishing someone would hand me a script. I was drawn to beautiful girls too. I liked to loiter around them. They just made the air nicer. I knew I wasn't one of them, but I didn't begrudge them that. By now, I knew it was useless questioning my place in the world; that in the same way some of us were born lumpy children and some of us sleek, agile cats, there were beautiful girls and there were girls with limp, lifeless hair and utterly forgettable faces. It was all just scientifically ordained. So I worked around them, gave them the space and respect their prettiness demanded, and sometimes, when they let me, I would bask in their glow.

One July, my parents sent me to a local summer camp to learn badminton and play rounders and get in water balloon fights. I know I went to this summer camp five days a week for two weeks a year, but I don't remember any of it. I do, though, remember the beautiful girl who sat on my bus on the ride home every day, and I remember how, for that summer, because there were only five other kids – a group of rowdy boys and a younger girl who grilled us for lists of our favourite things before turning back around and lapsing abruptly into silence – she became my friend. She had a high forehead and a pixie-like upturned nose. Her thick raven hair was gathered tidily back into a glossy ponytail that had an unrealistic buoyancy to it. And she always seemed, any time I saw her, to be sucking on some kind of hard-boiled sweet, which pursed up her lips in a way that gave her a perennial expression of mischievous smugness. She was friendly, too, and chatty. I sat in the seats opposite hers, tentatively, deferring to her to strike up the conversation if she so wished, and she did. We talked about summer camp and school. About our hobbies and the activities we were most looking forward to each day. I felt the warm glow of being singled out for company by someone who was clearly, visibly wonderful. On the second day, I was cautious, tentative again, waiting for her to resume conversation or to decide to rescind her warmth. But she was chattier still, and we talked about our love of *Pokémon* and *Sabrina the Teenage Witch*. By the third day, I strode confidently up the aisle and sat beside her. We chatted animatedly and made some Pokémon card trades, ones that worked far better in her favour, but that I made happily. At the end of the two weeks, we waved our goodbyes and I asked her eagerly was she planning to start tennis lessons at the local club, which she had expressed a passing interest in. She gave a vague 'maybe' and a noncommittal shrug, but I clung to this one wild hope for cementing our friendship. As country children of the nineties, we didn't know about any such modern custom as 'keeping in touch'. After summer camp, you all just toddled back to your respective sleepy corners of the earth, substituting new friends for old dolls.

I made a passionate plea to my parents to sign me up for tennis lessons, citing a newfound interest in 'keeping fit' and 'getting out there' more, and my perplexed mother assented. My older sister, Emily, was already a member of the tennis club, so I went along with her. For the next few weeks, I tried to like tennis, but my new friend never showed. By the end of term, I was still missing most of the balls and my forearms seized up in protest after just a few minutes' play. Emily whipped serves of terrifying velocity over the net, and at home she studied her favourite players' movements in forensic detail. *I might as well not be here*, I decided, thinking my new friend had probably long forgotten me.

A year later, I returned to the same summer camp. I held my breath as I got on the bus, thinking she wouldn't be here, but that she might. She was sitting in the exact same spot, halfway down the bus on the right and gazing out the window. She was still sporting that glorious shiny ponytail, but now she had two poker-straight, deliberately placed pieces of hair framing either side of her face, and she'd traded in her hard boiled sweets for chewing gum, her jaw working mechanically. I walked awkwardly down the bus aisle, sort of wishing she wasn't there, because it had been a year, and the feeling of emptiness had worn me down further, and I knew there was no way she'd possibly remember me, and I just didn't have the energy anymore to find words to introduce myself. But just as I was about to slide into a seat near the front of the bus, she looked up, and caught my gaze, so I had to approach.

'Hi . . .' I said, stupidly, stumbling down the aisle with my two shoulder bags swinging wildly at my hips, like some sort of graceless, lopsided camel. 'I . . . I'm Evanna . . . we used to talk on the bus . . . about *Pokémon* and . . . and . . . tennis,' I finished feebly, desperately reaching for words to define me that just weren't there, anything I could cling to that she might remember me by. I was about to start describing the bright pink denim jacket I used to wear, which was far more distinctive than my personality, when she laughed, apparently amused, and said, 'Yeah, I know who you are. I remember.' She was chewing and smiling bemusedly like I must be a bit daft.

'Oh,' I said, flummoxed, falling into the seat opposite hers. 'Yeah. Cool.'

We chatted about what we'd done at summer camp that day, about how much we were dreading going back to school and about our favourite TV shows. She was still friendly and sweet, but she didn't watch *Pokémon* anymore, and the chewing gum was giving her an intimidating air of sophistication, that of someone who is going to thrive and become more confident the more she grows up. After a while, we both fell silent. She gazed dreamily out the window, her profile cartoonishly perfect. I sat staring at the headrest in front of me, my mind working, wondering, desperately searching for who I was, for what about me she could have possibly remembered.

But all of these feelings – the stress, the anxiety, the growing existential dread – evaporated the moment I opened the kitchen door and set eyes upon my mum. Five-foot-nothing in heels, with slender freckled arms and delicate wrists, she had always been a petite woman, but she might as well have been Mother Earth for all the warmth and love that seemed to emanate from her compact frame. She has a kind smile and fine, curly hair framing her heart-shaped face, and she favours a charmingly mismatched ensemble of bright wool jumpers, printed blouses and loose cotton trousers patterned in dizzying paisley or a maze of swirls that you could get lost in, absent-mindedly tracing them over and over with an index finger. Whether I came from a fight with one of my siblings or having fallen off a bike and skinned both knees, she'd be there at home, decorating buns in bright yellow or pink icing, or deftly knitting a hat for a friend's new baby, or darning a neat patch over the hole in someone's trousers. She'd stroke my hair and dissolve my sadness with an icy bun and a colouring book. Whatever had happened, she'd hug me, say that it didn't matter anymore, and then she'd ask me to help her with her baking, or to run upstairs and get my art supplies so we could make some Halloween decorations. She'd nudge me back into the sanctuary of my imagination, where I didn't need to be anyone, where there were just endless exciting patterns to uncover, and where I was too busy digging for treasure to remember why I'd been sad a few moments before. And she was right. It didn't matter. As we sat there, snipping, cutting, pasting, painting, it didn't matter that I wasn't very good at tennis or piano, that I wasn't super smart or quick-witted, that I didn't have fairy-tale prettiness or a disarming charisma. All that mattered was that we could sit down at this colourful, quiet space at the kitchen table, and that there was something to create.

Mum's love was the centre of my whole universe. It was strange, then, to see the same quiet disappointment cross her face when she met her own reflection that I was beginning to feel when I met mine.

Her eyes would skate quickly over and look past the surface of any mirror. She'd tuck her curls behind her ears, smooth her blouse, straighten her necklace, and then sometimes her lips would press together in a half-hearted attempt at a smile before she'd drop her gaze down and quickly turn away from the mirror to whichever one of her four children was tugging at her trouser leg. She never really talked about herself, never mentioned her weight or her clothes, and she never shared what she wanted or dreamed about, so I didn't really know what she thought of herself, but I saw it in the way she acted. She was shy, agreeable, and apologised profusely for being in the way of people. She was a competent driver but could never drive to the airport alone, her nerves so shot by the fear of 'getting in the wrong lane' and provoking the ire of more confident drivers. A devoted learning support and resource teacher, she didn't push back or defend herself when colleagues or parents of students made criticisms of her work. She'd come home wringing her hands, anxiety etching new lines on her forehead because of some subtle snub made by another teacher, and she'd wrack her brains all evening, combing through their interactions of the past week for any microscopic detail, any small way by which she might have offended them.

'Maybe,' my dad would say, with a shrug and an air of finality, grinding a corner of butter into his mashed potatoes, 'that fella is just an arsehole.'

But my mum could not accept this. There must have been something she'd said, something she'd done, something about her that she needed to apologise for, if only she could identify what it was. She was quick to forgive everyone but herself, whenever she discovered that the source of a colleague's irate mood was due to some external factor and not actually because of an innate fault in her personality.

'Do I?' she'd ask, her eyes brightening, when one of her daughters said she looked pretty in her new floral dress as she got ready for a cousin's Holy Communion. But then she'd look at herself in the mirror again, a look of sad resignation clouding her expression.

'Well, it's a good thing this dress hides my varicose veins.' Then she'd smile. 'Have to try and keep up with all those Glamazons outside the church.'

We were just different, Mum and I, I was beginning to realise. There was just something the matter with us, something we couldn't escape. It was nothing obviously discernible, nothing that stuck out too much, and nothing you'd notice from a quick, cursory glance. And though it was nothing tangible, nothing that could be put into words and easily remedied, other people were beginning to see it too.

'What's wrong with me?' I mumble sadly to my mum as I trudge after her around the local supermarket one day after drama class. The drama classes are a new thing, my thing. My sisters have no interest in performance, and nobody can really imagine me – shy, retiring and increasingly awkward me – standing on a stage under bright lights and reciting monologues to total strangers. But there is something so appealing about finding my own private feelings reflected in a character who lives worlds away, and being given the space to stand up and share these pernicious feelings under the guise of someone else – their clothes, their story – someone who people want to look at. The relief of it is too great to resist. I love these classes, and I eagerly wait for 4pm on Wednesday to roll around again each week, but it has only taken a few weeks of the classes for the loud, cheeky, popular boy to sniff out the thing about me I've been trying to stifle, and to make a point of reminding me that, try as I might, there is something inherently embarrassing about me that cannot be hidden. He is stealthy in his methods of torment, whispering taunts in my right ear as the teacher calls the roll from the other end of the room. He is well liked by students and teachers alike, and cannot afford to become a public bully, so he does it quietly, with finesse.

'Big fucking Nike Maxes on ya,' he'd hissed in my ear, laughing. 'Hear you coming a mile off.' I'd looked down at the Nike shoes, that were indeed almost two sizes too big for me. They came in a blue-and-white striped canvas bag, filled with hand-me-down clothes from my impossibly trendy older cousin. My cousin, who is always five steps ahead of everyone else in the fashion game, and who drops so many obscure musical references it is like she is speaking a foreign language. I am in awe of her. These bags arrive maybe twice a year, and I unpack them with the same delicacy and care you might employ trying to fix an antique clock. Her clothes are always bright – exotic colours, expensive fabrics, nothing faded – and decorated in fine strings of beads or embroidered with obscure French words. I can't believe I am related to her, let alone that I am lucky enough to be the benefactor of her seasonal cast-offs. If *she'd* worn them, they were cool, no question, and so *I* would wear them too. I'd pulled on the Nike runners eagerly, ignoring Mum's protests that they were far too big, and that I already had a brand new pair of runners that fit me perfectly. But that day, sitting on a black painted wooden box in my drama class and listening to the jibes of this snide boy, I'd been reminded that I am not my cool, trend-setting cousin, and I look silly. Hot tears clouded my vision as the boy started taking thunderous, full-bodied steps across the room, in what was clearly meant to be a cruel parody of me in my too-big shoes, while his long-haired, Slipknot-T-shirt-wearing mates sniggered in the corner.

'Maybe he fancies you,' Mum suggests, grinning mischievously at me as she lightly fingers the crumpled top of a bag of potatoes. 'Maybe he doesn't know how to talk to you, so he teases you instead.' Her hand is now clutching the bag of potatoes hesitantly. I can tell she is considering buying them, wondering will she get away with passing them off as my dad's homegrown spuds, which this year are small, green-tinged and covered in knobbly growths that look like clusters of warts, but are still a source of enormous pride to my dad. She throws a fearful glance over one shoulder, as though expecting to see his crestfallen form framed by the vegetable aisle.

'No way!' I tell her, blood rushing hotly to my cheeks. I find myself glancing around self-consciously as she had done a moment ago. 'That's not what it is,' I insist. 'He doesn't even like me. Why would he ever fancy me?' I hate myself for even asking the question.

'Well, it certainly sounds like he's paying a lot of attention to you,' she says, still grinning and shrugging her shoulders. 'Now, you won't tell Dad I've bought these potatoes,' she tells me, hoisting the bag of potatoes on to her hip like an unruly toddler. 'He's not the one who has to peel them.'

All week long, I quietly ponder Mum's theory, which makes me equal parts uncomfortable and intrigued. Why *does* he pay me so much attention, I wonder. Why does he spend so much time pestering me? I'm not sure I could like him, though: he is mean and arrogant and not the kind of blue-eyed, curtain-haired soulful boy I've started to admire from afar. But I've felt considerably warmer towards him ever since Mum posited this unlikely scenario, and I decide to keep an open mind. I dress carefully before drama class the next week. I ignore the big Nikes, along with the leopard-print faux-fur jacket I'd worn a few weeks previously, and which he'd immediately spotted, announcing to the class: 'Make way for the Queen of England.' I'd bowed my head, mortified, as he'd accompanied my journey across the room to the theatre seats with an imitation trumpet rendition of 'God Save the Queen', and the entire class had erupted in laughter. I leave off anything boldly printed or statement-making that he could single out for ridicule. (In retrospect, and in fairness to him, I have to admit that my sartorial choices were eyebrow-raising, and I didn't have the bold personality to back them up. But I was trying to show up as the person I wanted to be. It just so happened that this boy saw right through this pitiable facade to the lost, empty space I was trying to fill.)

That day, I dress like everyone else: no studs, no faux fur, nothing cat print, and wear well-fitted flat shoes. I wonder what he'll find to mock about me today, or if we might instead have a proper conversation. He ignores me, though. He doesn't say one word, or glance my way, or make any jokes at my expense. He spends all his time in the far corner, making the shiny-haired, glossy-lipped girl gang laugh and twirl their hair coquettishly at his wisecracks. I feel mostly relieved as I make my way up the street after class to where Mum has parked, but also a small, secret bit disappointed.

'Hi, pet,' Mum says, as I get into the car. 'How was class?'

'It was good, thanks. We're working on new monologues next week.'

'Oh, fantastic!' Mum exclaims. She's about to turn the key and start the car, when she looks up and pauses. 'Isn't that girl very pretty?' she remarks, and I turn to follow her gaze, which is fixed on one of the shiny-haired girls from class, who is standing amid the attractive, loud or rich kids that make up the popular group. She is undeniably beautiful. Her hair is like sunlight that's been woven into a sheet of silk, and she has a smiling, symmetrical, open face: the kind of beauty that invites people in and makes them feel lighter. She's the best dancer in the school, and her natural grace and ease in her own body is evident even in the way she leans casually against the wall. The mean boy is chatting to her now, his hands in his pockets, his whole body facing her, talking quickly in a manner that suggests he wants to keep her there, laughing at things he says. He doesn't have to slyly communicate with her through barbed comments from the side of his mouth. He doesn't ignore her on certain days and jeer at her the next, depending on her outfits, depending on the strength of the whiff of insecurity and self-hate he is getting off her. He just likes her.

For a long moment, I study my mother's profile as she admires this attractive girl, that gentle, unselfconscious smile of looking at something that is simply and unfairly aesthetically pleasing playing about her lips, and I wonder, with a stab of longing, what she sees when she looks at me. If this girl is 'very pretty', what am I? Am I nice to look at? Do I have some more subtle charms? Would Mum ever have chosen me if she hadn't been landed with me? I am too afraid I know the answer to venture the question. I turn my gaze back to the girl as she laughs sunnily and tosses a few strands of hair over her shoulder, and I feel like I'm dissolving, like I don't know where any of my edges are, as indeterminate as water that's been poured from its container. The constant feeling of faint desolation that has noiselessly crept into my life over the past year seems to corkscrew its way a little deeper into my bones as I look at the girl. It might as well be a metaphor for the whole of our lives, because this was how it always felt: Mum and I sitting quietly and looking out at other girls and women who were more beautiful, more interesting, more witty, more worthy. More, just more.

But it doesn't matter, I tell myself firmly, later that evening as I sit on my bed and cry over things that I know don't matter. A mean boy who I don't even like. A pretty girl who I've barely spoken to. It doesn't matter. I don't need to be any of these things, be it cool, or pretty, or super smart or *gifted* – all of that is just stuff other people have, and none of it matters so long as I stay torso-deep in the dressing-up box looking for my fairy wings, or on my bedroom floor unpicking flakes of glitter glue from all the way up my arms, or in my corner, designing alternate worlds I'd like to step into. In my corner, I am busy, self-reliant and content. *They* can all grow into buxom women and make their desperate bids for power and husbands. They can grow up and leave me be. Lock Rapunzel in her tower and bury the key.

Try as I might to keep my eyes averted, to stay determinedly the same, I could see that things were changing around me. Change was happening to my sisters as they grew up just ahead of me, and I watched at a safe but ominous distance. It was becoming clear that girls didn't simply blossom one day into smooth-legged, clear-skinned, graceful women. Women weren't born, sliding easily in a cloud of perfume and pollen from the inside of a flower; they were *sculpted*: by life, by their mothers, by misfortune, but mostly, pathetically, by the stupid, hapless girls they had been before. I was starting to see that it was an ugly and ungainly process, and there was absolutely no guarantee that one would emerge from the whole awful, gut-wrenching process somehow more proficient at womanhood than she had been at youth. The unspoken, horrifying truth was that so many girls were actually worse off as women, contending with all sorts of new, inescapable afflictions that you didn't see in magazines. Innocent young girls went to Pleasure Island picturing themselves morphing into long-necked swans, but returned dazed and stumbling about as swollen-bodied, fleshy-necked turkeys. Emily, my eldest sister, the piano/tennis/everything prodigy, was not taking as naturally to womanhood as she did academia. She was bullied badly at school and would come home sobbing and disconsolate. She'd take to her bed, burying herself beneath her duvet, and Mum would follow her in, sitting on the edge of the bed, stroking her hair and crooning loving words in a routine that became so frequent it came to be known collectively by the entire family as 'counselling sessions'. My other sister, Mairéad, and I would creep silently to the bedroom door and crouch outside to eavesdrop. Why were the other girls so bitchy to her, Emily would beg of Mum. Why couldn't she find a boyfriend? And honestly, truthfully, was she fat?

'Nooooo,' Mum would cry, in a gentle, soothing tone. 'You're LOVELY.'

'Lovely,' Mairéad informed me, a wicked grin lighting up her freckled face, 'is just the diplomatic word for "fat".'

Mairéad embraced the changes a lot more willingly. A stubborn, hot-tempered tomboy since childhood, an unexpected and disconcerting wave of feminine energy seized her in her early teens, and she positively gloated to Emily and me about the suddenly noticeable curves she triumphantly (and generously) called 'C-cups!'. One day after school, she returned home late with Mum, swinging a brown paper Tully's bag from her fist, the contents of which remained a mystery for approximately three seconds before she proudly whipped out two pristine pink-and-white polka-dot bras that were lined with a frivolous lace trim. She wasted no time in stepping into her new bra-clad self, refusing to take it off even at night ('My friend Aoife says if you don't wear your bra, your boobs will grow into your armpits'), and every evening that week she paraded around in the bedroom we shared in just her bra and pants, admiring her figure from every angle.

I watched from the top bunk with a kind of detached, reluctant fascination. It was shocking how suddenly a bra had taken a bruised-kneed, jersey-wearing, sweaty-faced girl and turned her into a pouting, preening shapely young woman. The bra seemed to imbue her with a special confidence, too, that she channelled towards the boys around her. The furry toy dogs that had filled her bed and threatened to smother her to death each night were relegated to the plastic storage boxes in the corner, and instead of planning our future animal shelter or scheming what kind of bird to convince our parents to get us next, I'd lie wordlessly, blinking up at the glow-in-the-dark stars on the ceiling, as she rhapsodised from the lower bunk, long after the lights had gone out, about the quiet boy with the number-two haircut who excelled on the football pitch and who possibly wasn't aware of her existence. She'd scour the local newspapers for mention of him in the sports section, and happily relay to the family how she envisioned their fairy-tale romance would play out, fully convinced by the strange power her new bra had lent her that this was an assured eventuality. And though she'd always been cheeky, the naughty one who told bold jokes and took risky dares, that cheekiness had a danger and a prominence to it now. She was no longer inconsequential, and the little woman she'd become embarrassed and alienated me. She caught my eye in the mirror as I peered warily at her in her bra over the top of a new *Art Attack*.

'Don't worry, Van-van,' she smugly told me, choosing one of her deliberately condescending nicknames, as she mistook my expression of blank horror for envy. 'You'll get one someday.'

The realisation hit me like a bus. Womanhood was coming for me, too, far, far sooner than I'd anticipated. And with it, all the horrible things that couldn't be hidden: the breasts, the bras, the bleeding, the blotchy skin, the body hair, the responsibilities, the exams, the expectations and the mounting, debilitating pressure to figure out exactly what kind of woman I'd be. *What are you going to be when you grow up?* What kind of woman-shaped specimen would I assume that would forgive me the litany of flaws and sins inherent in being a woman? I needed to figure this out, to come up with the answer soon, because beneath all this was the gnawing, terrible fear that someday, someone who wasn't my mother would have to love me, and I wasn't sure they ever would. And this was no longer an abstraction in the distance that I could muse at my leisure, as Mairéad, beaming from the mirror, had abruptly reminded me. It was an incontrovertible fact: whatever I did, whether I willed it to or not, proudly snapping on a bra like bronzed armour plates as Mairéad had done, or retreating to my duvet where I wouldn't have to look at myself like Emily, I was going to turn into a woman. My body would grow up – there was no point denying it anymore – but would *I*?

And then one day, amid this fervent search for myself, this growing existential dread, the sense that womanhood is about to come and claim me and make everything worse, I hear something that interests me. It's Sunday afternoon and all four siblings are crammed into the backseat of my dad's Toyota as we make our way home from Mass. Mass is a non-negotiable part of the week. My dad is the only sincere Catholic of the family, the rest of us having been lured there by marital duty or the promise of sweets or pocket money. A lifelong Catholic, my dad made it through seven years of 'priest college', right up to the vow of chastity, whereupon he realised his true, honest dream was to become a dad, not a 'Father'. He left to travel the world, then came back, became a teacher, met Mum and started a family, but the guilt of leaving the priesthood followed him, and for many years after, we all paid for his transgressions against God by sacrificing our Sunday mornings to the mind-numbing ritual of Mass.

I'm studying a teenage magazine in the backseat while Emily extracts the tennis news from the Sunday paper, while Mairéad and Patrick (my curly-mopped little brother, the youngest of the clan) are swapping Maltesers for red Skittles. I've switched to *Mizz* and *Elle Girl* lately, leaving behind poor, pure Neil Buchanan in his post-box-red jumpers and his papier-mâché world with the same ruthless decisiveness my dad demonstrated when he walked out on Jesus. I've started to take my urge to colour in and beautify closer to myself. It's like I'm suddenly aware I have a body, a face, hair – and they're all my responsibility. They are the things people look at to see me. So I paint tiny flowers on my nails and place shiny gemstones along my lash line. I pore over the hair crimping tutorials in these magazines that seem to have all the answers, taking notes as I go,. But oddly, I just can't get the parts of myself to adhere to the images in my head with the same ease and dexterity with which I could manipulate wire and string and coloured pencils. Whatever way I braid my hair or paint my eyelids, I still see me poking out. I just can't seem to cover her up or colour her in, but it is comforting to read there are ways and products and myriad tips and tricks to help me work on this. I'm examining an article on how to achieve the perfect zig-zag parting that promises 'a funky and original new 'do in less than five minutes!' when I detect my parents conversing in sombre, weighty tones that speak of drama and things they hope won't meet our ears.

'. . . just dreadful,' Mum is saying, her brow furrowed in concern in the mirror of the passenger seat.

'Yeah, yeah,' my dad agrees, nodding solemnly, his eyes fixed on the road ahead.

'Poor Darina,' Mum continues. 'Anorexia is a terrible disease.'

They fall silent for a moment, letting an aura of inevitable tragedy settle on their conversation. I look sideways at Emily, who is nodding sagely along with Mum's statement, the worldly eldest child, and at Mairéad and Patrick, entirely oblivious to the discussion as they dig each other in the ribs, trying to snatch each other's sweets.

'What is . . . an-or-exia?' I enquire, feeling an odd satisfaction at sounding it out. There is a danger and exoticism to the word that I enjoy. My parents remain silent, but I can feel Mum's mind working carefully and my dad concentrating more intently on the road, tuning out of a question that is better left to mothers. Then Mum turns around and looks at me with a curious expression that is at once conspiratorial and sympathetic.

'It's an illness, pet. It's when someone refuses to eat and gets extremely thin. Doireann O'Sullivan, Darina's daughter, has it and she's very unwell.' Mum speaks without breaking eye contact, as though trying emphatically to warn me away from a place no one should ever go. She turns back in her seat, but I'm not satisfied by this tidily sanitised explanation of a secret that is evidently dripping in darkness and I'm tired of being dismissed as a child and told not to peer too far down into the cavernous depths of this darkness when I can already feel it seeping its way into the edges of my own mind, and I just want to know what it is, because maybe then I'll be able to manage it.

'How thin does she get?' I probe, hungry for details and determined to get a proper answer from my mother this time. 'Doesn't she get hungry?' The car is quiet now and saturated by an atmosphere of discomfort, the sense that there is something horribly perverse about my curiosity.

'I'm sure she does get hungry,' Mum replies in a strained voice, not turning back to meet my eyes this time. 'But she's afraid of getting bigger, so she represses her appetite. It's a horrible disease,' she says firmly. 'People can die from it.'

'Does she want to die?' I blurt out in shock, but Emily rustles the paper noisily in agitation, and Mum murmurs that we shouldn't be gossiping about other people's private lives, and everyone lapses into contemplative silence for the rest of the car journey.

We all pile out at home, Patrick sprinting towards his football nets, Mum loading her arms with shopping bags, with Emily helping. I quietly slip away to the top left corner of the house where my bed is. I sit on the bed, the magazine laid out in front of me as I leaf through articles about hair chalk and nail-art transfers and quizzes that tell you how well you know your best friend, but I can't concentrate on anything. I keep thinking of the girl that my parents were whispering about. Questions plague my mind, which is crowded by the enigmatic presence of the girl with the strange problem. Who is she? Why does she want to be thin so badly? Is she a supermodel?

What was that in my parents' voices when they spoke of her? Was it pity, concern, horror, shame, envy, awe or reverence? Was it all of those things? But most of all, what does she want? It seems to be thinness, but there is something else beneath that, something deeper, because apparently she can never be thin enough. There is seemingly no end goal other than death – is *that* what she wants? And yet, there is something sparkling in her iron resolve, her gritty determination and brutal stubbornness that suggests a fierce, burning energy for life. She is obsessed with and yet defying her own body, the force of change, nature itself. She sounds like nobody I've ever heard of before and yet somehow she is also familiar, somehow deep down I understand her quest. '*She's afraid of getting bigger.*' I hear Mum's words repeating, and a spark of recognition seems to ignite within me. This girl has stepped neatly sideways, removing herself entirely from the unrelenting cycle of life that is pulling the rest of us forwards without resistance. She isn't a woman or a child or beautiful or ugly or desirable or anything at all except *Thin*.

My gaze drifts to the floor, where a saucer filled with beads and a half-started rainbow bird lie. I think I already know that I'm never going to finish this bird. I don't know who I am or what kind of woman I'll be or how to stop it, and I don't know how to do a fucking zig-zag parting in a way that looks 'trendy and original' rather than unkempt and mildly demented, but I know with absolute certainty that I no longer have time to hunt down toilet rolls or make Christmas cards for second cousins or weave tiny rainbow-patterned feathers on to ornamental birds that aren't even very good. There is too much about me I need to fix. And all these creations, the birds and the bugs and the toilet-roll people, they are all so silly and they are wasting my time. Maybe Mum will always treasure and celebrate each beaded bird in turn, but other people make birds and fairies far more fabulous and intricate, better than mine. It seems that, day by day, the older I get, the more people I meet, the more abundantly clear it is that I have nothing special, nothing exceptional, nothing that anchors me to life and love. Nothing for which anyone would want me. And creativity, which has always been my sanctuary, my way of communicating to the world all the images whirling around my mind, now frustrates and haunts me. It is all just teeming with imperfections I can't abide. The birds could always be more beautiful: I will never and can never be finished with them. Everywhere in my creations, I see mistakes rather than beauty, expressions of my innately flawed interior. What is the point in spending my life on things that can never be done, on something that won't save me from my inherent unworthiness? I need something more concrete, more worthy: something impenetrably perfect.

2

I hate this chapter of eating disorder memoirs. *The Descent!* The melodramatic and often boastful chapter chronicling the tragic downfall of a poor young girl as she whittles herself away, disfigured by her own self-hate, becoming a mere shadow of her former vivacious self! As if we all should weep bitterly over the fact that one self-obsessed, cosseted young girl is flinging a plate of lovingly prepared lasagne out the bathroom window where the cats will slurp up the evidence. I can't help but roll my eyes when she starts documenting the bird-sized portions of food she survived on while she ran marathons and sobbed through aerobics DVDs; when she cites the plummeting numbers on the scale, as if she isn't swelling with pride as she tells you her most dangerously low weight; when she recalls the solemn tones of the medical professionals echoing in the background, declaring how close she is to death, how a mere cold could polish her off! Gritty scenes of her running uphill as the rain lashes her face or of a wasted, hollowed-out body scrutinising a discordantly curvaceous reflection and pinching imaginary fat deposits in the mirror are underscored with the most painfully emo songs you can think of, maybe Christina Aguilera's 'Beautiful' or Radiohead's 'Creep'.

I am being harsh, I know. But I am weary (and wary) of these sensational accounts of the descent into eating disorders because during my recovery, these memoirs were triggering, and during my eating disorder, they were inspiring. These books read as manuals to my worsening disorder: *How to Be the Best Skinny Bitch Around and Not Get Caught by Your Parents!* Others read as cautionary tales, where the determined, energetic teen is flattened by a soul-crushing series of recovery programmes: *How Recovery is Just Another Word for 'Giving Up' and Why You Must Resist It!* The problem with this chapter of eating disorder memoirs is that it's very difficult to write about anorexia without *bragging* about anorexia, and an account of that specific, intense time in the grip of anorexia plays too neatly into the egoic thirst of the disorder – however long it's lain dormant. It is a condition that is in and of itself a total submission to the ego. And what a lot of people fail to notice about recovered anorexics is that, rather than being ashamed of or horrified by their past, they are often proud. They still get a thrill out of telling you their lowest weight or how many rice cakes used to sustain them for the day, and they might even keep a secret folder containing photos of them at their most impressively sick-looking. So, while my eating disorder has been waiting for years for me to write a book to shock and impress you with her numbers, her regimen, her daily calorie count, the thrilling countdowns the doctors used to pin on her declining life expectancy, while she would *love* me to include her skinny pictures, I'm not going to give her that. Because this book – spoiler warning – is not about how great I was at anorexia for a while. It's about how the relentless pursuit of perfection is a sad way to spend a life, and why you should wake up and pull yourself out of that downward spiral as soon as you possibly can. And the numbers on the scale, the diets, the shock stats, the details – they're all just symptoms that everyone gets distracted by while the real problem drifts sinisterly by under the surface, morphing and growing into other self-destructive behaviours. The skinniness and the weight and the medical issues are all just superficial aspects that are so alarming – and, yes, intriguing – that we tend to miss the deeper layer they are masking, which is what I'd rather talk about. All that said, I'm trying to paint a detailed portrait of anorexia, a condition that is most known and sensationalised for its fixation on thinness, but is in fact fuelled by something else. I'm trying to show you what a rollercoaster it is: how satisfying, exhausting, addictive and comforting it is, all at once, so you might also understand what may be going on under the surface. In the interest of presenting a thorough insight, then, I have to sketch in *some* of those gory details.

So, let's just get this bit over with.

You don't 'catch' anorexia. If I gave you that impression in the last chapter, that's incorrect. I don't believe you can catch it from someone else or manifest it within after reading an article about it. What is infectious is the feeling of inherent unworthiness that so many people carry with them and trail around in their wake. That dawning sensation that we are shameful, excessive, embarrassing or just innately worthless is the perfect soil in which an eating disorder can take root. In truth, I can't definitively say where eating disorders come from, or why they affect some people so seriously, while others merely flirt with them. An eating disorder is not something that can be calculated or conjured when you feel like it. It just *happens* to some people.

For me, there was no prompt or incident or moment of decision. It was more like, one day, I just sort of . . . found it. Somewhere shortly after my eleventh birthday, between being a child and knowing I wouldn't always be, I started a diet I'd found on the back of a cereal box. I was small already, a fact people would comment on from time to time, but I'd never thought much about my weight or felt any dissatisfaction about it. But I was observant, attentive and had noticed that everywhere, people talked about how desirable thinness was, how mythical. Nobody could seem to get thin, stay thin, be thin enough. Nobody managed it. 'Thin' seemed a completely elusive, unattainable state, which made you want to reach for it. There was a reverence for and a fascination with thinness that nothing else in life seemed to garner. So when I started my new diet, I hoped I could learn to manage my weight, but I didn't really believe I'd have much of an aptitude for thinness.

I started by saying no to cake. Cake was an important feature of life in our household. Hardly an evening went by when the worktops weren't covered with a dusting of flour, an array of cookie cutters, greased baking trays, apple peels and pots of chubby glistening glacé cherries, with Mum darting around the kitchen kneading raisin-speckled dough on one surface, before dashing back to the cooker where the dinner was threatening to boil over. And after dinner, when everyone was slumped on the couch or belly-down on the rug by the fire watching TV, she'd emerge beaming from the kitchen, laden with a tray of scones spread with butter and jam, or steaming plates of apple tart with generous dollops of cream and sugar, and she'd visit each of us in turn with these treats. After a long day at school, it was customary for each of us to make straight for the biscuit tin, where perhaps the last few chocolate-chip cookies dwindled, the ones from the batch that had disappointed her with their crispy burned edges. Even my friends at school all agreed that receiving an invitation to play at my house was a welcome occasion 'because of the food'. But it was Mum who derived the most delight from feeding people treats, lighting up when she saw a visitor's hand reaching for a second slice of fruit cake, or practically lunging across the table to serve them when they cheerfully accepted 'just another sliver' of apple and blackberry tart. Cake was my mother's love language. But I managed to say no to seconds, and soon I began refusing it entirely. I didn't feel that I deserved cake or love anymore, and felt a thrum of satisfaction, a faint and interesting pleasure in rejecting them. I told everyone I was on a 'health kick', giving up cakes for a little while, and was encouraged and praised for it. Each evening I'd announce how many days it had been of my health kick, how long since I'd eaten an icy bun or a muffin, and murmurs of admiration would follow. Mairéad joined me after a few days, studying the back of the Special K box with a sceptical expression, saying she thought we all could do with a health kick, but not two days had passed before she stormed in from school, making straight for the biscuit tin.

'Life is bloody difficult enough already without chocolate,' she said, snatching up a Kit Kat. I stood rooted to the floor, staring at the biscuit tin I had no intention of opening, my insides glowing with a feeling of pride and a sense of purpose. Had I finally found something I was best at? That evening, Mum made cherry cake, my favourite, slipping into the darkening living room as Emily and I watched *Friends*, bearing two generous slices of cake.

'Here,' she said, smiling, happily presenting me the extra-thick slice of cake on a fancy china plate. 'You've definitely earned this,' she insisted. I looked at the cake, with the bright glossy cherries poking out, the smell of warm cinnamon and sponge cake meeting my nostrils, and I almost took it from her, unthinkingly. But then I remembered how many days I'd been doing my health kick, how good I felt, how awed everyone was by it, how that would all be wiped away and forgotten, and I would go back to being an unremarkable, inexcusable heap of flesh. The moment I bit into that cake, all that effort would have been for nothing.

'I can't have that,' I told Mum firmly, looking away from the cake. 'My health kick, remember?' Her face fell, her hands still proffering the cake on its dainty china dish. She looked disproportionately sad, like I'd taken something precious from her. But it was nothing to be alarmed about: it could only be a positive thing to be invested in one's health, and it's good at any age to create healthy habits. At this stage, it was only her feelings I'd hurt.

'Oh, right, OK,' she conceded, nodding glumly. I felt a sense of guilt and remorse as I watched her quietly retreating to the kitchen in her flour-spattered apron, clutching the little plate with the still steaming piece of cake. I didn't mean to make her sad. I just liked how I was feeling, felt like I was doing something worthwhile, building towards something. *She shouldn't take cake so personally*, I thought, frustration setting in as I turned my attention back to the TV. Someone else would eat the cake.

After cakes, it was biscuits. Then chocolate, then sweets, then all sugar. Then complex carbohydrates. I started reading about nutrition and weight-loss, snagged every woman's magazine in the house, rapidly assimilating the information on optimal dieting, taking every minor critique of certain food groups as a challenge to my willpower, a test of my commitment to self-improvement. '*Our nutrition expert advises readers eat hydrogenated fats sparingly*' – but these articles were written for average, desperate women, a state I was trying to circumnavigate, so I cut those things out completely, wiping entire shelves of the food pyramid from my life, and felt powerful for it. That feeling of power and superiority fuelled my determination to do better, to keep on improving. And where I used to tail after Mum as she made her rounds of the supermarket, dreamily eyeing and sighing loudly over the expensive chocolate yoghurt pots while she reached for the cheap, own-brand family-pack, now I stayed in the magazine aisle, rifling through *Women's Health* and *Shape* for pictures of thin, veiny women and the all-important fact file comprising details of all the things they didn't eat in a day.

Then I started exercising. I took up yoga and running and cycling. A lifelong, decidedly indoorsy child, I didn't enjoy the discomfort of burning lungs or the wind raging against me as I struggled up a hill with my bike in first gear, but there was satisfaction and peace to be found in the mundanity of physical exertion. You could perfect a sit-up in a way you never could a painting. And maybe I did actually enjoy the physical aches and pains, derived some pleasure from the punishment. Maybe I felt I was finally treating my body the way it deserved, and that helped me sleep easier at night. Soon every spare moment not spent exercising felt wasteful, gluttonous, felt like I loved myself too much, like I was saying I was OK with exactly the way I was. To sit and watch TV or eat a little more cereal would be equivalent to saying, 'I am enough' – and I simply wasn't. Every waking minute was an opportunity for self-improvement. Why be driven when I could cycle to school? Why sit when I could stand? Why watch TV with my siblings when I could be in my room doing sit-ups? There could be nothing more absurd than stopping to eat a snack when I had so much room for self-improvement, so much fat to burn. The opportunity to ceaselessly improve and better myself was comforting. And relentless.

Life continued like this for some time – weeks, a couple months maybe – with me refining my diet day by day, substituting tasty white foods for knobbly, wholegrain varieties that boasted lower and lower fat quantities, politely declining biscuit tins and boxes of sweets passed around at parties, Mum becoming increasingly tense, rolling her eyes when again I refused even a bite of a cake she had made, brightly telling her that I wanted to keep up the health kick just a little bit longer, maybe just another week. I don't think there ever came a moment where I realised there was a problem – and, even all these years later, there is a small but sincere belief inside me that I really was fine, just fine, until everyone got involved – but if there was a moment it shifted into something more dysfunctional than a health regime, it was probably somewhere around the time where I instinctively knew to stop bragging about my dietary triumphs, and where my whole routine attained a deliberate layer of *secrecy*.

One evening, Mum is passing around dinner plates, the kitchen steamy, my siblings seating themselves in their usual spots. Dad is home early from school today, in a cheery mood, having had no detentions to conduct for a change. I'm sitting quietly in my place, an empty plate in front of me, my mind working furiously as I run through all the food items I've consumed today, comparing it to my caloric intake of yesterday. It's always preferable if I can manage to improve on my regime from the day before, but it's tolerable as long as I can maintain progress. I just can't go backwards, that's my rule. Constant improvement and refinement. I have found I am beginning to feel spurts of panic and fear on those evenings when I look back and realise with a jolt of horror that I'd eaten one sandwich less the day before: I can't just shrug it off and pledge to do better tomorrow. I lie there sleepless with anxiety before switching back on the light, hitting the floor and cranking out a hundred sit-ups, a hasty apology note to a persistent voice in my mind.

This evening at dinner, I cannot remember if I put skimmed or semi-skimmed milk on my cereal that morning, and am wondering if I have earned the right to dinner at all. Mum delivers my dinner first: brown rice, peas and a dry turkey burger. I'm still eating white meat because all the health magazines endorse it. Immediately, I see that the burger is coated in batter, fat and calories I hadn't bargained for, but Mum's patience is already running short with my rapidly fluctuating diet and having to cook me a separate special meal, so I don't say anything and murmur a quiet 'Thanks'. Mum heaps cheesy squares of lasagne on to everyone else's plates, adding a heap of potatoes to my dad's because he harbours the staunch belief that a dinner without potatoes does not count as dinner. She sits down finally, smiling around at everyone, the table full, the mood light. I keep my head down, nibbling at the peas, trying to stay calm as I search for an excuse to not eat the burger that won't disrupt the cheery mood or deflate Mum's happiness.

Patrick is swirling a chicken dipper in copious amounts of tomato ketchup and then mostly missing the small hole of his mouth, dollops of sauce smearing across his cheeks in poppy-like blotches. Emily is gabbling excitedly about her moody new music teacher, who has singled her out to accompany him in class with her violin as he plays the piano. She's leaning further, more comfortably, into her role of teacher's pet these days. Mairéad is imitating Emily over her shoulder, her mouth gabbling soundlessly, her expression imperious, Dad chuckling quietly. And I am panicking now, nudging my rice and peas away from the offending burger, shrinking away from it myself and wondering if you can inhale fat cells. I simply can't eat this, I know that; I don't know the precise nutritional statistics of this burger, and can't account for it in my day. But I can feel Mum throwing glances in my direction, and I know that she's watching for signs of something more sinister than an interest in health food. She is not a naturally suspicious person, but she's starting to look more closely at me lately. So I start to quarter the burger with my fork, carefully slicing it into smaller and smaller pieces. Heat is rising in my cheeks as I look at the fried white bread coating the stringy meat. I can't remember the last time I've eaten something made with white flour, a food all fitness magazines and diet books seemed to unanimously agree is a poison. I just can't live with myself if I eat this piece of crusted meat.

At that moment, I feel a soft, insistent weight in my lap. Our dog, Lucky, has just placed her silken white head on my knees under the table, her doe-brown eyes looking lovingly up at me: a solution so wonderfully simple, delivered right in my lap. I look back at that trusting furry face, but I know Mum is watching me again, waiting to see what I'll do with the piece of burger that is speared on my fork. Then my dad interrupts, diverting her attention.

'Are these our own potatoes, Margie?' he asks, gesturing to his plate with a fork, in a tone that is casual but measured, measured in a way to disguise the hint of challenge in his voice. It reminds me of men on soap operas hammering their fists against blockaded doors as they demand a paternity test from a panic-stricken wife. I quickly slide the burger from my fork, passing it to the wet nose under the table for perusal, whereupon it disappears immediately. It's been another turbulent crop season for my dad's vegetable garden, another round locked in fierce combat with the wireworm, another week of turning a blind eye to Mum's dalliances in the produce aisle. She stares, caught like a deer in the headlights, at the spuds on his plate, and hesitates a beat too long. Despite all her diligent efforts to cover her tracks, implicating her children in the process, she could never lie about the provenance of potatoes when confronted.

'. . . Ahhhm, no, Donal, they're Flanagan's, I'm afraid,' she admits. 'I was worried we didn't have enough with yours.'

I grasp another large piece of burger with the very tips of my fingers and noiselessly pass it to the waiting mouth under the table. Mum can't quite meet Dad's eyes, and is still peering at the potatoes as though hoping they'll pipe up in her defence. *Try as she might, your offerings wouldn't even coat the base of the casserole dish!*

'Ohhh-ummmph,' he grunts, his blue-green gaze searching her, his cheeks bulging with another man's potatoes. Mum is looking ashamed, and a shade annoyed. When did feeding one's family become such a political obstacle course?

I guide a heap of rice shielding two more pieces of burger to the edge of my plate, gently knocking the pieces over the edge and into my lap, where they are snapped up instantaneously. I shovel some of the rice into my mouth and give Mum a supportive smile.

'Well, why don't *you* cook the potatoes next time, if it means so much to you?' she rallies, her elbow propped somewhat sullenly on the table as she goes back to her own dinner.

I pick up the very last piece of burger, a feeling of euphoria growing in my belly, and pretend to pass it from hand to mouth before dropping it below the table, right into the bottomless pit that is sweet Lucky. I ruffle the top of her head with a grateful hand. *Good dog.*

'Ahh,' my dad grunts dismissively, before admitting: 'I wouldn't know where to begin with cooking.' He returns gloomily to the potatoes, his pride wounded, but wisely sensing he's probed too far into the corners of an otherwise happy and amicable marriage.

Mum looks tired all of a sudden, but I am feeling elated and generous towards those around me, so I smile warmly at her. 'Thank you for dinner!' I say, jumping up to put my clean plate in the dishwasher.

'Oh, you ate it all – good girl,' she says, her expression brightening as her gaze follows me, surprised at the empty plate. 'I'll have to get more of those burgers,' she adds.

'Yes, sure,' I tell her heartily, and if I could have winked at Lucky as she washed her paws under the table, I would have – but alas, I do not have the eyelid dexterity.

Yes, reader, as you may have guessed, sleight of hand and a robust family dog are excellent accessories to a burgeoning anorexic. It all really snowballed after that. Lucky and I had a strong telepathic link that winter, her sitting under the table by my chair, me funnelling turkey burgers and pasta shells from my sleeve to her jaws like a life-support drip. I found other ways too, in situations where she was outside and not available to act as my personal compost heap. I'd tear off a piece of kitchen roll before dinner, placing it on my lap as a serviette, classy lady that I was, and then ball up little piles of potatoes, beans, bread, bananas, any kind of scrunchable food, siphoning it all neatly into a tight kitchen paper bundle. I'd retire to the garden after dinner 'for some fresh air' and pretend to gaze meditatively out at the setting sun on the glorious country horizon, but I actually went out there to fling fistfuls of dinner into the field behind our house. Hey, at least I was providing sustenance to the local wildlife! The feeling of euphoria and triumph when I'd managed to get away with eating even less food was intoxicating and sustained me through loud and lengthy hunger pangs. It was no longer about specific food groups, swearing off sugary breakfast cereals or giving up animal flesh. The more foods I cut out from my normal daily routine, the more I tested the limits of my willpower and body. How much food did I really need to eat? Did I *need* to eat any of it, at all?

But after some time, almost from one week to the very next, my 'health kick' went from being something that everyone praised and indulged to a distinct and openly acknowledged problem.

'What have you got there?' Mum asks, startling me one evening after dinner as I make my way to the back door to deliver another secret care package to the cows. I've managed to crumble more than half a mushroom pie into a now-sodden sheet of kitchen paper, which I am cradling protectively in the front pocket of my hoodie. Mum has started buying me Weight Watchers meals lately, having seemingly decided to play along with my regime, plucking packaged ready meals from plastic shopping bags and emphatically pointing out the nutritional tables that boast only point-something grams of fat per serving. I had been intrigued by these meals at first, with their bold assertions to enable consistent weight-loss all while eating modest but satisfactory dinners, but I am suspicious of the fact that they are tailor-made for clinically recognised overweight people – surely

I should be eating less than these for dinner. I've told Mum I like the ones with crusts, the pies or quiches, because they're easier to scrunch and mould into little balls of dense, easily portable snacks for my wildlife friends. I'm taking greater risks lately, arriving at the dinner table before everyone else while Mum is still busy at the cooker, to stuff handfuls of rice and chicken from my plate into my sleeves before placidly eating the remaining third in full view of everyone else. It's not always possible, though. Sometimes Emily is already sitting at the kitchen table, glaring intently at her maths homework, but still sharp enough to notice me claw half a turkey burger off the table. On these occasions, I slowly pick my way through dinner, gathering minuscule bites at the tip of my fork and feigning heightened exhaustion as I peck at the edges of my food for a long time, before setting doleful eyes on my mother and attesting that I'm simply not very hungry today, and today – just today – may I be excused? But, for the most part, I manage to palm larger and larger portions of the meals from plate to dog or sleeve or, sometimes, though I really do try to avoid it, the very bottom of the rubbish bin.

Until today, when Mum makes her way to the freezer at the same moment I'm sneaking out the back door, and finally she sees something. She's standing facing me, a quizzical but searching look on her face, holding herself so absolutely still with attentiveness that I wonder if she has known all along, deep down. Perhaps now is the moment we drop the facade and I confirm what she already suspects. I cradle the kitchen paper bundle closer to me, like I used to do with newly born kittens when I'd steal them away from their mother's warm, furry belly nest to admire and kiss their tiny pink paws, their intricately patterned velvet coats. Somehow, this secret feels much more dangerous than borrowing a kitten. I'm frozen to the spot, dumbstruck, with fear gripping my insides, as if I've been caught in a dreadful crime and am now facing life in a cell. What will she do when I reveal my indiscretions? Slap me? Rage at me? Certainly not – she doesn't have the temperament. But she might sit me back down at the table, unpack the soggy bundle on a plate while conjuring images of starving, swollen-bellied third-world children, the ones she pays €7 per month to feed, before making me consume the entire thing. Would prison really be worse?

'Nothing,' I stammer, unconvincingly. 'Nothing . . . just something for the cats.'

She studies my face, hesitating. She is not inclined to take her children for liars, and yet . . .

'No, come on. Show me what you have there,' she says, and takes a half-step towards me, her hand reaching for my secret. Reluctantly, I hand it over and feel my cheeks redden as she examines the squashed-up pie, a mixture of alarm and grim resignation playing on her face.

'I just . . . wasn't very hungry . . .' I splutter. 'I didn't want you to get upset. I just wrapped it up so I can eat it later. I will eat it . . . just . . . later.'

'Ah, no,' she says quietly, looking up at me, her expression frank, like it is impossible for me to deny the obvious a moment longer. 'This is most of your dinner,' she tells me, as if I had perhaps done it by accident. Then, her eyes flicking to the back door and back to me again, she asks: 'Were you about to throw this out?'

'No!' I answer quickly, acting scandalised. 'No, I was just going for a walk.'

'I thought you said you liked these pies!'

'I do! I just . . . I'm not hungry right now and I didn't want to upset you. I'll eat it tomorrow.'

She looks at me a long moment, her face full of doubt, waiting for me to say more, to confess, to drop the act, but I hold her gaze, trying to communicate utter sincerity with my eyes, though neither of us believe me.

'OK, well, if you're really not hungry.' She sighs, her mouth a small line of displeasure. 'I'll put it in the fridge then. You can have it tomorrow.'

I slink back to my room, inwardly fretting over the awareness that it's going to be harder to squirrel handfuls of food away now: that she's going to be watching me carefully, that there is a silent chess match, an unspoken subterfuge at play, it's one that we are both still refusing to acknowledge, but are equally determined to win.

'I'm bringing you to a dietitian,' Mum says firmly the next day after school as I sit in the front seat of her car. I freeze in the act of putting on my seatbelt, looking at her in disbelief. She very rarely puts her foot down: she tends to leave the strict disciplining to my dad, hovering guiltily in the background as he loudly chastises us over the mess of the living room and threatens to dispose of all our possessions unless we tidy them away. But now she stares straight ahead, her hands clamping the steering wheel, as though she is afraid that if she meets my eyes, I'll talk her out of it. She has been impressively strategic too, choosing a day when Emily is staying late for homework club, Mairéad has football practice and Patrick is at a friend's house. It's just me and her and the unspoken war we are waging.

'What?!' I huff, rolling my eyes. 'You're being ridiculous.' I'm already calculating how much time this appointment will leave me to go for a run before sunset, but I'm also mildly intrigued by the idea of a nutritional expert surveying my virtuous diet and vigilant exercise routine, and I wonder at this dietitian's reaction. Perhaps she might share her expert fat-loss tips.

'Well, I've booked this appointment, so we're going,' Mum insists, nodding curtly. 'I can't get you to eat, but maybe you'll listen to this lady.'

The dietitian's office is located on the ground floor of St Kevin's Hospital in the ER department. We're told to sit in the waiting area and that the dietitian will come and get us in a minute. We sit on the olive-green padded chairs, surveying jowly, purple-faced old men wavering slightly in their seats and restless noisy children with arms and fingers in casts. It's my first time in an emergency room, and I'm surprised by the lack of bloodshed, decapitated limbs and dying car-crash victims on gurneys. It's disappointing really: none of us look to be in a critical state, more just numbly *fading* from the tedium of our own lives and the aura of non-optimal health that seems to press down on this room. I glance sideways at Mum, who is perched nervously on the edge of her seat as she scrutinises the hospital signs, her fingers clenched anxiously on her handbag in her lap, distinctly uncomfortable. She does not want to become comfortable in this place.

A short, middle-aged woman with curly hair appears in the office door to our left and calls my name. She introduces herself as Deirdre, my new dietitian, and we follow her into the small, brightly lit office, seating ourselves in two chairs opposite her desk. Deirdre is an attractive, well-presented woman who smells like lavender powder. She has a look of the Whos of Whoville about her, an upturned nose and a slight overbite, but sadly not their festive spirit. She is a nice, softly spoken woman, but there lingers an air of sadness about her, an atmosphere of perpetual emotional weariness. I like her, she is kind, though I don't find her a particularly invigorating presence.

'Nice to meet you both,' Deirdre begins, settling herself behind her desk. 'Evanna, your mam has told me lots about you.'

I side-eye Mum.

'Maybe you could tell me a bit about what you're going through at the moment?' Deirdre says, smiling with an expression of watery sympathy entirely disproportionate to my situation.

Once more, I look at Mum, who is watching me hesitantly, and then I turn back to Deirdre. I'm thrown by the question, but I decide to answer it as honestly and simply as I can, to quickly allay this woman's suspicions so we can all go home and stop wasting time.

'I'm fine,' I tell her bluntly. 'I'm not really "going through" anything. I just started eating healthily and exercising a bit, and Mum got all worried for some reason. I'm fine,' I repeat, shrugging at her.

Deirdre looks back at me for a moment and purses her lips.

'*I'll* tell her what's going on,' Mum butts in, some vigour in her voice now. 'She's *not* fine,' she tells Deirdre fiercely. 'She's become absolutely obsessed with losing weight. She barely eats. She hides food from me and lies about it. She freaks out if there is so much as a drop of oil or butter on her food. She exercises several times a day. She seems to think about nothing else except her diet and her weight and her exercise regime, and she is looking paler and thinner every week, and I don't know what to do about it.' She finishes, looking slightly flushed, refusing to meet my eyes again. This is about as honest as our family get with one other. I'm not sure whether I feel embarrassed or impressed by her outburst. I look back plainly at Deirdre, not really feeling the need to challenge any of Mum's statements. Though heavily dramatised, that was the gist of it.

'OK, well, let's just have a chat to start, shall we?' Deirdre asks us placidly, opening a well-thumbed hardback notebook and writing a note at the top of a blank page. 'I'd like to get a clearer view of your diet, Evanna. Would you be willing to talk me through what you eat in an average day?' She looks at me, her pen poised above the page. I shrug at her noncommittally, but she continues to stare at me with an unblinking intensity that seems to demand a verbal answer, so I tell her 'Sure.'

Obligingly I talk her through my usual breakfast, lunch and dinner, and she writes each thing down, her face impassive. She insists I be very precise, interrupting me to ask the specific brand and flavour of anything that isn't a piece of fruit, and then notes that down too. Mum interjects too, to say no, that's incorrect, that I've stopped eating even the fat-free yoghurts lately, and that Deirdre shouldn't take my word for it.

'Is that true?' Deirdre asks, fixing me with another penetrating stare.

'No,' I reply, stubbornly, fuming with Mum. 'It's not.' If she has just come here to tell tales on me, I might not continue to be so cooperative. 'I still eat them *sometimes*,' I insist.

Deirdre nods and writes down the yoghurt. Agitation creases Mum's brow as she scrutinises Deirdre's upside-down scrawl, as though afraid I might have convinced this medical professional that everything is quite normal and that she is the one who is overreacting, and that she will have to go home and continue waging this silent war unabetted. I'm beginning to suspect I may have accomplished this too as I scan Deirdre's face for any hint of concern or displeasure as she calmly reviews my diet.

'OK,' she says, placing the notebook aside. 'Thank you for doing that. Now, I think it's important that we get your weight. Would you be OK with that?' she asks, looking at me again. She is not exactly condescending in the way she talks to me, but she speaks in a way that suggests we are co-conspirators. It's a tad overfamiliar for someone I've just met, but I'm fine to let her keep thinking this way, if only for her own benefit. As for being weighed, I'm uncomfortable though not appalled by the suggestion. Weight is just an innately shameful thing, isn't it? Any weight at all, no matter how skinny you are. It's embarrassing to take up space and have that space allocated a personal number that denotes your earthly bulk. I'm too young at eleven to examine why that might be, to realise how irrational and emotional that sentiment is. All I know is that weight is shameful.

'You can weigh me,' I say to Deirdre. Then I address Mum, telling her squarely: 'But you're not allowed to look.'

Mum looks back at me reproachfully, sensing boundaries being drawn as a punishment to her for taking me to a dietitian, for this sneaky and forceful move I hadn't anticipated.

'That's fine,' Deirdre affirms, getting up to pull out a strange plat-formed contraption from its place against the wall. 'We'll just keep it between us for now.' She asks me to remove my shoes and jacket, though lets me keep the rest of my uniform on. The weighing scale is one of those curious, clunky medical scales with a rubber-coated platform to stand on and a large measuring stick fixed perpendicular and at navel-height to the occupant. I can't read it, so I watch Deirdre's face as she adjusts the marking device, nudging it down to the left a little bit at a time. She continues to nudge it left, a few centimetres, then millimetres, her face unreadable, until the scale wobbles slightly before finally becoming still and perfectly balanced. Deirdre squints at the markings on the scale for several moments before straightening up.

'You can put your things back on, thanks,' she tells me, returning to her desk chair and pulling the notebook towards her again where she makes a subtle note, shielded by her hand. I sit back down beside Mum, who searches my face questioningly. But then Deirdre commands her attention, reaching for a thick purple folder filled with laminated pages. She lets it fall open to a large, coloured table with the words 'BMI Chart' over it, numbers lining the sides and crowding the hundreds of squares making up the chart. She pushes the folder in front of me.

'Do you know what a BMI is?' Deirdre asks me directly.

I shrug again. This is all such a fuss.

'. . . Sort of,' I answer.

'BMI is your Body Mass Index. It's a table that determines whether you're a healthy weight for your height.' She takes her pen and taps it on a cluster of green squares under my nose. 'See this?' she says. 'This is the healthy range for someone of your height.' I survey it disinterestedly. Mum leans forward attentively in her seat. 'And this,' Deirdre says, her pen moving backwards down the chart to some blue squares, 'this is where you are. You're in the "underweight" range.' I lean forwards to where her pen is pointing to admire my number. *Thank you*, I almost say to her, but I look up in time to catch her serious expression and I have the sense to repress this urge. She flips forward another few pages to another chart, with silhouettes of boys and girls of varying heights and ages, and a few paragraphs underneath.

'And this . . .' she points to a number in one of the paragraphs. '. . . is the average weight and BMI for someone of your age and height. You are significantly below the average weight for someone your age.'

My insides glitter with excitement as I hear these words, and I look closely at the noticeable gap between my own BMI and that of my so-called 'average' counterpart.

Deirdre clears her throat in an officious manner. 'Now,' she says, pulling a wad of tissue from a sleeve and dabbing at her nose. 'You're probably aware there are serious health risks to being so underweight at your age, but you might not know the specific conditions you're risking.' She proceeds to educate me on a catalogue of dreadful maladies resulting from malnutrition: stunted growth, infertility, osteoporosis, hair loss, kidney failure, death, etc., etc.

I blink back at her, nonplussed, as she lists off this series of potentially unfortunate events. But none of them do anything to disturb my mental equilibrium. Standing just under five foot, I am almost the same height as my tiny mother, and a career as a fashion model has never been in my future. As for infertility, *Bring it on*, I think. I can't imagine anything more repugnant than having a baby stretch and distort my body out of all recognition. Hard pass on pregnancy – today, and for the rest of my life. Even osteoporosis, with the graphic description Deirdre gives of bones hollowing out porously, starved of nutrition, and your skeleton crumbling inwards until you are hunched over and balancing on rods of metal rather than your own shin bones, has no effect on me. What do I care if my skinny aspirations at eleven result in my vertebrae crumbling down on top of one another one day in the distant future, at the age of sixty-five rather than eighty, making my latter years in the nursing home just slightly more uncomfortable? This is all so far from relevant to me. Sure, they were accurate, historically documented health risks associated with under-eating to cite and perhaps she was obliged to draw my attention to them but as a child you don't really think of a future beyond the next Christmas season and all her cautions might just as well have been speculative fiction as far as I was concerned. She just wasn't making a compelling case for giving up my self-betterment crusade. My mother, on the other hand, looks horrified, her mouth tense as she bends over an illustration of a bone interior that looks like honeycomb.

'Look,' says Deirdre, interlacing her fingers on her desk. 'I know your health is very important to you and you don't want to get fat.' I flinch at these words, which are too bare, too crude. It's not that I'm just trying to avoid the unbearable eventuality of being 'fat'; that is unthinkable. It's that I don't want to have any fat on me at all. I want to lead an entirely fat-less life, to be completely free of fat or, another word for it, mistakes. Maybe then I will be able to relax, take a breath, and try for a while to accept myself. I can't confide this to Deirdre, though, so I stay silent.

'So let's just focus on stabilising your weight for now,' says Deirdre, opening her notebook again and flicking to the page with my food diary. 'You're not currently consuming enough calories to sustain your weight with such an active lifestyle. So how about we add in the yoghurt *here* . . .' She taps her pen on my lunch items and then writes '+ yoghurt'. 'And then add in two slices of toast with jam *here*.' She adds the toast as a new meal labelled 'Supper' at 8pm. 'How would that be?' she asks, setting down her pen and peering intently at me. 'Would you agree to do that this week?'

60

Do I have a choice, I think bitterly, as Mum and Deirdre watch me expectantly. I have no intention of gaining weight, and I am not done trying to fix my body either, but I can almost see the porous bone diagrams and a neon red sign screaming 'OSTEOPOROSIS!' reflected in Mum's pupils. I know she is going to be on high alert for the next few weeks, and that maintaining my current weight is perhaps the most prudent thing I can do for now to assuage her fears and get her to stop paying such close attention.

'No butter with the jam,' I answer firmly, striking a less than satisfactory bargain.

'Understood,' says Deirdre, taking this as consent and making another note in her diary. She copies out my diet on a fresh page, then tears it out and hands it to Mum, who folds it carefully.

Deirdre leans forward in her seat then, her tone conspiratorial again as she addresses me. 'Can you and I make a deal?' she says, looking me in the eyes.

There's a pointless question if ever I heard one. It almost didn't warrant an answer.

'Ehm . . . it depends on the deal,' I reply, reasonably.

A shadow of a smile crosses Deirdre's face. 'Yes, well . . . can we make a deal that you won't lose any more weight while we're working together?'

Working together? I think. I've been practically shunted into this office. When has my grudging tolerance been taken as tacit complicity? None of this has been for me. Neither of them has considered or even bothered to ask what *I* want. I feel a rush of anger towards the two of them, but especially my mother, who seems to take it for granted that strange adults with medical charts have more right to decide what goes into my body than I do. That they know what's right for my body better than I do; that they ought to decide what size it should be. I feel no ethical qualms about the lies I'm going to tell them from here on out. They don't want to know what's really going on with me, so I might as well just say the things they want to hear.

'OK. I won't gain weight, but I won't lose it either,' I agree.

Deirdre looks satisfied and holds out her hand to shake over the table. I grasp her fingers briefly. Mum appears pleased by this little ceremony. She looks brighter, hopeful. She naively expects it will be this simple, but my mind is already fixing my impressively low BMI neatly in my mind. I am thinking fondly of all the other average, lumpy children my age and realising that I am unique in my aptitude for thinness. I walk a little taller exiting Deirdre's office, eyeing all the grey-faced, sick people expiring slowly while I thrive on my disease of scrupulous self-improvement.

After that, I saw a different doctor every week. Mum made something of a hobby of it, flicking through the Yellow Pages in the evenings and studiously copying names, contact details and qualifications of doctors, psychiatrists and therapists into her little address book. Sometimes, friends of friends would call her up, parents of other children who had 'issues', with testimonials about expert psychiatrists who'd helped them. I would grit my teeth as I caught a snippet of her conversation, mumbling on the phone in sombre tones to perfect strangers, oversharing details of her problem child's lifestyle. It was all so ridiculous to me, such an overreaction, but for the most part I let her carry on with this hobby uninterrupted, because it kept her entertained and often diverted her attention from me as I snuck out the back door to squeeze in another quick run.

As for the doctors, they were all the same really. Po-faced, whisk-ered men with large, cold hands, sitting behind handsome oak desks framed by oddly sexual sculptural lamps. They'd sit me down, ask for a few sparse personal details, and then peer into my ears or throat or listen to my heart with an ice-cold stethoscope, their expressionless eyes looking out the window as we waited, their slow blinks the only thing moving in a clean, lifeless office. Doctors who looked like they hadn't seen the sunlight in years would grill me on my diet, my exercise regime, my image of my own body, and then slowly recount the multitude of illnesses I was risking. Osteoporosis was the firm favourite and they always had diagrams. But what obsessed them all even more than osteoporosis was the question of whether or not I thought I was 'fat'. Afterwards, a permed secretary would casually demand €120, an obscene amount for my parents, and I'd avert my eyes, burning with guilt and shame as my dad fumbled a handful of crisp new twenties and slid them over to the impassive receptionist.

I don't think, over the dozens of appointments, sessions and meet-ings with medical professionals, that one of them ever sat opposite me, looked me in the eyes and truly asked how *I* was. I don't think they really looked beyond what they saw at first glance – a stubborn, shy eleven-year-old girl and an eating disorder – to the person who was desperately trying to look after herself as best she knew how. So, they focused their brilliant minds and professional expertise on the easy, evident problem, my medical particulars, which were plenty distracting and which had easy remedies – food, supplements, rest – and they asked how I was as a passing afterthought, something non-critical that could be dealt with someday in the fullness of time after they'd addressed my weight problem.

Occasionally, one of them might ask me if I was depressed, and

I would shrug, uncomfortable, and tell them 'not particularly'. I'm not saying that any of these doctors or therapists were negligent or incompetent but I am suggesting that the medical system got it wrong in their methods of treating the superficial symptoms of starvation to heal the eating disorder, and I'm not sure their approach has evolved much since. I'm saying that they were asking all the wrong questions.

Socially and medically speaking, when compared to anyone else, I knew I wasn't 'fat', but I still looked down at my own body every day and felt an overwhelming swell of revulsion and nausea at the bits of soft flesh clinging to my legs and abdomen. I still fantasised about taking a knife to my inner thighs and attempting to squeeze the remaining fat cells out. A fat person and a fat cell were two entirely different things; one was just an abstract social construct; the other one I loathed and wanted to scourge from my body. And as for being depressed, I hadn't lied about that either. *Before* I adopted my health regime, before I began to control my weight, I had been adrift, lost, stressed, lonely – and, for a short while until I found a way to help myself, depressed. I'd been intermittently grappling with this horribly urgent question of who I was and coming face to face with the realisation that I didn't have a place in the world, that my life was probably meaningless and I had no inherent worth to pay for my existence. But then I'd found something that muted that pain and took my mind entirely off it. So maybe I was still depressed, deep down, but I had this *thing* now, and with this thing I was too focused, too driven, too busy, too obsessed, too tired, too numb to feel anything deeper.

'Do you know how much weight you've lost since you started coming to me? Since we made that deal?' Deirdre asks, leaning forward and looking at me intently. It's been two months since I first entered her office, and my weight has taken a steady downwards trajectory since our handshake.

'No.' I shake my head, truthfully. *Tellll meeee*, my mind purrs.

Deirdre's answer shocks and thrills me. It is much more weight than I'd planned or expected to lose. I feel a flutter of pride, a rare moment of self-satisfaction. I don't weigh myself at home, terrified of the resultant panic of seeing the numbers creeping upwards, and strangely, I don't ever *feel* like I've lost weight. I only notice small things, like my school skirt becoming looser, the tendons on the backs of my knees feeling sharper as I press my hands into their hollow crevices for warmth. Deirdre looks at me meaningfully, searching for any indication that I recognise the seriousness of this news, so I try very hard to suppress my delight and to arrange my features into an expression of sombre acknowledgement.

Mum puts her head in her hands, curling over her knees, and lets out a throaty sound that is somewhere between a sigh and a sob. I don't know if you ever saw your parent crumple in front of you as a child, but there is something uniquely repulsive about it. Rather than elicit sympathy or a rush of compassion towards a tender show of their own bare humanity, it provokes a kind of horror at the fact that this fragile, pitiful person has somehow wound up being your parent. This is the helpless sapling meant to protect and guide you through life, to educate you in the ways of this world. Instinctively, I cross my arms and legs as she breathes heavily.

'I don't know what to do,' she confesses, and whether she is speaking to me, Deirdre, herself, or an indistinct celestial being, it is unclear. She continues, ranting into her knees. She's just venting nonsensically now, emotion thickening her voice. 'I take her to every doctor . . . every therapist. I buy her any food she'll eat. I don't force her. I try to encourage her. I try to talk to her. We try so hard with her. I don't know what I'm doing wrong . . . I don't know . . .'

Deirdre lays a hand on her forearm, quietening her. 'I know, Marguerite. You're not doing anything wrong. We'll figure it out.'

I watch the two of them commiserating quietly over this fiction they have concocted, this tragic tale they have spun around me using BMI charts and their own overactive imaginations. Feeling disembodied from this whole experience, feeling like it doesn't even concern me, I shrink away from the two of them in disgust.

But while everyone around me documented and scrutinised my diet and diminishing frame in minute detail, they didn't notice that I was losing something much bigger than weight; I was losing my creativity. My regime was more than a superficial obsession with my body; it was an overall obsession with productivity. Every moment of every day was a new opportunity to prove myself worthy of the space I took up.

And though I tried to hang on to the things I used to love – painting pictures, drawing, sewing, dancing – gradually, those things started to feel like frivolous indulgences I could not justify. It was so much easier to accept and live with myself when I was focusing all my resources, mind, body and soul, on simply burning fat. Art was still important to me – I couldn't quite stop myself reaching for intricately patterned fabrics or glittering tubes of beads – so I tried to find space for it by squashing my creativity into small, square boxes of time, assigning myself thirty minutes of drawing or beading at the very end of my list of objectives for the day, after school, after several hours of exercise and food prep, the two hours of homework and the inevitable serious chat with Mum. Then, and only then, I would sit down and try to force the breath of creativity from my numb, exhausted body. But creativity, she doesn't fit in a box. She's a wild, fluid, uncontrollable energy that spreads out sensuously from a curious, wide open mind, in large expanses of aimless time on dreamy liminal train journeys or in subtle moments between waking and sleep. She can't be pushed or coughed up or beaten into submission by a brutal and unmerciful regime. She needs light and breath and space, and then, maybe, if the mood takes her, she'll unfurl her wings and let her colours run into the atmosphere. And this energy – this wild, fun, unpredictable magic that I'd played with so happily as a child, that had flowed through me like it was my very life force up until this point – I didn't understand it anymore. Creativity was this swirling, wild, mysterious language, but now I lived in a colourless, angular world that promised me a certainty I valued above all else. And where before I was just scribbling, writing, moving for the mere joy of it, now I tried to commodify my creativity. I tried to squeeze it out and make it *do* something worthwhile, be special, be important, be good. I could no longer see the point of art if it wasn't good. But that's the tricky thing about art: it's never strictly good or bad, it's just expression or excretion. It couldn't be measured by scales or charts or contained in small manageable segments of the day. It was always, by its very nature, *so* imperfect – and the imperfections drove me mad. The anxiety and frustration with my creative endeavours turned into an actual fear of blank pages and palettes of paint. There was too much potential and too much room to fail, so, day by day, I chose perfection over creativity; I chose no more creativity and no more mistakes. There are things that eating disorders take from you that are more important – much greater and more profound a loss, and much, much more difficult to recover and restore completely – than body fat, and that reckless urge to create just for the pure, senseless joy of it would become the one I missed the most.

Am I suggesting it would have been a more effective treatment to send me to an endless succession of art, dance and drama classes than on a national tour of Ireland's most prestigious mental health professionals? Not really. Sometimes I think there is an inevitability to eating disorders: a fierce, focused, burning force, that nothing can alter or stop, a fire that won't just be snuffed out. I'm simply pointing out that an eating disorder is a mental condition, and that the physical problems that occur are side effects, and so it will never work to use the strategy of trying to seize and pull apart the problem in one's hands, by carefully monitoring a body, by trying to stuff that body with food and squash the eating disorder out. It was never simply an eating problem to begin with. What I am suggesting is that the more everyone zeroed in on my eating problem, measuring my body, monitoring my diet, balking at my compulsive exercising or the peculiar behaviours I collected as easily as Pokémon cards, the more my environment seemed to suit my eating disorder. My world was getting smaller and smaller the more everyone tried to fix my problem. It was becoming easier and easier to keep up my routine, and only my routine. I didn't have to make up so many excuses, keep up a careful semblance of normality. It was almost as though by watching me and keeping me under careful scrutiny, they were all expecting me to lose weight, setting me new, more ambitious targets to beat each week – and I wasn't about to disappoint. It was becoming more awkward to maintain friendships too. The other kids wanted to play and gossip, whereas all I wanted was to get things done. I stopped accepting invitations to friends' houses, and gradually they stopped asking. I didn't really miss my friends, either, because I didn't have time to think about them. I had sit-ups to do, another hour of cardio, journaling about my fitness plan for the week ahead, and I was exhausted and cold, and I had nothing to talk about.

Maybe it is asking too much of a parent to smile and relax and treat their daughter as their daughter, and not as a sick, vindictive demon that has ensnared their child, when they can't look at her without being appalled by the physical changes they see. Maybe that's just too hard. But I'll always object to the depiction of eating disorders as an evil parasitic presence, because it doesn't feel like that, and it doesn't help for everyone around you to treat you as that. My 'problem' felt too much like my solution, my strength, the part of me that was saving me from just being depressed, from giving up on everything. But the more they focused on this thing they had termed my 'problem', the more it felt like it was my entire identity. The more life became a series of doctor's appointments, psychiatric interrogations, heated arguments, and a sea of angry or anxious faces everywhere I went, the easier it was for the person who had been there before to slink away, and the more she became just a memory. And the harder it was to find her, to even believe in her, when I finally started to want her back.

All of this time, however, nobody had given a name to what was going on. My life, which was comprised almost entirely of medical appointments, dieting and tense exchanges with my family, was vastly different from the lives of all the other eleven-year-olds in my periphery, but the way I saw it, these were just the tedious new precautions of an overly anxious mother, just a phase we were going through as my parents learned to adapt to my new ambitions, the divergent path I was treading. They were modest, self-deprecating folk who just couldn't understand a child with the ruthless determination to not settle for herself. This was just a common parent–child miscommunication, and we didn't need a word for it. Until, one day, my sister blurted it out.

It's Sunday afternoon and the family are rushing around the house, wiping off worktops and hastily applying mascara in the dusty mirror over the fireplace. It's a few days after Christmas, and today is the annual family gathering, where all Mum's side of the family get together to weigh each other down with dense fruit cakes and buttery chocolate logs, and then to sleepily ruminate on political scandals and family affairs around the fire. I am not looking forward to this. In years previous, I would giddily anticipate this day, overdosing on sugar, swooning at beautifully wrapped presents, and then snuggling up to my older cousins and gazing adoringly up at them with their edgy eye make-up and anecdotes of teenage revelry. But a lot has changed in a year, and a day of overindulgence and aimless lounging comprises all my greatest fears now. I'm in the kitchen, slathering cupcakes with green-and-red lemon frosting, painting on elegant candy canes and holly sprigs in glitter-pen icing, but mentally, I am running through all the delicious, rich, indulgent foods I'm going to have to avoid. A familiar undertone of dread and panic is tugging at my mental clarity. Mum knows my diet and routine: we have an understanding, a system that is perfectly normal and functional, but I know it won't appear that way to anyone else, that they won't get it. They'll ask questions and give me sidelong glances, and I'll have to stand there feeling awkward and distinctly uncomfortable. I'm bending over a cupcake, my fist clenched tight around the icing pen as I work to finish an elegant, cursive '*Happy Christmas!*' on one of the cupcakes. Strangely, I've become totally obsessed with *making* food lately. I've always liked baking, but it's become almost compulsive, my need to empty bags of caster sugar and little packets of chocolate chips into mixing bowls, to whip them up into delectable-looking desserts, and it monopolises my attention when I'm sitting in class or cycling home. When I'm not fastidiously totting up the calorie content of Ryvita crackers in my head or plotting my weekly work-outs, I'm poring, open-mouthed and glazed-eyed, over colourful baking books with gorgeous confectionery, making endless lists of all the things I'm going to bake. I love passing these treats around to family and friends, get a warm rush of pleasure from seeing them sink their teeth into thick pink icing and demolishing the cupcakes crumb by crumb. Mum thinks it comes from a tendency towards sadism – 'You enjoy watching your friends getting fatter while you waste away' – but it actually isn't that. It's that watching other people lick and swallow their way through sumptuous-looking treats that I long to taste is the closest I can get to actually eating them. Mum comes in from outside, where she's been feeding the cats an early supper, shaking some raindrops out of her hair.

'Mum,' I say, in a quiet, tentative voice. 'I don't think I can come today.' I don't meet her eyes, focusing instead on the cupcakes, quietly nudging them into tidy lines of four by six, enough to go around the whole family, with a few spares. She stops moving and stands, just looking at me. I think she may have anticipated this.

'No,' she says, firmly. 'You have to come today.'

She never says no. Her flat refusal steels something inside me.

'I'm sorry, I just have too much to do. I don't think I'd be good company anyway,' I push back, carefully picking some hardened icing off the palms of my hands.

'No,' she repeats. 'You have to come. It would be very rude not to. And your aunts have bought you Christmas presents. You can't *not* turn up.'

'It's OK,' I insist, my voice louder now. 'They can just keep them. I don't need them.'

'That's a very ungrateful thing to say,' she snaps back. 'So, what, are you going to spend your holidays running in circles round the football pitch while your family enjoys a nice Christmas together?' she demands, sarcasm colouring her rising tone.

I keep my eyes downcast and answer her as calmly as I can, just willing this exchange to be over, for us to peacefully agree to leave me to my own devices. 'No, I just really need to do *some* form of exercise today and I won't get time if I go to Dublin. You know I don't enjoy sitting on couches and stuffing myself with pudding and I'd just be a nuisance anyway with my diet.'

'Your diet, your *DIET*,' she scoffs, smacking the bag of cat food down on to the table. 'I am sick to death of your diet. You're the last person in this house who needs to be on a diet, and now you won't even join your family for one day on Christmas.' Her voice breaks and she strides out of the kitchen to the living room, where I hear her whispering in urgent tones to my dad. I close my eyes, readying myself for battle as I hear him storming into the kitchen.

'*No*, I'm not having this,' he growls, his face flushed with anger already. He's a soft-hearted, cheerful country man on any given day, smiling at everyone and enquiring about their parents' health, but the strict, unyielding vice principal who keeps wayward teenage girls in line and oversees biweekly detentions comes out when pushed, and he can be scary. 'Do you have any idea what you're doing to your mother? Do you have any regard for us at all?' Mum is standing in the background, meekly clutching her own elbows. The guilt-tripping is what gets me.

'I'm doing *NOTHING* to her,' I shout, standing up to face him. 'She's the one who keeps pestering me with her doctors and dietitians. I didn't ask you to get me all this *help*.' I spit the last word in disgust.

His face is scarlet now, his mouth pinched in an angry line. 'You're a right brat, you know that!' he answers jutting his index finger at me, and I feel a well of despair and pain rise up against this assault, my chin wobbling. 'We don't deserve this treatment at all.'

'If you hate me so much, then why don't you just leave me alone like I'm asking you to?!' I scream at him, and then, unable to withstand any more blows, run around the kitchen table, through the living room, hearing Mum quietly counsel, 'Just leave her . . .' I head to my room, my bed, where I wrap myself in a dark, impenetrable cocoon and cry. Ten minutes later, I hear them collecting in the hall, debating where to put Lucky, reminding each other to bring this box of chocolates, that bottle of wine, the Christmas cards, as they make their way out the door.

'Where's Evanna?' my little brother pipes up. He is eight, and all of this chaos and familial tension breezes swiftly over his curly head.

'She's not coming,' Mairéad answers in a cold voice. My sisters are always angry at me lately. I'm taking up all my parents' attention these days, and hundreds of euros per week of their modest teacher salaries for counselling sessions that are not yet yielding results. From their perspective, all I had to do to cheer up my parents and restore the balance and humour that I'd cruelly stolen from our lives, was to eat something. And then, in a deliberately raised voice, so she knew

I would overhear, Mairéad says: 'She's staying at home to live out her MISERABLE, *ANOREXIC* life alone.'

The door slams, and moments later I hear the car tyres crunch on the gravelly driveway, Lucky barking them off on their journey. I cry in my bed for a little bit longer, then get up, wipe my face and make my way down to the kitchen. Mum has left two cupcakes, one red, one green – the one that says '*Happy Christmas!*' – and a short note telling me where to find the rice and beans she's left for me, and to please be careful and take Lucky if I go out on the roads. She signs it off with a multitude of 'x's and 'o's that prompt another stream of silent tears from me for some reason. But even though I feel terribly lonely and a bit heartbroken, my overwhelming feeling as I stand there, breathing in the serenity and calm of an empty house, broken only by the comforting, methodical ticking of the clock, is *relief*. Trixie, my favourite cat, winds her velvety body around my ankles, and I smile at her and go to shake out a few more biscuits into her bowl, the little morsels hitting perky musical notes in the silence as they bounce off the bottom. Now they are gone, and I can just spend the whole afternoon and evening exercising and organising my life and carefully planning out the precise portions of food needed to sustain me for the week ahead. It is my idea of a perfect day.

Anorexic, my sister had said. The word hadn't stopped ringing in my head since she said it. The memory of that mysterious, intriguing girl my parents had mentioned a year back, the one I'd pictured as a supermodel or a kind of otherworldly alien-woman, flitted to my mind. It had been a long time since I'd wondered about her and what she was searching for. Was this where we were? Had I come that far from myself – was I there already? When I first heard about anorexia, I never planned for it to become my *thing*. I didn't connect to it or dwell on it or decide to try it out for a while. All I'd known was that I was empty, unremarkable, unexceptional at everything, and that it would be hard to find love, friends, work, a place in the world at all, if I didn't find something by which to define myself – and then I'd found *it*. I think to me, being unremarkable was the same thing as being unlovable, and if I didn't have love, I wouldn't want to live, and if I didn't want to live, I'd eventually die. And I really wanted to find a way to fight that urge to die. People see eating disorders as slow self-destruction, but the intention is quite the opposite. It's a stab at life, at asserting oneself. It's a fierce, warlike struggle to battle all the voices – internal and external – telling you you'd be better off dead. I hadn't planned for this to be my path – was shocked to hear that dangerous, spiky word affixed to me by my sister – but OK, now I'd found it, and here we were, and I didn't know how – nor did I care – to find a way out of it.

'You're a horrible, selfish person!' Emily screams at me, her cheeks red, her eyes blazing and filling with tears. She is blocking my exit to the front door, instructed by Mum to make sure I don't go out for a cycle while she makes a quick trip to the shops.

Mum has started actively banning me from exercising now, asserting that I'm too thin and it's dangerous for someone that weak to go out on a bike on narrow country roads. Weak! On the contrary, her regime has provoked a fierce, rebellious streak in me, a surge of energy that I channel into openly resisting and defying her demands. I don't feel pity for the cute little cakes she tries to guilt me into eating anymore, or for the mask of anxiety and fear she seems to never take off around me. I feel contempt for her interference, for her pathetic displays of weakness, weeping on the phone to her friends or appealing to my sisters for help in handling me. I scoff at Emily's responsible-older-child act.

'This has nothing to do with you,' I spit back at her. '*You* don't tell me what to do! I'll just go out the window!' I grin, dashing through the door to the sitting room and fumbling with the catch on the window.

'I hate you!' Emily screams, pursuing me. 'The only person you care about is yourself!'

'I just want to be left ALONE!' I roar, forcing Emily to step back, my temper snapping, my heart thumping, as I try to smother something raw and tender below all that red-hot anger. I cannot understand what they're all talking about with their melodramatic assertions that I'm 'dangerously thin', that I'm risking my life with my diet, when right now I've never felt more energised, more driven – and even though sometimes the hunger pangs cause spells of lethargy and I can't ever seem to get warm anymore, no matter how many cardigans I pile on, right now I feel like I could fight anyone off with my bare hands. *Too thin*. It feels like they are mocking me when they say these things, pantomiming some other sick, vulnerable girl's life, someone who is *actually* close to death and in need of medical attention, when behind closed doors they are throwing back their heads and laughing at this elaborate ploy to drag me back down into being my fat, useless old self. I just can't see myself in the things they say about me, refuse to indulge this ridiculous atmosphere of danger and urgency they've concocted around me, when right now I feel vibrant with health and more purposeful than I ever have before. From the corner of my eye, I see Mum's car pulling into the driveway.

'You're ruining Mam and Dad's lives!' Emily throws at me, sniffling, before she turns on her heel and runs off to get Mum's help. I don't waste a moment, bolting out the window, racing to the garage, wrenching out my bike and making straight for the road, not looking back. Tears are streaming down my cheeks now, and I tilt my head to hide my face as cars pass, trying to look like a normal, happy person on a bicycle, not a hysterical, anorexic nutcase. Lucky has joined me on the road, prancing along beside my bike, tail waving frantically, tongue lolling happily, the sole supporter and ally of my outdoor sports career. Watching this happy, buoyant presence calms and soothes me. Animals. They are so simple, so nice. They don't care if you eat breakfast or not, if you gain five pounds or lose fifteen; they don't even care if you eat other animals. And they won't abandon you when you're being a selfish, ruthless, conniving bitch, ruining the lives of everyone who loves you. They'll just continue lolloping along, asking for nothing more than your presence and kindness, a few squeezes of affection. Lucky is practically beaming as we race down the other side of the hill, the wind smoothing the tears off my face, the tension off my back. I look back briefly at the white house perched on the hill. It looks so cosy, so warm, a swirl of smoke spiralling out of the chimney into the deepening dark blue sky. No one has chosen to follow me. I've won this battle.

Ruining Mam and Dad's lives. Emily's words echo in my mind as I pedal further and further away from them. It's true: I am. Consuming their happiness, throwing out their food, absorbing all their thoughts and peace and hard-earned comfort.

Or – my mind fights back angrily against this blanket, unfair accusation – are they just overreacting? Am I really asking for that much? To have the freedom to look after myself, to go for a cycle, to eat what I want, to sort out my own life? Aren't I simply asking to be left alone? Isn't it my life, *my* unfortunate body? They have their own lives and bodies, and I have never tried to interfere with those.

I continue on my cycle, focusing on the calming, exhausting ritual of pedalling one foot after the other with a body that is already sore and tired, depleted from hunger and lack of rest. As tired and drained as I feel, physically, it is always far easier to keep going than to confront the anxiety, the cacophony of panic and criticism that will start up the moment I choose to stop burning calories I'd promised to be rid of. This is the only way to achieve calm, to feel OK, to keep finding that lovely, elusive feeling of momentarily being enough.

An hour later, I wheel my bike back into the garage and then slip quietly through the back door and into the utility room. I can see my sisters working studiously in the kitchen, the surface of the table entirely covered by the contents of their schoolbags: thick, dog-eared textbooks, calculators, dictionaries, copybooks, Shakespearean texts. Perfect children hunched over complex words and numbers, their faces masks of concentration, their minds teeming with deeply serious and important worldly matters. I try to slip by unnoticed, but Mairéad glances up, her expression hardening when our eyes meet, and then returns to her Geography homework. Emily refuses to look at me, but I see her anger in her reddened cheeks, her furious concentration on her calculator. Anger and disdain radiate from both sisters.

'Hi,' Mum says just as I reach the door to the living room. She is distant with me, sad, though offers a weak smile as she rinses some vegetables by the sink.

'Hi,' I answer stiffly, unsmiling, then hurry to my room.

My sisters' fury is weighing on me. They seem to really hate me most days, and though I maintain a needle-pointed focus on my goals, let nothing and nobody deter or distract me from my daily routine, the atmosphere of collective vitriol they create still seeps in through the cracks of my armoured defences and hurts the vulnerable softness underneath. *Selfish*, that is their primary complaint. That I don't care about the family or the stress I've brought into their lives, or the aura of fear and anxiety that hangs about my parents all day, every day. I am a spoiled, self-centred brat, as far as they are concerned. And while, in some ways, they are right about that – I don't have the space in my mind or my day to sit and think about other people or what they need, and this is an entirely selfish, isolated way to live – in another way, I'm not asking for anything at all, and isn't that the opposite of selfish? I don't want people's food or attention or sympathy or help. I don't expect people to like or love me, and I don't waste my time looking for it. If they could only feel all the self-loathing coursing through me, the visceral self-disgust, the ardent wish to be rescued from the unrelentingly awful reality of being in this body, maybe they'd be selfish too. All I want is to quietly with-draw from life – which is too difficult, too painful, too much for me to get a handle on – and all I am asking is that they leave me to it, to the safe, comfortable anaesthetising routine I've developed that feels much easier than living fully. Is it so selfish to self-preserve?

I put my sisters' scowling faces out of my mind as I nestle into a corner of my bed, and crack open *Goblet of Fire* for the third time that year. My *Harry Potter* books are the only things that stop my mind obsessively running through the calorie count of foods I've eaten that day or devising clever methods of avoiding eating certain meals at friends' parties. The magical world is the single place I can go where I'm not confronted by images of glamorously wasted young women, girls as skinny and malnourished as I am, but who have made a career out of it. The books give me a break from the atmosphere of tension and unrest that pervades any time I enter a room. Nothing else seems to still the relentless whirring of my mind in the same way *Harry Potter* does. And where my art, my friends, my dreams have faded and fallen out of my life, somehow *Harry Potter* remains. I read them over and over during this period, picking up *Philosopher's Stone* to start the series all over again as soon as I have finished the last page of *Goblet of Fire*. Mum tries to diversify my reading materials every now and then, bringing home books with brightly patterned covers and cheesy titles like *Nobody's Perfect* or *Love Yourself First!*, written by 'girls with similar problems', but she ceases these efforts when I start citing the calorie-burning tips and extreme crash diets I've picked up from these memoirs.

Half an hour into the second task of the Triwizard tournament, I hear a soft knock on my bedroom door and permit Mum to come in. I don't lower the book as she perches at the foot of my bed and looks at me.

'How's your book?' she asks, her voice soft and tentative.

'Great,' I reply.

'You must have read it ten times by now,' she says, conversationally.

'Almost,' I tell her, lowering the book. 'I think it's more like eight.'

She nods and smiles, amused. 'Well, you'll be more than ready for the fifth one to come out then.' It's the winter of 2002, and the next book in the series is due to be published on 21 June 2003. I'd reserved a copy in Eason's, our local bookshop, the day after it had been announced.

'Yes, I'm going to be the first person in line to get it this summer,'

I tell her happily. Something about what I've said seems to bother her, though, and I watch her relaxed smile become corrupted by that familiar grimace of anxiety.

'Will you have something to eat?' she asks.

'No, thank you,' I tell her, returning to my book.

'Just a small bowl of cereal?' she says, a note of pleading in her voice.

'I'm not hungry,' I answer firmly.

'Nothing?'

I am so *tired* of this game, the constant bargaining, the seemingly hourly negotiations to eat or not to eat. I just want to retire from eating, be done with the whole messy, unpalatable affair. Why do people have to eat so often, upwards of three, four, five times a day? Do they have nothing more interesting to do? Do people eat to live or live to eat?

'I'll have an apple,' I tell her, grudgingly.

For a moment, it looks as though she's about to start ranting hysterically, or worse, to wilt and do that unbearable broken-parent act, but then she seems to swallow her emotions, nodding agreeably and telling me she'll be back in a moment. She returns five minutes later, places a small bowl on my bedside table and bids me goodnight. I continue reading for another few minutes, stubbornly ignoring the bowl, until eventually my curiosity, more than the aching hunger that I've grown used to, which feels more like a companion, a tangible affirmation of self-worth than an inconvenience, urges me to reach for it.

I stare down at the little bowl in my hands: white, with dainty blue and red flowers decorating the edges. She has peeled a perfect Golden Delicious, sliced it thinly and then arranged the pieces in a small flower shape, the slices overlapping each other like petals. I'd taken away her favourite love language, banished all the cakes and biscuits, the Penguin bars and Jaffa cakes, the little jam tart treats she'd sneak into our lunchboxes as a surprise. No sugar, no butter, no light and fluffy thickly iced buns. I'd denied anything she made with her hands, with thought and love, and allowed only cold, hard flavourless whole foods from the ground to pass my lips. I had barricaded myself away from love, stripping away life's most simple, frivolous pleasures one by one, until my world was completely boarded up from the affections of others, impenetrable and unforthcoming. I'd told everyone to leave me alone, to stop trying to help, that I didn't need them or ask them to care about me. I'd told them to go about their lives and forget I was there. I'd denied and refused my mother's love for months, coldly pushing it back towards her across the table. I had tried to get rid of it so it would be easier and less complicated to continue my efforts to slowly, peacefully shrink. And yet here it still was, bare, simple, stripped of its frills but neatly arranged in the shape of a yellow flower made of carefully sliced apple pieces, my mother's love still trying to get through the cracks of the fortress I'd built against it.

3

After a while, everyone just sort of accepted it. Things calmed down at home somewhat. Mum continued to ferry me to weekly appointments with any medical professional who'd see me, but we didn't argue relentlessly over food portions at dinner, and I'd stopped contradicting my sisters when they scathingly referred to my exercise regime as an eating disorder, though I really did believe, right until the bitter end (and this is something you have to understand about eating disorders) that I had everything under control. From time to time, I struck loose-ended new bargains with Deirdre or my parents to not lose any more weight, but I'd become adept at outsmarting the scales, chugging water for hours before a weigh-in, and wrapping batteries in socks before tucking them discreetly into my skirt pockets, and this worked to allay their panic – for a while, anyway. We talked about anorexia quite openly at home now, though I couldn't say the word. I still find it hard to say it, to even write it, like I'm in the presence of royalty, a mysterious darkness, a powerful force of which I'm not worthy. But everyone acknowledged I had it, resigned themselves to its presence and, as with any pervasive horribleness for which nobody can find a resolution, soon we found the comedy in the situation and it became something we all made dark jokes about.

So it was that it became normal for my siblings and I to sit around the TV in the evenings and irreverently discuss my diminishing physique.

'How many of your vertebrae can I count now? I want to check!' Emily would declare, jumping out of her seat as I shivered through a thin cotton nightie that exposed my spine.

'Your back is getting hairier than your arms, did you notice?' Mairéad would point out in disgust, squinting at me from her place on the couch.

Far from being offended, I was always thrilled by these observations, encouraging them to elaborate. I think they meant to mock me, to slyly deride and punish me for the havoc I was wreaking on my parents' mental health, but I found their barbed comments and contemptuous stares deeply flattering, and always considered our sisterly bond greatly strengthened by these conversations.

One evening as my mum, sisters and I are sitting around the fire watching a *Lord of the Rings* DVD, a certain character prompts a stark comparison from my sisters that satisfies me immensely.

'Gollum! That's it! That's who you look like! You're as bad as him,' Emily exclaims triumphantly, pointing emphatically at the TV screen. I'm sitting on a pouffe in front of the roaring fire, combing my dripping wet hair, my feet tucked into fluffy slippers. I've taken to stationing myself in front of the fire each evening after I've finished my exercise routine and showered, sitting so close that the skin on my upper arms and face glow ruby red. It's the only time I manage to snatch a few moments of physical comfort, the only way I can stop feeling cold nowadays.

Mairéad, the resident *Lord of the Rings* fangirl, cocks her head at the TV before agreeing. 'Oh yeah, that's you all over.' She nods. 'You have the same body type. There now,' she says to me, grinning widely. 'You have a celebrity doppelgänger!'

Mum, who has been sitting in an armchair near the fire and studying a knitting magazine, looks up at this conversation, frowning slightly at the television and at Mairéad and Emily sniggering on the couch.

'I don't!' I protest, only half-heartedly, because I am looking at the knobbly creature on the screen, with his crazed, orb-like eyes, and feeling faintly flattered by this comparison. *That's what I look like to them?* I wonder, in disbelief, looking at him more closely. He's grotesque, sure, sort of endearingly gross, but that's not what I see. I see his entire skeleton! He's all sinewy, twig-like arms and bony femurs bound tightly by ropey muscles. There is not a pick of fat on him, bones jutting starkly out beyond skin at every angle. Huge, hungry eyes bulge out of a hollowed-out, angular face that is more skull than flesh. Those cheekbones, that xylophone ribcage, darling! His looks like a body that hasn't known any type of physical pleasure or indulgence in a lifetime, toughened and beaten into a gnarled, worn shape: a body that knows only how to endure suffering. It's a body that doesn't know what it feels like to indulge in rest or love or self-acceptance. He looks *great,* in my opinion. Not beautiful, but he has achieved some sort of aesthetic physical perfection. I feel elated by the insinuation that I bear any resemblance to this rippling specimen, as he scales the side of a slimy rock face, muttering furiously to himself, the vertebrae of his entire spine shimmering. '. . . do I?' I ask, tearing my eyes from the screen to interrogate my sisters.

'Yeah, look,' Emily says, a mixture of distaste and bemusement colouring her features as she watches the screen. 'You even act like him.' On the TV, Gollum is having a conversation with himself, intermittently weeping and lapsing into vicious tirades of self-flagellation. 'You don't have any friends,' he snarls at himself. 'Nobody likes youuu!'

'Uncanny,' deadpans Emily, as Gollum writhes around in agony, cowering from his own insults. As pathetic and pitiful as this tortured creature looks, I can't help but admire his spiky shoulder girdle. 'I hate you. I *hate* you,' he croons, tenderly cradling his own face. I admit, I find him somewhat relatable.

'Stop that,' Mum pipes up sharply from her knitting magazine, berating my sisters. 'She doesn't look like Gollum, go away out of that.'

My sisters continue to giggle, Emily offering a small conspiratorial shrug to Mum.

'He's a horrible, ugly little demon-man, and you're an attractive young girl,' Mum affirms in my direction.

I grimace inwardly at the feeble compliment. I was much more comfortable being likened to a horrible little demon-man.

'Sure, you don't want to look like him, do you?' Mum says, and it's hard to tell if it's a rhetorical question, a note of alarm creeping into her voice. I am silent a moment as I watch Gollum scampering away into the darkness on all four of his wiry limbs.

'I actually think he looks quite *good*,' I say in a very low voice, knowing immediately those were words I should not have dared breathe aloud. I can feel Mum staring at me, freaked out by her freaky daughter.

'*Jesus*,' *Emily* mutters under her breath, the laughter gone now.

But I am unperturbed, feeling buoyed, inspired even, by my apparent resemblance to this wasted little imp man.

These are the things you don't say to people with anorexia. It only encourages them. It feeds the eating disorder and quiets the person beneath it. People think they are doing something productive about your problem, pointing out how frail or scary you look, recoiling at your exposed arms in PE class and gasping at your spindly legs in a mini skirt, but actually they are just airing their own anxieties and insecurities, and reinforcing the idea that, first and foremost, the world sees an eating disorder when it sees you. I became accustomed, almost every day, to hearing a version of 'You look sick' or 'You're killing yourself' or 'You look like a corpse', but rather than jolt or upset me, as was perhaps intended, I enjoyed these comments. I sought them out, enjoying the shock and attention my thinness attracted everywhere I went. I loved to hear Deirdre recite what weight percentile I'd dropped to, loved the look of worry etched on Mum's face as she exclaimed at the way my new jeans were 'falling off' me, loved when my sisters took bets for how long it would be before they could fit one hand all the way around my upper arms. I know on some level they were trying to shake me out of my reverie, trying to reach me, or maybe they just couldn't help themselves, but these comments were counterproductive to their aims. To my mind, 'You look like you're going to die,' sounded more like they were telling me I was special or strong, maybe even perfect.

If you really want to be a positive influence in an anorexic's life, if you want to help them out of this darkness rather than allowing them to sink deeper into it, it's better to talk about any-thing else with them than their bodies. Talk about the weather. The news. Naked mole rats. That crazy conspiracy theory about the Hollywood elite torturing virgins in order to harvest and drink the adrenochrome from their blood. Talk to them about literally anything other than how bad they look. Don't count their ribs or grimace when they remove their coat, and definitely don't refer to them as 'an anorexic'. I know I have routinely used this term a lot throughout this book, and I know that this chapter is riddled with it, but I'm only doing so out of convenience, as a way to collectively refer to people who are struggling with a condition I'm trying to explore, and partly because the only way I know how to deal with writing in vivid detail about experiences that were my darkest and saddest is to do so irreverently. But I would not reduce a person to an illness, no matter how sick or faded they are from it, because I know how hard it is to disentangle oneself from the label. Anorexia is a problem, not a person. When you find yourself forgetting this distinction, when anorexia almost completely takes over, resist. I strongly believe in maintaining a firm verbal separation between the person and the problem, because, as I remember it, it was at about the time when people started habitually referring to me as 'anorexic' that the eating disorder became more prominent to everyone else than *I* was: that was when mentally, emotionally, spiritually, I almost completely checked out. I didn't have much of a personality anymore, or a life. I'd become more like a machine than a human, lifelessly drifting from one activity to the next. I wasn't depressed or unhappy during this time; I was just completely driven and completely numb. In some ways, I was the happiest I'd ever been. Maybe not happy, but content, certain. I had achieved some previously elusive anaesthetised state of mental calm. In some ways, I think the only way to be truly at peace is to turn your capacity to feel way down, to not really be fully alive.

And yet . . . I still had dreams. Small, quiet dreams that I secretly nurtured in a hidden enclave of my mind when nobody else was around. Dreams that felt silly and childish, that I didn't dare express openly, but that refused to be extinguished. And I still attended drama and dance class every Wednesday evening from 4–6pm. Like everything else in my life, the atmosphere around me in drama classes had changed as my disorder intensified. The boy who used to taunt me under his breath and snigger at my outfits took to ignoring me completely, and the cool girls gave me a wide berth. Also, I had two new friends, Clara and Caragh, confident townies who had recently joined the drama class, who weren't exactly shunned by the popular group, but who were too proudly nonconformist to fit in with them. I was always good at picking up the dance steps and eagerly shared my techniques with them. I had also learned over time how to dim my eccentricities enough that I didn't make a spectacle of myself with every outfit. These attributes combined meant that, over time, Clara and Caragh accepted me into their fold. They'd been best friends since childhood and so had an intimidating shorthand and archive of in-jokes to pull from that alienated but fascinated me. I'd watch them gabbling animatedly to each other, rapt, wondering what it felt like to be so vital in another's life, to have your thoughts so intertwined, your presence justified by the other's presence. Sometimes, I would contribute to conversations about our favourite pop stars and *Pokémon*, but for the most part I stayed quiet, watching and listening, and mentally practising the dance steps in my head: my social currency. The only time my presence really garnered any direct attention was during breaktimes, when occasionally one of my friends would dare me to eat some of their snacks for money.

'I can't remember the last time I saw you eat anything at breaktime!' Clara, the obvious leader of our group, exclaims loudly one day between classes. 'You're so skinny, I bet you don't eat any sweets at all!' she continues, her mouth crammed with Tayto crisps, her fingers coated in a greasy layer of salt. Clara is loud, pretty and naturally skinny, thin-limbed with a taut, perpetually bare midriff, à la noughties-era Britney Spears. She has the kind of metabolism whereby it doesn't matter how many fizzy drinks she knocks back or how many orange cheese puffs she gorges on: her lithe physique remains unaltered. For months, I've envied her jutting hip bones and twig-like arms, and now here she is, anointing me the skinny one of the group.

'Yeah, except apples. I seen her eat apples,' Caragh agrees. Caragh, in contrast to Clara, is a naturally plump girl, which she carries well, always swaddled in velvet Juicy Couture tracksuits that lend a maturity to her shapeliness, and swishing around a thick brunette ponytail of hair so shiny you can practically check your reflection in it.

'I dare you to eat this Freddo bar!' Clara says, pulling a Cadbury's chocolate smiling frog man out of her pink plastic handbag and shaking him under my nose. 'I'll even pay you two euro to eat it!' she adds, producing a coin.

'No thanks,' I answer, shaking my head and giggling, but grasping my elbows tensely.

'Come on!' chimes in Caragh. 'That's a good deal!'

I continue to shake my head politely.

'Fine – five euro to eat the head, final offer!' says Clara, whipping a clean €5 note out of her back pocket. The two girls watch me, agog. But I don't relent.

I never do. I enjoy these exchanges. It feels nice to be receiving attention for a covetous talent – thinness – rather than being the awkward, oddly dressed and just generally peculiar girl in the corner. People treat me like I am something fragile and unusual, not pathetic and embarrassing. It's a kind of scrutiny I can endure.

The attitude of my peers wasn't the only thing that changed about drama classes, though. For the first time since I'd ventured into that small black box theatre with the multicoloured lights, I was no longer getting picked to play the lead roles. Previously, I'd been one of the students that teachers trusted with large blocks of text, multiple entrances and quick costume changes. But that all stopped as I leaned further into my eating disorder. I still got high marks in the drama exams, still showed up every Wednesday with my monologues and poems neatly annotated and learned by heart, but apparently I no longer looked like I could handle things.

Still, I nurtured this acting dream, albeit privately. But you have to have remarkably high self-esteem to state aloud these kinds of lofty aspirations, especially in sleepy, rural Ireland, and I thought so little of myself. I felt so small and insignificant in the face of these dreams, so my pursuits were only half-hearted. When the cool, confident, beautiful kids cottoned on to the fact that drama classes weren't just for weird, bookish losers and that it was potentially a path to fame, so joined drama class and started sweeping up the best parts, I didn't try very hard to compete. Instead, I just intensified my exercise regime, my diet, drifting and drifting, cutting out more and more, feeling less and less, until it seemed like I was living on the peripheries of the lives of everyone around me.

A new word had entered my remit lately: recovery. Everywhere I went, people seemed to venture this unappealing word. Before I even knew what it meant, before anyone bothered to explain, the concept of recovery was forced upon me. *Your recovery,* they called it. *My* recovery wasn't going well. *My* recovery was going to take some time. *My* recovery demanded my total cooperation. They spoke about it like it was inevitable, like it was a given that I would consent to it. But recovery of what? That was the thing nobody explained. They gave vague, nondescript answers, like my 'health', my 'future', my 'career', but I was already going to school, my classes, cycling hither and thither with my disorder neatly intact. What would I even be recovering? My previous sad, insecure, lumpy self, without her steely armour of thinness? I didn't *want* her back. I didn't *need* recovery from this thing that was helping me fit in and stand out in ways I liked. They had all colluded in it, too, stressing and obsessing and focusing on my disorder above every other thing about me. What would recovery look like when it would annihilate the thing I'd built my identity on? Was there anything worth salvaging, worth *recovering* about me beyond my disorder? I didn't know at this point, and was not remotely curious to find out. It gets to a point where to kill off the eating disorder would feel like self-annihilation, and you don't actually want to die, so instead you just keep starving yourself. Where did I see this ending? I didn't. At eleven, you don't plan your life much further than two weeks into the future. Everything else just seems too far away, practically a fantasy. All I knew was that I was *fine*. I was coping. I wasn't drowning in self-hatred anymore;

I knew at the end of each day, as I lay there exhausted, spent, my insides growling with hunger, that I'd done everything I could to fix myself, and that knowledge alone lulled me into a deep, dreamless sleep. What was I waiting for? Nothing, really. I couldn't picture a future anymore, be it as a cat or a pony or an actress or simply a happy person. I was just *waiting*. For life to spontaneously change, to improve, or else to just quietly end.

But one person refuses to submit so easily to my disorder. Mum approaches me one evening as I'm crouched over the heater in the living room, struggling to write an English essay on the ironing board. She generally hates it when I spend my evenings hugging the heater – it reminds her how sick and strange I am, as my siblings' shouts and squeals of laughter permeate from outside where they are playing football on the front lawn in the brisk cold, normal healthy children enjoying the outdoors – but she smiles amiably as she approaches me. It is a tentative approach, her expression friendly, hands clasped in front of her, and I know a proposition is playing at her lips, one I'm not going to like.

'I've just got off the phone with a very nice lady,' she tells me in a bright, melodic voice, before hesitating. '. . . A psychotherapist.'

I scoff in reply, and hunch further over my copybook, wrapping my huge cardigan around my sides.

'No, no, I really think you'll like this lady,' she asserts, pressing on. 'She's a psychotherapist who has just moved to Drogheda, and she's very excited to meet you. She has struggled with anorexia and bulimia herself, so she knows exactly what you're going through. I thought you could just meet her and have a chat . . .'

'I don't think so,' I answer flatly, blinking at my copybook.

Mum twists her hands around one another tensely. 'Now, just hang on a minute, this lady really is different,' she continues. 'She's *young* and she's *alternative*; she isn't going to weigh you or show you all those charts.'

My expression remains impassive, but frankly, a therapist who isn't going to weigh me and list a litany of conditions that might polish me off is a dramatic swerve in the direction of my mother's doctor-browsing results. All the same, I am just done with them all.

'I don't want to go,' I tell Mum firmly. 'I'm sick of your doctors. She'll just try to get me to talk about my hidden traumas, and she'll get you all flustered, and anyway we both know the aim of these appointments is to get me to gain weight, no matter how you sell it to me.' I return to my essay, agitated. 'And I bet she does have charts,' I add.

Mum stands there, hands still clasped, looking deflated, but she doesn't budge. And then she seems to gather herself, her face resolute. 'Well, I've already made an appointment,' she says firmly, as I '*Ugh*' loudly, annoyed but unsurprised. She continues: '. . . And you don't have to go if you really don't want to, but if you don't go, then I'm afraid . . . I won't bring you to your drama class tomorrow.'

I look up at her in shock, totally taken aback by this new, hard-nosed, ultimatum-dealing swindler, standing where my sweet, wholesome, agreeable mother had been moments previous. Indeed, she herself looked quite shell-shocked at the words that had just left her mouth, shifting from foot to foot as though expecting me to laugh at her. '. . . And Dad has said he won't bring you either, so . . . that's that. We have an appointment at six-thirty tomorrow, so if you agree to go, I'll pick you up from drama class at six, and we'll go straight there.' She nods, pleased with herself for having effectively delivered this clearly rehearsed speech. 'I'll let you get back to your essay,' she finishes, before retreating to the kitchen and pulling the door closed.

My drama classes. It's clever of her, and I didn't see it coming. There are pivotal moments like this when in the grip of anorexia, when your mind must conduct a fierce, back-and-forth negotiation between your dreams and your disorder. It isn't safe for my disorder to meet yet another therapist, to be scrutinised under a medical lens, to be poked and prodded, both mentally and physically, to be elbowed into a forced confession of disordered eating habits and toxic self-talk. To maybe actually receive effective therapy that might encourage me to gain weight, and then to wake up one day horror-struck at my body and how drastically I've let some psychotherapist brainwash me. These doctors will never be a safe place for my eating disorder. At the same time, my drama classes are the safe place I go to to nurture my dreams, and I do not want to relinquish them either. To protect the dream or the disorder: this will become the most difficult of choices that I will routinely have to grapple with, a choice I will have to make over and over. But today, it is just *one* small micro-decision, as I scribble angry doodles in the back of my copybook, fuming with my mother for putting me in this impossible position.

'OK, fine,' I bark, throwing the kitchen door open and addressing Mum, who is sitting at the kitchen table leafing through a *Woman's Weekly*. 'I'll go see your *lady*,' I tell her, rolling my eyes pointedly. 'Just for this week.'

'Wonderful,' Mum answers, beaming, a naive, foolish, almost childlike expression of hope lighting up her face.

95

'Are you sure we have the right address?' I ask Mum the following evening at 6.30pm as we shiver on the doorstep of a modest semi-detached house that shows no signs of being the office of a respected psychotherapist. Mum is looking concerned as she squints at the doorbell and then twists her head around to glance up and down the quiet residential street, but there are no impressive gold plaques listing medical credentials, and no stray dog-walkers to interrogate.

Frowning, Mum digs in her bag and produces a small, folded piece of paper. She squints at it. 'Yes, we're definitely at the right address,' she says, shrugging. '. . . But maybe I got the appointment time wrong,' she adds doubtfully, furrowing her brow.

'Maybe *she's* forgotten about our appointment,' I suggest hopefully. 'Let's just leave it,' I say, jerking my head back towards the safe warm car, my mood brightening.

'No, no, this is definitely the house, let me just try one more time,' Mum insists, pressing the bell with greater purpose this time and stepping back. I shiver and look back towards the car longingly, and just as I can see Mum about to give up too, we hear movement within the house, the sound of feet barrelling down the stairs, and a cheerful, ebullient voice crying, 'SorrydarlingsSORRY!'

Mum glances at me briefly, an expression playing on her face that is half curiously intrigued, half deeply wary, and I can tell that she has no more idea what we're in for with this psychotherapist than I do. But the front door snaps open just then, and a tall, blonde, radiant woman stands there beaming at us, and bellows to the whole street: 'SORRY darlings, I need to get that doorbell fixed, I can never hear it properly over my meditation music!'

Dr Natasha Tighe. She's unlike anyone I've ever encountered before. She's loud, majestic, oozing charisma, and even though she has a PhD to her name, she is dressed like a regal fairy queen, draped in turquoise and gold-spangled shawls, a sensuous silky maxi dress, and sparkly thong sandals. She is the Elle Woods of psychotherapists. She has caramel-hued skin, bright, *bright* blond hair framing a handsome, square-jawed face, and wide, soulful eyes of a deep sea-blue that have been decorated liberally with a layer of glittery silver eyeshadow. In fact, everything about her seems to sparkle: her eyes, her glossy pink lips, her multi-layered gauzy outfit, her *spirit*. The effect is somewhat dazzling, or dizzying, in a way where the eye is unsure where to settle, which glitzy detail to try and take in. But there's no time to take her in; no sooner has she opened the door than she descends on Mum – 'Hello Marguerite!' – planting an audible kiss on each cheek, and then turns to me, exclaiming 'Hello beautiful!', printing the same lip-glossy kisses on either of my cheeks and wrapping me in a hug so tight I almost cough. She smells of rosewater and fake tan. I feel warmed, but distinctly embarrassed by her welcome, casting my eyes quickly about me as if expecting one of the neighbours to spring out from behind a bush and sneer at the fact that this tall, glowing angel-lady just addressed me as 'beautiful'. I glance at Mum, who is looking similarly ruffled, and repress a giggle as I sight two lurid, shiny pink lip-gloss marks printed on her pale cheeks, giving the impression of a rosy-cheeked girl with pigtails in a 1950s storybook. A modest, diminutive, Irish Catholic lady, Mum does not trust effusive public displays of affection – or women who wear fake tan. I can see she is already questioning the authenticity of Natasha's degree, and missing the familiar formalities of dead-eyed secretaries and airless waiting rooms papered in stark anatomical diagrams. But Natasha is beckoning us warmly into her home, and with one last look of trepidation in my direction, Mum steps inside.

We follow Natasha into a cosy living room that feels exactly like the interior of a fairy's secret woodland sanctuary, albeit with a few electrical enhancements. The room is dimly but magically lit by tasteful yellow fairy lights stretching across the mantelpiece and snaking around golden picture frames. They could also conceivably be Christmas lights that have simply been left up two months late; Natasha seems like that kind of person. The beige carpet is thickly cushioned and springy to walk on, enhancing the feeling that we're treading on the mossy floors of a hollowed-out oak tree, and the navy couches are plump and inviting, their surfaces draped in countless sumptuous velvet, fleece and satin throws and quilts. They're the kind of couches you can only collapse in to, and later have to hoist yourself out of with a great deal of effort so Mum and I perch ourselves cautiously on one couch edge after Natasha gestures for us to sit. And instead of degrees and osteoporosis diagrams, the walls are filled with stoic, proud-shouldered angels with majestically unfurled wings, and scantily clad fairies lounging on toadstools. Fairies and angels, in fact, populate every surface in the room: the mantelpiece, the top of the TV, the cluster of small tables in the corners, all of them lounging, luxuriating and basking unapologetically, interspersed with the odd family photograph. I am nervously eyeing a bare-chested, Rapunzel-haired smouldering male angel, when Natasha appears at my side, still beaming, and throws a cream-coloured shaggy blanket around my shoulders. She wraps it around me once, twice, until I am fully bundled up, just a pair of eyes peering out of a faux-fur cocoon.

'Now, darling, just want to make sure you're comfortable,' she mutters, squeezing my shoulders, and then reaches behind me, seizing another blanket, this one an emerald-green velvet. She throws this around the shoulders of my unsuspecting mother, who looks quite uncomfortable as Natasha encases her in velvet. Finally, Natasha grabs a pack of matches and lights a pink incense stick held aloft by a small ornamental fairy child, before settling herself in a cross-legged position on the carpet in the middle of the hearth, whereupon she sets her twinkling eyes upon us, and smiles kindly.

'I'm delighted to meet you,' she says, addressing me, as though I am an important guest, a much-anticipated VIP, her eyes holding my gaze the whole time. 'Your mam has told me so much about you; I'm really happy you've come to see me.' She is familiar and friendly in breaking the ice, not cautious and careful the way I usually prefer, but I don't mind, because, for once, this strange lady is looking at *me*, is seeing me, is speaking to me like I'm an adult, or just a whole person worthy of respect. Her gaze is arresting and alive, demanding my full presence. And when she asks me to tell her in my own words what's been going on, she seems like she is genuinely, honestly asking me a question and is interested in getting to know me.

But I don't trust glamorous women either. I've never found them kind or sincere. They always seem too aware of their beauty and power to fully invest themselves in another person, to surrender to the act of truly listening to someone else's troubles. They don't need to, either; it isn't a fight or even an effort for them to justify the space they take up. And I come from a family of teachers, who spend their evenings poring over copybooks or historical fiction novels, who only ever glance at the mirror perfunctorily, to flatten their curls or pick lint off a jacket – never to admire, to enjoy the sight of their own reflection. It seems socially impossible that one could be smart, well-read, *and* have time to administer a smooth, even layer of St Tropez to every square inch of skin. It seems unfair too, and self-indulgent. These are all prejudices of course, based on the fact that I feel self-conscious, insignificant and completely exposed, my every flaw thrown into relief, under the unwavering gaze of this strong, beautiful woman who clearly loves and cherishes herself.

'Well . . . it was Mum's idea . . .' I say awkwardly. I look at Mum imploringly, but she doesn't take over, just sits there staring at me intently from her blanket. 'I don't really need help . . .' I continue, suddenly noticing all types of intricate, distracting details on my own palms. 'I just don't want to gain weight . . .' I blurt out, my face feeling hot. I'm embarrassed at my inarticulacy and how childish I sound. I twiddle the tufted blanket between my fingers, nervous. I'm usually so able to deal with these therapists. Deflecting them archly with a series of sarcastic, monosyllabic replies, the disdain and aggravation I feel towards them forming an impenetrable barrier. But for some reason, I can't summon any anger towards this woman. She doesn't feel like an enemy. She is offering and commanding respect. And today my laconicism is not coming from a place of simple, stubborn resistance, but from this feeling of defencelessness and total vulnerability that her attention elicits; from genuinely not having the words to answer her question.

'That's OK, angel.' Natasha smiles, answering a question I didn't need to speak, and then asks Mum to share how things have been for her. Mum shoulders her way out of the velvet blanket in a small, irksome movement, and sitting determinedly at the edge of the cloud-like sofa, proceeds to tell the familiar sob story in a grave, formal tone that I've come to know as the serious-adult voice she adopts to impress new doctors. Natasha makes sympathetic noises and nods along as Mum speaks, not taking notes, but listening intently, her palms open on her knees like a Buddhist in meditation. Every now and then, her glance flickers over to me, smiling so warmly, but not in the mischievous, faux-conspiratorial way of previous doctors trying to get me on-side, trying to fool me into thinking we have a secret alliance; she's just looking at me, checking on me, letting me know that I'm part of this conversation too. Mum is recounting our most recent visit to Deirdre, who is losing patience with the both of us and threatening hospitalisation if things don't improve. A note of despair in her voice now, Mum is airing concerns that if I'm hospitalised, I'll fall behind on my education and not progress to secondary school along with my classmates, when Natasha interrupts her politely.

'I understand, Marguerite, but I think we're getting a bit ahead of ourselves,' she says gently.

I pull my attention away from the window I'd been gazing out of; I tend to zone out completely when Mum allows her imagination free rein to follow every paranoid train of thought, right to the end of its track.

'If it's OK with the two of you,' Natasha continues, 'I'd like to talk to Evanna alone for a bit.' She looks between us both, enquiringly.

I shrug towards Mum and give Natasha a small nod. Mum looks anxious, hesitant, as though she'd like to confer with me and verify all the details I'm going to divulge about myself and her, before sharing them with this bronzed heathen, but seeing no other option than to comply, she nods too, and stands nervously.

'Wonderful,' Natasha declares, springing to her shoeless feet. She grabs a white-and-gold covered book entitled *Angel Magic* off the top of a pile of books beside her, along with the green velvet blanket. 'I'll show you into the front room.' She leads the way out into the hall, and Mum, throwing one last worried look at me, as though anxiously envisioning the kind of terrible, psychologically manipulative, abusive witch-mother I might depict her as in her absence, follows her out. I hear Natasha tell Mum, 'You might like to read this . . . pass the time,' and Mum mumbling something about having schoolwork to finish, but a minute later, Natasha returns without the blanket or the book, and I enjoy the mental visual of Mum in a quiet room swaddled in velvet again, clutching the New Age book and probably trying to avoid the sensual stare of a nude archangel Michael.

'So delighted to meet you, angel,' Natasha says again, squeezing my hands firmly before sitting down again in her cross-legged position on the floor and fixing me with those penetrating eyes. 'I just want to get to know you a little better. And, darling, before we continue, I want to tell you that anything we talk about in this room remains strictly between us. You don't have to share anything we discuss with anyone else, not your doctor, not your family, not even your mam. And similarly, I won't share anything we've discussed with your parents, unless I've reason to be concerned for your safety at any point. So, *this* –' she gestures to the twinkling room around us '– is our sacred space. Cool?' she asks, raising a thin, arched eyebrow and waiting for my reply.

'Cool,' I confirm, in a small voice.

'Fabulous,' Natasha says, smiling widely again. And then she plunges in with a question so direct, so simple, so normal, it catches me off guard. 'So, darling, how are you doing?'

I fidget with a tassel on the fluffy blanket and try to recall my day at school, to dredge up the ordinary rituals I fill my time with, and that one usually uses to fend off this apparently superficial but all too complex question.

'I'm . . . I've . . . well, I . . . I'm . . .' In a flash, Natasha has produced a large box of tissues, before I even realise that I'm crying. Not crying – weeping, I am full-on *weeping*. In another instant, Natasha is by my side on the couch, hugging me firmly and pressing wads of tissue into my hands. She is squeezing my shoulder and saying in a soft voice, 'It's OK, darling, it's OK. Just get it all out.' She doesn't seem to care that I am snotty and leaking a river of tears on to her lovely, warm, perfumed shoulder, or that I might smudge her tan. She doesn't care that I am an awkward child whom she barely knows, and she hugs me like I'm a person who needs a hug, not a delicate china doll she's afraid might shatter. She seems to emanate love as she rocks me, this person I didn't know twenty-five minutes ago, and tells me in a gentle voice to keep crying as much as I want. I cry and cry and cry, soaking through fistfuls of tissues, and she doesn't do anything except hold me for a long time, until eventually I start to feel somewhat soothed and, through gulps and sniffles, in a strangled voice, I tell her *Thank you.*

I should point out here that you won't find many therapists who hug and rock you for a solid ten minutes as part of the therapy, and nor should you expect it; it's definitely unorthodox in the field of psychotherapy to be so tactile with a patient, but Natasha is a maverick in her line of work and refuses to play to the system's rules. She once recounted to me her own first experience of psychotherapy, how cold, clinical and impersonal it was and how it only made her retreat into herself deeper. It crystallised in her the firm intention to offer precisely the opposite energy in her work, to emanate love and warmth to every lost soul who showed up on her doorstep. I'm sure she would be criticised and frowned on by her peers, and indeed it would not have felt OK if any one of the greying, mustachioed doctors I'd encountered before had pulled me into a bear hug, but Natasha was working from her heart and intuition and in that moment she knew I needed a hug. She continues hugging me tightly, and just as I begin to wonder is this some kind of ultra-alternative New Age therapy where we spend the entire hour hugging rather than talking, she gives me one last squeeze, fixes the blanket around my shoulders again, and returns to her spot on the floor, looking at me with a tender expression.

I don't know what it was. She hadn't done anything except ask me how I was. And with anyone else in the world, I would have shrugged, answered that I was 'fine', and I would have believed that I was. But for some reason, looking into these kind, loving, deep-blue eyes, for the first time in a while, I seem to breathe out and realise that I do not feel fine at all. I'm just *sad*, I tell her. I'm lonely. I'm tired. I'm bored of my life and sick of the constant exhausting cycle of exercising and thinking about food and navigating my family and the doctors and my own obsessive thoughts, and then waking up the next morning, still exhausted, with a feeling of dread, knowing that I have to repeat the cycle all over again, but also knowing that eating like a normal person would feel so much worse than any of that. I have big, ludicrous dreams of being an actress or an artist or a dancer, but I am too shy and awkward and plain, and people will just laugh at me if I speak these dreams aloud. I want real friends, but I don't have the time to spend on other people, and everyone thinks I'm a freak anyway, so why bother? I want a different life, but I do not want to break this safe, familiar cycle. I want to be someone else, but I don't believe I can be, and I don't want to risk sacrificing my comforting state of thinness to try that out, only to realise that I've lost my armour and confirmed my worthlessness. Deep down, I want to be free of my obsession with thinness, but nothing in my reach seems worth it. And, I tell her, the only time I ever feel anything approaching happiness is at the end of the day when I get into bed and there is nothing else in the way of me succumbing to exhaustion, and maybe for a few fleeting moments when I step on the scales and see that my weight has dropped before my mind starts panicking and planning how I'm going to maintain this new low weight. And *maybe*, I add, maybe sometimes for a few minutes a day, when I'm reading a *Harry Potter* book, though even that is fading lately and losing its power to distract me.

I talk more to this kind stranger than I have done to anyone else in a year. For her part, Natasha doesn't do a whole lot, just sits there nodding encouragingly, taking everything in, reminding me to breathe when I get too worked up, but her presence is entirely unusual. No matter what I tell her, the ugliest, meanest, worst thoughts, she doesn't seem shocked or offended, or to like me any less. She actually seems to *understand* everything I tell her. I don't know or trust that it isn't an act: I'm well aware that I'm unworthy of her attention, and that she may just be tolerating me for the €60 an hour that Mum is paying, but she has such compassionate eyes, and she listens with an attentiveness that seems to imply she actually wants to know me better, and understands completely. Too soon, she thanks me for my honesty, laying her hand gently on my twisting, tightly clasped fingers, and then tells me she'd like to lead me through a meditation. I've never meditated in my life; I hardly know what it means. It conjures images of crinkle-faced, bearded monks on snow-capped mountains, and I'm highly suspicious of anything that claims to improve people as they lie, inert, on a sofa. I only know how to achieve through bitter, painful graft and action. Nevertheless, I comply, too discombobulated and confused to object, and lie supine on the couch as Natasha busies herself, burying me in a mound of blankets and quilts, tucking the edges in beneath my elbows, and then adjusting the CD so it begins to play what sounds like a choir of virgins crooning mournfully to the Irish sea. She instructs me to close my eyes, places her hand on my forehead and tells me to imagine myself in a forest by a waterfall, proceeding to talk me through a visualisation where I meet some sort of white light and step into its embrace. A stream of tears trickles down the side of my face, like something deep within has become unstoppered. The virgins continue to wail, but the tears have nothing to do with their melancholic chant or the bright light; I'm just leaking emotions, for no discernible reason. I try to go with the meditation, to lose myself in the enchanted mists of this magical forest, but I am enjoying the comforting nest of this blanket cocoon in the corporeal world, and Natasha's firm, reassuring touch on my forehead, and I don't think I ever really penetrate the spiritual plane. When Natasha calls me 'back into the room' a few minutes later, I sit up immediately, probably too quickly, clumsily trying to wipe the wetness from my cheeks and hair. The sky is pitch black outside the window, and Natasha gives me one of her warm smiles before reaching for a small pink-and-navy box to her right.

'Well done, angel. That was a lot,' she says, nodding sincerely. She removes a stack of navy cards from the little box and begins shuffling them easily. 'We got through so much today. Thank you for your honesty.'

I'm not sure I agree. All we've 'got through' was me verbally vomiting a stream of incredibly toxic thoughts, none of which were a surprise to me. Now this nastiness I've been cultivating privately for months is out in the atmosphere, percolating within another person. I don't see how that could possibly be progress. I feel nicer in her presence, safe, but I do not feel like I have changed remotely. An hour has passed, we've traversed some sort of magical spiritual garden, but still I know I will go home and resume my fierce, unrelenting routine. Nothing has changed. I am at once profoundly relieved and disappointed.

'Pick a card,' she tells me, splaying them out in front of me. I see that each one of them is printed with a whimsical picture of a golden-haired mermaid sitting on a rock, under the light of a full moon and a star-spangled midnight-blue sky, as a small, graceful fairy with elegant, iridescent pink-and-yellow wings reaches out a hand to touch the mermaid. It is either enchanting or horribly saccharine. But in the light of the sparkling fairy lights and the haze of the post-meditation glow, my cynicism has evaporated and it feels like this moment is mired in significance.

'How do I know the right one to pick?' I ask Natasha, immobilised by indecision.

'Whatever you choose will be right for you,' she says, smiling serenely. She can't possibly be right about that – there are so many cards, and I'm being guided by worldly whims, not supernatural forces – but she's smiling at me kindly, waiting for me to choose a card, so I grab one from somewhere in the middle and turn it over.

'*Dream big,*' it says. '*Let go of small thoughts about yourself! See yourself succeeding.*' On the card is a picture of a dark-skinned mermaid with a glistening green bandeau top, lying against a moss-coated rock. She looks lost in thought, dreaming, or longing.

'What a gorgeous card!' Natasha exclaims, delightedly. 'Let me read you the inscription.' She pulls out a small notebook from the card box and reads. The inscription tells me that I need to 'release any thoughts or feelings of inferiority' and urges me to believe I am qualified 'for any endeavour you can dream about'. As though she is reciting from a divine, ancient oracle, Natasha tells me, with a look of pronounced wonder on her face, that I need to write down my fears and then drown them in a bucket of water, before revitalising myself with a cleansing shower or bath. I smile weakly at her, knowing I will do no such thing. I hate taking off my clothes and having to confront my body, and I always shower and dress myself as quickly as humanly possible. There will be no revitalising or dousing or cleansing happening for me. Natasha leaves me to ponder the card as she gets to her feet and goes to fetch Mum, and I can't help but admire the artwork of the lovely, dreamy mermaid resting against a rock. As trite and vague as the advice to 'dream big' sounds, it is also oddly comforting.

Natasha returns a moment later, gliding, glowing, followed by Mum. Mum looks at me and I can see how undone I look by her startled expression as she perches carefully on the edge of the couch. She keeps throwing nervous glances between me, Natasha and the mermaid cards in my hand.

'Well, we have a lot of work to do,' Natasha tells us, happily. 'I'm really glad you came to me. I'd love to continue working with Evanna if you both decide that's right.'

Mum throws a curious glance at me. 'Thank you for seeing us,' Mum answers, formally, and then cuts right to the chase: 'What do you think about the weight issue? What would be a reasonable goal for weight gain from week to week?' I turn the mermaid card back over, returning it neatly to its deck.

Natasha shakes her head firmly at Mum's question before continuing. 'I don't deal with weight and numbers,' she says, and I raise my eyebrows, disbelieving. 'That's all just the superficial stuff. That's not going to help us. My only interest is in dealing with the *root issue,'* she says, emphatically pronouncing the last two words. 'I want to address the *root issue* before we even mention food and weight. In my professional opinion, that's the least of our problems.' In an instant, she has switched from kind, angelic benevolence to a regal, unyielding force – not unkind, but not to be fucked with. She's take it or leave it.

As she says these words, an image of a simple birch tree swims to mind, stripped of its leaves, but with a tangled network of roots sprawling and twisting in the dark undergrowth, miles beneath the surface, diverging in a hundred different directions, and I feel a swell of hopelessness in the pit of my stomach. Natasha is expecting something complicated about me, hidden depths, a secret buried deep, to be delicately excavated. I wish I had something tangible to offer, something interesting, that she could unveil and bring to light. But there's nothing there. I've never been physically or psychologically abused; no dodgy second cousin has ever tried to snake his hand up my thigh while tying my laces. No one I love has cancer or is a criminal. My parents are neither alcoholics nor drug addicts, and are in the most steadfast – if somewhat sleepy – marriage known to mankind. They never threaten separation or divorce, not even at the very apex of a heated argument over who was responsible for the family's tardiness at Mass. Sometimes I fantasise about discovering I'm secretly adopted: my sisters eagerly endorse this theory and point out our noticeably different hair textures as concrete biological evidence of two enigmatic, absent parents who tragically hadn't loved me, but my birth cert and irate mother have already put those rumours to rest. I have no trauma. There is no buried treasure for Natasha to find at the end of a lengthy course of psychotherapy sessions. I have no damn right and no excuse to feel this awful.

With a knotted feeling of dread, I suddenly foresee a nightmarish scenario somewhere in the not-too-distant future: Natasha towering over me with an expression of blithe incredulity, shrugging as she tells me that she has looked inside me, plunged into the very depths of my soul, and found that there's actually nothing wrong with me, that there is nothing to work on, that there is no root issue and that there is in fact *nothing there*. I splutter to her that I've known this all along, that I don't have a reason for being so difficult, that it was never anything more or less than the fact that I found being alive – the simple fact of existing – quite painful, and everyone already knows there is no cure for that. I *wish*, with a desperate kind of longing, that I had a root issue.

'OK, well, thank you very much for seeing us,' Mum says politely, gathering her handbag to her. I can tell she's disconcerted and unconvinced by this wholly impractical, intuitive approach. 'We'll have a think and I'll call you tomorrow,' she informs Natasha, who nods genially and springs to her feet again to show us out. Mum fumbles a few €20 notes from her handbag, placing them on the small table in the hall and discreetly gesturing to Natasha, as though passing the money from hand to hand is an indecency best avoided. I feel a wave of guilt and sadness seeing Mum fork out more money – Mum, who works tirelessly helping children with learning difficulties all day at school, Mum, who never spends any money on helping herself – and I have an irrational urge to tell her that I'm going to get better, that Natasha has fixed me, to promise her that I'll start eating normally for the sake of this €60 that she has handed over without deliberation. But this urge evaporates almost instantly, and privately, regretfully, I concede that these efforts are fruitless, that I'll never surrender or change my ways, that sadly I don't have a root issue, that she's just wasting her time and money. Natasha bends low to hug Mum, and then gathers me in her arms, whispering, 'So nice to meet you, angel.' Then she waves us off into the brisk, frosty night. And even though I already know that Natasha, for all her magic and charm, doesn't have the answer to my problems, that she will quickly uncover my lack of complexity and absence of a root problem, I feel a little bit brighter now than I did one hour previous on that doorstep when I'd tried to convince Mum to turn around and just go home.

'So . . .' Mum asks, hesitantly, driving carefully as she navigates the frost-covered roads. 'What did you think of her?' In profile, I can read her scepticism about this evening's escapade.

'I liked her,' I tell her simply. 'She was really nice. We talked a lot . . . I'd like to see her again.'

For a moment, a look of hurt and dejection crosses Mum's face as she studies the road in front of her. What is Natasha offering that she can't give?

'OK,' she says, finally, with a small, resigned nod. 'Let's see how it goes.'

Before long, my sessions with Natasha become my most favourite part of the week. I look forward to them even more than my acting classes, anxiously checking my watch on Wednesday evenings at 6pm as I wait for Mum's car to pull up to the kerb. We don't talk about my weight or the 'root issue', and Natasha never asks me for a food diary. We talk about everything else, though. Very soon, Natasha's cosy, warm, angel-encrusted living room becomes the place I can go to quietly discuss my dreams, where they are safe to be uttered aloud and to exist again, if only as inconsequential thoughts and words.

Natasha doesn't question them or balk at the comical discordancy between this small, meek girl and these wild, unrealistic dreams. She listens and lets them be, coaxes the images from my imagination and enthuses over the details with me. It is so unusual to share these dreams with someone who sees only possibilities, who never snuffs them out with a sceptical frown or points out the statistical unlikelihood of a shy, inexperienced, unexceptional girl making a name for herself in the acting world. Some days, we do talk about food, like when a failed audition for a televised talent show triggers a meltdown and a fresh burst of aggression into what is undeniably no longer a diet but an experiment in starvation. Some days, I just cry and tell her that I've given up, that I am done.

A few weeks into our sessions, she asks me to buy two journals and to write down a short entry at the end of each day about whatever is going on in my mind. Each week, I trade the journal I've been writing in for the one she's just reviewed. It's hard to stop writing once I start. An endless stream of toxicity and pain pours itself out over pages and pages. It is mostly mind-numbing, obsessive jabbering about the fat content of Ryvita crackers and a disturbingly in-depth analysis rating the pros and cons of white vs brown rice, the way most prepubescent girls might compare the various floppy-haired members of a teen boyband. I fill ten pages with anxiety over a friend's upcoming birthday, the mounds of fatty, indulgent foods I'll have to avoid, and the ensuing awkwardness as I sit there avoiding everyone's eyes and the limp fruit salad on my plate. But in between the lists and meltdowns and the scrupulously plotted timetables, my dreams are glinting from the pages too. They are not raging and spreading out with the same roaring voracity as my eating disorder, but quietly, consistently, they continue to show up. They are simply there, written down, offering themselves as humble suggestions to be considered at a later date.

Natasha never asked for my current weight or a food diary. I learned later that this became a point of contention between my parents and Natasha. 'I won't ask her to gain a pound,' Mum recalls her saying, 'until I've gained her trust.' Building trust was a delicate matter, Natasha affirmed, and she was not going to be pressured into jeopardising that bond. The way I see it, she was right. I would have sensed it the moment our therapy sessions became an agenda to make me gain weight. I would have lost respect and admiration for her, and would have immediately shut her out the way I had every other person who tried to cajole me into relinquishing my eating disorder. As for my weight, it continued to drop, but not at such a dramatic pace, and some weeks it stayed the same, on the point of stabilising. But it wasn't enough for my parents, and it wasn't enough for Deirdre, who was keeping a hawkish eye on me now. Though Mum could see that Natasha was helping me mentally, that I was finally cooperating with a therapist, the sessions weren't yielding tangible results quickly enough, and she still had to look at my diminishing physique and see a bad mother reflected back.

What nobody seemed to notice, unable to look past the obvious problem, what only *I* could feel, was that, with Natasha's help, I was beginning to be able to see a future again. I was becoming curious about what might happen next. I looked forward to the moment, at the end of every session, when Natasha produced the magical mermaid cards, with the same eagerness a child looks forward to a large bag of sweets after a tedious sermon at Mass on Sunday. And looking at the enchanting images of mermaids draped restfully in a crescent moon, or swimming joyfully with dolphins, or gazing dreamily at castles in the distance obscured by a layer of purple mist, I felt tiny seeds of hope start to sprout in my heart. I felt that I was gazing through a window that reminded me there was beauty, colour, magic and wonder available to me out there, if only I would just step over the precipice.

One day, spontaneously, and totally unprompted by anyone, I decide I am going to eat a full meal at an arts and culture festival that Mum and I frequent. It's always one of my favourite days, taking place one weekend of the year on the estate of a famous Georgian house in Co. Louth, where several tents are erected for the weekend and various arts and crafts stations are set up, along with rows of tables holding beautiful handmade goods, from patterned scarves to carved stone necklaces, intricately wound dreamcatchers and multicoloured felt purses. I don't know why, but I just decide that today, I am going to take a break from my eating disorder. I am going to eat an entire sandwich and some cake, and I am going to be fine with it. And I do exactly that, making my way through a whole tuna sandwich and a large chocolate muffin. It is *absurd*, after a year of avoiding these foods like they were actual poisons. These are normal-people, sinful, bad foods, but for some reason, I decide that today, just today, I will eat like a normal person.

Mum does her best to act casual, to not whoop delightedly as we pick our way through lunch with flimsy plastic cutlery and casually review our purchases, but she keeps throwing nervous sidelong glances my way. She is being *so* polite, and walks as if treading on eggshells all day, as though afraid that if she so much as sneezes, I might jolt myself out of some trance and immediately barf up the sandwich.

I resume my regular habits the following day, forcing myself out on my bike first thing in the morning and continuing my restrictive eating patterns, but I don't disproportionately punish myself for that day of sinfulness. I don't really know what possessed me. A spontaneous moment of madness, an irrepressible urge.

But it was nothing to get excited about, there was nothing significant about that day. I had not decided on recovery; it was not a path I *ever* foresaw myself choosing and pursuing. I'd just had this gnawing curiosity to remember what a normal day felt like. I wanted to know how I'd feel if I ate what I wanted, just for one day. It was a risk I could take, just for one day. It was a momentary indiscretion, a borrowed fantasy: Cinderella going to the ball and then, as the moonlight and magic dissolved into nothingness, soberly deciding to stay put in the safe monotony of her cellar, busying herself with chores and blocking out the summons of an unpredictable world. The recovery journey is not a linear one, and it would be a very long time before I ate another sandwich of my own volition. Even with Natasha's help, my weight continued its downward creep, and I was only half-heartedly trying to resist it, still refusing to choose recovery.

So, eventually, maybe three weeks after the sandwich day, my parents decided it was time to take decisive action. I woke up on a Friday towards the end of May 2003 and got ready for school, but my parents suggested we go to the hospital instead. *You just need a rest*, they said, ever so gently. *We'll just go for the weekend*. I didn't put up much of a fight. I just felt so *tired*, as I sat at the kitchen table passively listening to their proposition. It was the day of my class's annual 'school tour', where students forewent school uniforms and trekked around some family-run outdoor entertainment venue, maybe a water sports park, but more likely a farm, mindlessly munching through plump bags of gummy sweets as we stared blankly back into the glassy amber eyes of bearded goats. I wasn't exactly feeling ecstatic about the day ahead, or the increasingly arduous and exhausting uphill cycle to school before it. Every day was just so uncomfortable by now, so cold and tiring and socially awkward, and ultimately it came down to a choice between quietly following my parents to the hospital and slipping obediently into a starchy, unfamiliar bed – or the goats. For future reference, and to neatly summarise the message of this book, if you want to avoid all pain and trauma and growth and change, *always choose the goats.* This was the pivotal moment, the moment I would rue and rage at for weeks afterwards, fuming and sobbing in the corner bed of a stifling children's ward as the days ticked aimlessly by and nobody would give me what I wanted. This was the moment I would relive with a painful longing, and wish with all my heart that I'd chosen the goats.

4

I slept for a full forty-eight hours upon admission to the hospital. My memory of that first day is so foggy. I have a very vague recollection of being weighed and measured by a nurse – stand on this cold white thing; lie on this hard bed and stare into the light while cold clammy hands press into your abdomen like it's playdough; open wide and try not to cough; breathe here and bleed there – but after that, I just kind of melted on to a bed, fully clothed and unprotesting. I woke up a few times, the sky outside the window seeming to flicker between colours each time I blinked, from bright, clear blue to a pink-and-orange sunset, to a deep, soothing navy. I knew I needed to get up, to hit the floor and do 500 sit-ups and race up and down the stairs for a quick blast of cardio, but every time I was on the point of rousing myself, I just slipped into an even deeper sleep. Each one of my limbs seemed to have switched off, lying there stonily and bluntly ignoring my mind. A few times I woke to hear whispered voices, my mum or dad quietly conversing with various nurses by my bedside, though they sounded faraway, distorted, as if in a dream or a parallel universe.

On Sunday night, I wake up, suddenly fully awake and alert, to a dark hospital ward. The only sounds are the steady beeping of machines and the raspy breathing of other sleeping patients. There is nobody else around me, no nurses or parents, just a green reusable shopping bag that wasn't there before, sitting upright on the chair beside my bed, crammed with neatly folded T-shirts and pyjamas from my wardrobe. The light from the corridor outside is leaking in through the open doors of the ward, and I can see the top of someone's fluffy yellow head poking out over the top of the reception desk, so I tiptoe out into the hall. A tall nurse in a blue tunic with stripy highlights and a friendly face springs up from a seat by the wall and bustles over to meet me.

'You're awake,' she says, in a whisper. 'Your mam left you some pyjamas. She'll be back in the morning.'

I nod, shyly.

'Now, I have to get you something to eat. The dinner ladies are gone home, but you need to eat something.' She has a warm, maternal demeanour that puts me at ease. She keeps her hands in her tunic pocket as she surveys me. I see the name on her badge reads Áine.

'Do you have Rice Krispies?' I enquire, cooperatively. I follow her down the corridor into a small blue-and-white kitchen, where she pours some Rice Krispies and milk into a little plastic bowl and hands it to me with a spoon. I slurp my way through it obediently as she tells me how lovely my parents are, that my mum has been calling every couple hours, that I've come at a quiet time and that it might even be a nice break from school to be in hospital. She ushers me back into bed then, pulling a curtain for privacy as I change into my pyjamas.

'No fun to be in hospital, lovie,' she says sympathetically as she helps me straighten out the tangled bedcovers. 'Especially when you're young.'

'Yes,' I agree, clambering back on to the bed and pulling the covers over my knees. 'But it's not been so bad,' I add, stoically. 'And I do feel much better now. It'll be nice to get home to my own bed tomorrow.'

Áine shoots me a confused look, but doesn't say anything, smoothing out the bedcovers and bidding me goodnight.

By morning, I am sitting up perkily in bed and feeling as though I've just returned from a weekend at a luxury five-star spa resort. I am totally refreshed and feeling considerably positive about life. I even comply with the nurse's prompts to choose something from the breakfast trolley when it rattles into the room a few minutes after 7am, and eat my second bowl of Rice Krispies in twelve hours. Rice Krispies aren't on my safe foods list, but I'm trying to feign a convincing level of normality to the nurses, so everyone has no choice but to conclude that there has been some sort of mistake and there is absolutely nothing the matter with me. All in all, it hasn't been so terrible to succumb to a sojourn in the hospital. Two days of sleep and two bowls of Rice Krispies, and I am ready to get back out there. I can't help but commend myself, as I scoop up the last few Rice Krispies swirling around in a pool of milk, on my incredibly magnanimous compromise that would no doubt go a long way towards alleviating my parents' guilt and anxiety and reward them with a peace of mind that had eluded them for months. It has been a pure, sincere act of altruism that speaks of great maturity, and that will no doubt assuage any worries that I am in the grip of some sort of dangerous, uncontrollable mental illness. They can go back to feeling like good parents again, and I can carry on with my life. By 8am, I am fully dressed, sitting on the edge of the bed and chatting animatedly to Áine about nail art as I wait for my mum to arrive. It turns out Áine keeps her hands shoved firmly in the depths of her tunic pockets because she is hiding a fondness for long, garish talons and glamorous French manicures that she is forbidden from indulging on the hospital ward, but that she routinely indulges in anyway, especially when she has a date. I'm showing her the quick and wondrous invention of nail-art transfers, when both my parents shuffle quietly on to the ward, looking exhausted but carefully put together, their faces drawn, their eyes darting nervously all around them, as though searching for an imposing figure of authority to tell them exactly what to do.

'Ah, there they are now,' Áine says, getting up from the edge of the bed and greeting them. Mum smiles, looking slightly more comfortable, presumably reassured by Áine's considerable height – she towers a good foot above my mother – and her laid-back friendliness, which is so incongruent with the aura of dread that hangs about a room designed to remind people that children die too. 'Well, I'll leave you to it, lovies, I'm off home now to my bed,' Áine trills, waving cheerfully and heading for the door.

'It was nice to meet you,' I call after her, surprised at her abrupt departure. 'Good luck on your date later.'

She acknowledges me with a small smile, then exchanges a curious look with my mum that is something akin to pity. I'd thought we'd had a nice connection, thought she'd want to say a proper goodbye, but she must see hundreds of children drifting in and out of sickness and health, leaving before she's fully memorised their names.

My parents are sitting in the two chairs by the wall beside my bed, looking very much like they could do with taking a short hospital retreat themselves. Mum's sickly-sweet perfume crowds the air around us, and she keeps tucking her hair unnecessarily behind her ears, her hands and feet gathered tightly together. Dad, on the other hand, looks like a fish who's only just realised he's not in water, his expression blank and confused, his elbows poised tensely on the arms of the chair, as though frozen in the act of deciding whether to stand up or sit back. He's used to striding purposefully down school corridors with armfuls of copybooks, sharply telling bolshy teenage girls off for being late to class or patrolling the school grounds to catch smokers. I smile sympathetically at them both. I guess I have to be the soothing adult presence here; the two of them just look so stressed.

'I'm feeling much better,' I tell them, cheerfully, and then, because I want to make amends, not because I really mean it, I decide to compliment their parental choices. 'It was probably a good idea to come here.'

Mum nods and gives me a half-hearted smile, but Dad just presses his lips together in a strange grimace and looks away.

'I ate a lot of Rice Krispies,' I offer, but neither of them responds. They're both somewhere else mentally, still casting their eyes here and there as though bracing themselves for a surprise doctor attack. I sigh heavily, finding them both quite tedious now. 'So, how long 'til we can go home?'

Mum glances at my dad, who is studiously examining the palms of his hands. 'We have to see the doctor first,' she tells me. 'He should be here any minute. He's going to assess your details and review your case.' She tucks both sides of her short curly hair behind her ears again.

'But . . . why?' I ask blankly. 'They already checked my weight. What does he need to assess?'

But exactly what that is, I never find out, because at that moment, a short, male doctor with an intense brow and a large cloud of bushy black hair streaked with silver enters the room and introduces himself as Dr Nolan. My parents bolt up out of their chairs in perfect unison to shake his hand and nervously straighten their jackets. They chat for a full two minutes about the weather, and make some feeble jokes about my dad not being missed at school by the students who were to have a history test this morning, before Dr Nolan finally turns his attention on me, addressing me in a slow, cautious tone, the kind you might adopt when addressing an exotic, feral pet.

'Nice to meet you,' he says, smiling, and though he's looking directly at me, his eyes never settle on one point, and it feels more like he is trying to peer *through* me, squinting to make out some far more interesting shape on the wall behind me. It's like talking to someone through a screen or a thick pane of glass, where you can't tell if they can fully see you, and you're tempted to flail about wildly just to check. 'Let me take you into another room where we can get some privacy,' he continues, and then leads the way out into the hall. I scramble to pick up my various belongings, but Mum whispers, 'Just leave it for now,' and ushers me out after Dr Nolan. We follow him into a spacious, brightly lit room with just two beds and countless clunky, plastic contraptions and medical machines shunted into each corner. Dr Nolan politely gestures for my parents to take the two chairs by the beds as I hover awkwardly beside them.

'You just sit up on the bed there, good girl,' my mum whispers to me. I narrow my eyes at her cautiously, my suspicions raised by this unnervingly quiet room and her reluctance to speak in anything louder than a breathy undertone, but I sit on the bed and wait quietly for someone else to speak.

Then Dr Nolan proceeds to read us the riot act. Situation much more dire than suspected. Dangerously low BMI. Could collapse at any moment. Stunted growth! Serious malnutrition! A cold could be fatal! At risk of infection! Of infertility! Of heart failure! Death! This damn doctor could write his own gripping medical TV drama – emphasis on the drama. I sit with my arms and legs crossed firmly, openly glaring at him, thinking only that this brazen, puffy-haired man in a white coat is doing nothing to allay my parents' worries or make my life any easier.

'I don't want to worry you,' he says, and I almost scoff, 'but it's a good thing you brought her here when you did. I don't like to think what would have happened if you'd delayed this by a few more days.'

He stops speaking and surveys my parents sombrely, letting the silence hang, and it's only now I notice my dad's breathing has become shaky. I turn with a start to see that he is crying, tears streaming endlessly down the saddest face I've ever seen. It knocks the wind out of me. I've never seen him cry before. I have never known solid proof that men over the age of fifty even have tear ducts! My dad – this blocky, reliable, uncomplicated, country man who likes Mass, history, hurling, potatoes, and not much else – weeping like a scared toddler. Dad, who revamps his style about as often as Homer Simpson, buying himself the same maroon woollen jumper, half-off in the Arnotts January sales each year, maybe sometimes with a brown diamond pattern or a green stripe, but nothing more adventurous. My hardy dad, who doesn't bother with useless frivol- ities like daily teeth-brushing or a comb, and whose entire self-care routine consists of a quick shave and an icy blast of water to the face. Everything about him has always seemed to say 'Sturdy'. And here he is, this solid, sturdy dad, looking small and helpless, his mouth comically downturned, his eyes overflowing with tears, totally undone by the fact that his youngest, silliest daughter has got a bit too skinny. It's like he's only just realised what's been happening, and it occurs to me now that maybe he hadn't known. I think back to our interactions over the past year, his furtive, nervous glances in my direction, and the awkward silence between us in waiting rooms when my mum disappeared to the bathroom. The way he'd avoided my eyes and skirted past me in the living room as I sat sniffling and hugging the heater after another argument with Mum, and his wordless acquiescence as he'd driven us to doctors and backed up whatever Mum said. Maybe he really hadn't had any idea what was going on. I gaze at him, perplexed, spooked and saddened. It feels so different to the time my mum had crumpled weakly in the dietitian's office and I had had to turn away, repulsed. I want simultaneously to reach out and pat his big, hairy dad-hands, and to step back in awe and gawk. Dads aren't meant to fall apart and cry. Something feels seriously wrong now.

Mum, on the other hand, is unexpectedly composed, nodding along with the doctor's grave assessment. When she speaks, her voice is measured and strong, and I realise that she is relieved. The situation isn't just dawning on her like it is my dad. She's been struggling and stressing and wrangling for answers from medical professionals for months, and now here we are: she has trapped me in a hospital, with a grave-faced doctor shining a stark light on the problem that everyone else has been batting away. She's no longer alone at home, whispering her pleas like prayers to the Yellow Pages, grasping for help from anyone who'll take a cheque and being routinely gaslit by an enraged anorexic. Here is a professional, upstanding doctor confirming to her that her daughter is definitely on the verge of passing out and maybe of dying from malnutrition, and I can tell, though she is still concerned, that she is feeling vindicated, and possibly a bit thrilled. A problem shared and all that.

'Well, thank you very much, Doctor,' she says, emphasising his title as if it's a compliment. She fucking loves a male doctor with a pessimistic prognosis. I think to her, male doctors and paranoia are the two safest things in the world. 'I'm very glad we're here now,' she says, with a small insipid chuckle. 'So, what do you think is the best method of treatment?'

Dr Nolan returns to his medical drama script. Immediate medical attention! Strict refeeding programme! Careful psychiatric observation and evaluation. Biweekly weigh-ins and total bedrest. Mum nods along, enraptured, lapping up his every word, but my attention is not really on either of them. Dad is still pouring tears beside me, his eyes downcast. He is not really listening to Dr Nolan either, and I notice that he is stroking my calves, which are outstretched on the bed in front, in a swift, repetitive motion, like he is trying to sweep away the anorexia. In a croaky voice, I hear him whisper, 'You'll get better now, you'll get better now,' as he continues his sweeping motion, and it is so pathetic, so sad, and I can't bear the silent stream of tears dropping off his reddened face, so I whisper back: 'OK, I'll get better now.'

If only it was that easy.

I'm still distracted by the weepy little man beside me when my mum asks the operative question. 'So, Doctor, how long do you think this treatment will take?'

My eyes snap back up to Dr Nolan abruptly and I hold my breath.

'Well, that depends on you,' he says, inclining his head towards me with a conspiratorial smile that I do not return. 'It's however long it takes for you to gain the weight. We'll design a weight-gain schedule and diet, but it will be up to you to commit to it and meet your target weights. Ultimately, you can go home as soon as you've gained sufficient weight.'

'Sorry,' I interject loudly, finding my voice and what it is meant for. 'How much weight exactly do you expect me to gain?'

Dr Nolan blinks at me a moment as if the answer should be obvious. 'Well, enough weight to reach a normal, healthy BMI,' he answers plainly.

I blink back at him a moment more as the penny drops.

No, says every cell of my being. Normal? Healthy? It is so far from acceptable. I don't want to be normal or 'healthy'. I don't want to gain a few pounds, let alone fit the weight profile for the national average prepubescent lump. My ideal weight is loitering precariously on the very verge of passing out. Normal just isn't an option.

'No,' I state loudly to the room. 'No, I won't be doing that. No, no, I just want to go home now. I'll gain weight at home,' I insist, hopping down from the bed. 'Thanks,' I throw dismissively in Dr Nolan's direction, but nobody else moves. Dad has stopped crying now, dabbing at his nose with a tissue and looking at the floor, and Mum is looking anxious again, her eyes fixed on me fearfully.

'I'm afraid that isn't an option at this point,' Dr Nolan replies in an infuriatingly calm tone. 'You are dangerously underweight, and your health has been seriously compromised. It's not safe for you to be anywhere but in a hospital bed. That's our only option at this point.'

No, I think. But I can't reason with this stolid, detached doctor-man, so I round on my mother, who is looking small and scared again, not hopeful and assured.

'Take me home,' I tell her insistently. 'I'm not staying here. I'm not staying in this place. Take me home and I'll eat – I'll eat! – I don't care. I'm not staying in a hospital!'

But neither of my parents will meet my eyes now, grasping their own hands and fiddling with hankies.

'Come on, let's go,' I tell them bracingly.

'OK, I think it's time to call the nurses,' Dr Nolan says, making for the door and calling to someone out in the hall.

Two nurses appear, one with dark skin and a thick silky bun, the other with wispy blonde hair and round red cheeks. They hover by the door.

But in an instant I'm no longer angry and obstreperous, I'm desperate now, pleading with my mum, who I know won't desert me here. 'I can't stay here,' I beg, grasping her hands and hanging on firmly. 'I can't gain all that weight – you know I can't. You can't leave me in this place.'

'We're going to have to give you something to calm down if you're going to be like this,' says Dr Nolan authoritatively, and then I feel a firm pair of hands – not my parents' – grabbing me by the upper arms, and steering me back to the bed. Dr Nolan is telling my parents to leave, and they're heading to the door, my dad's head bowed, my mum saying over my cries that she'll be back later, the most useless apology I've ever heard, and then they're gone and the door swings shut and I collapse back into the bed away from the nurses and cry.

I cry for an hour. I wail and cry, but my parents don't come back. Dr Nolan has cleared off too. The nurses pass in and out, checking on me, leaving glasses of water on the nightstand and trying to offer some generic words of comfort. After a while, the blond-haired nurse returns, business-like, and tells me it's time to return to the ward. She tells me I'm being silly and that I'm acting like a baby, but I don't care, and I don't help her as she swings my legs down from the bed and half-carries me back out of the room, down the corridor, and returns me to my bed in the corner of the children's ward. My mum has forgotten to take her silk scarf, which lies atop the freshly made bed. I climb back into the bed, bury myself under the blankets and continue sniffling. After a few minutes, I get the sense that someone is watching me, and peek out of my blankets to have this sense confirmed by the appearance of an older woman sitting in the chair by my bed. She has black hair streaked dramatically with grey, like an actual badger, and is staring back at me from pouchy, yellow eyes and clutching a notebook.

'Who are you?' I ask, staring suspiciously at her.

'I'm Miriam,' she answers plainly, her husky voice betraying a deadly smoking habit. 'I've been sent to keep an eye on you while you adjust.'

I frown at her, critically, not liking any of this. 'What's that?' I demand, nodding to the notebook and not giving a damn who I'm rude to in this oppressive system that has stripped me of my freedom.

'Nothing for you to worry about,' she says bluntly. 'I'm just keeping record of your progress.'

'So, you're just going to sit there and stare at me?' I ask, scathingly, but Miriam has evidently decided to stop humouring me and just stares boldly back. 'What a great way to spend your day,' I tell her sarcastically, crossing my arms.

Miriam ignores my comment and chooses instead to write about it in her petty little journal. I spend the next few hours trying to give her something interesting to write about, things that will make Dr Nolan think I'm complicated and deeply troubled, whispering limericks to myself under my breath, and picking up my mum's discarded scarf, sniffing it mournfully and then flinging it fiercely to the floor. I hope Dr Nolan concludes my parents are to blame for all my problems. I hope he really makes them suffer. By the time lunch rolls around, I've decided to join Miriam in silent rebellion, and I'm now embarking on a full-blown hunger strike. The nurses try to sweet-talk me into eating as Miriam scribbles away excitedly in her chair. Even the dinner lady abandons her trolley after delivering all the meals, leaning chummily over my hospital table to try and coax me into eating just one pot of Petits Filous. She has poker-straight, chin-length, brassy yellow hair and a remarkably puckered mouth. She greatly resembles the grandma in Roald Dahl's *George's Marvellous Medicine*, except that she is kind and lives to feed ailing children. But I ignore them all, petulantly shaking my head and shrinking away defensively in a corner of the bed.

'You're a very bold girl,' Miriam chastises sharply, her pen and notebook poised threateningly as Dinner Lady rattles back down the corridor, leaving just the Petits Filous pot and a teaspoon. I glare back at Miriam provocatively. This evidently gives her a flash of literary inspiration, and she begins composing a lengthy paragraph about my lunchtime antics. The day passes horribly and slowly, my bitter mood darkening with the sky outside. Miriam tails me everywhere, even into the bathroom, her wheezy breath and smoker's cough the appropriately awful soundtrack to my awful day. She chronicles my every move and bowel movement, writing the most mundane and presumably unfavourable biography known to man. Eventually, I get bored of helping Miriam pad out her notebook with deliberately erratic behaviour, and instead pick up the pile of *Sabrina the Teenage Witch* magazines my mum has packed in the green bag. I try to distract myself with hair tutorials and 'ideal boyfriend' quizzes but Miriam can't stop coughing, leeching the contents of her poisoned lungs into my curtained-off corner of the ward, and I am so disgusted I yank the covers up over my head, curl into a ball and promptly fall asleep.

I wake up to the sound of clinking glasses and an almost empty ward. The sky outside the large window at the end of the ward is pitch black. Turning my head to the right, I see that Miriam and her notebook are gone, and there stands my mother, busy at my nightstand, her attention absorbed by a large handful of yellow irises that she is carefully arranging in a blue ceramic vase. She looks quite at home, her expression calm, her coat draped neatly over the back of the hospital chair. On the floor, I see a second bright green shopping bag with familiar possessions from my bedroom poking out the top: floral leggings and bright T-shirts with cats on them; more teen magazines with more hair tutorials; my yellowing copy of *Goblet of Fire*; and my soft black cat toy who's shared my bed as long as I can remember. But the momentary leap of my heart when I set eyes on my mum and see her tender expression as she tweaks the buttery yellow heads of the irises, the desperate childlike urge to reach out and grab her warm freckled wrist and bury my face in her multicoloured wool cardigan, is immediately quelled and drowned out by the bitter, simmering rage I feel as I remember that it is her fault I'm here, that she has taken away my autonomy over my own body, that she has left me here to suffer in this ugly, fluorescently lit, off-white world with strange smells and strange people, and that she is happy about it.

'Oh, you're awake!,' she says, starting as she turns and spots me watching her. She beams down at me and then gestures to the flowers. 'I brought these from the garden, aren't they lovely? I thought we could do with brightening up this place,' she adds, glancing around the unconscionably dull space with a weak titter. Everything in sight is grey or beige or white or off-white, everything but the irises and my mum and her assortment of goods. 'And your friends from school have written a card, isn't that nice?' she continues, handing me a card with a miserable teddy bear beneath a plain typescript with the vague offering: 'Sorry You're Unwell'. I read the inside of the card, which is peppered with the well wishes of my sixteen classmates, starkly delineated between the sexes: the boys' reluctant, perfunctory messages – variations on 'Good luck – Daithí O'Shea' – are on the left, while the bubbly, enthusiastic, heart-spattered well wishes from the girls are on the right, written in an entire rainbow of gel-pen colours. 'We miss you!!!' reads one pink, splotchy inscription. 'Get better soon!! ♥,' trills another, in luminous green. 'So jealous of ya, missin all d homewrk here!!' quips a third. I replace the card dispassionately on the table, refusing to meet my mum's eyes. She hesitates a moment, registering my foul mood, but then ploughs on, producing more cards and reading out the infuriatingly cheerful greetings from my teacher, our neighbours and an aunt. *Get Well! Get Better! Get Well Soon!* they chant, foisting this blanket status of 'invalid' on me, as I wonder at what point it had been unanimously decided that I was 'sick'. Apparently, all it took for me to cross the invisible threshold from health to sickness was a hospital bed and a quick once-over by a tyrannical doctor. Not three days ago, I was tearing determinedly up a hill on my bike in the lashing rain, as independent and able-bodied as any of these well-wishers. How was I here, stuck on this rickety bed under these nauseating yellow lights, surrounded by wailing, snot-faced children who trailed haggard teddies in one hand and intravenous drips in the other?

Mum settles herself in the chair, admiring the vibrant irises splaying out from the vase in all directions. I can see she is nervous, from the restless way she is twisting the gold chain at her collarbone, and I feel a thrum of satisfaction in letting her stew in the silence.

'How are you getting on?' she asks me, her tone falsely bright. I cross my arms and sink down in the bed, my gaze fixed stubbornly on the ceiling. Mum fiddles with the sleeves of her cardigan anxiously. 'Did the doctor come by?' she tries again, but I let the silence drag on. She casts her eyes about hopelessly, as though appealing for a nurse to come by and break the awful tension with mundane chit-chat about the weather, but the ward is almost deserted, and she turns back a moment later, apparently steeling herself against the icy front I'm presenting with a renewed resolve to be even more cheerful.

'I brought you your *Harry Potter* books!' she exclaims, springing to her feet, and pulling the chunky tome that is *Goblet of Fire* out of the green bag, followed by the rest of the collection, and laying them out in a row on my bed. 'And your beading set!' she adds, hoisting a tattered shoebox from the bag, which rattles with the dozens of pots of sequins and beads jostling around within as she handles it. She continues unpacking the bag, revealing all my most beloved possessions, planting them carefully over the bed, framing the outline of my legs, trying to bury my rage and pain beneath these carefully chosen treasures. She's bought new magazines with free butterfly clips and roll-on perfume, and various sparkly trinkets from Claire's Accessories that would have taken me weeks of saving to afford. She lays it all out, brightly introducing each item and appealing for feedback, but I can tell she's trying to break me down, to buy me off, to bribe me into good-natured acquiescence, my freedom for some plastic hair bobbles, so I lie there mutely, fuming, knowing this is the only way to hurt her as I was hurting. She sits down heavily on the side of the bed, among all the treasures, her shoulders sagging.

'I'm sorry,' she pleads, emotion thickening her voice. 'I know you hate me for this. I know how hard it is.'

'You don't,' I tell her bitterly, unable to hold back, tears pricking my eyes and leaking on to the pillow.

She is silent a moment, her back to me, before she speaks again. 'I actually do,' she says quietly, her voice tremulous. 'I went through the same thing you did when I was younger.'

'What are you talking about?,' I demand, sitting up in bed and glaring at her searchingly. I watch her face in profile, disbelieving but intrigued, despite myself.

'Yes,' she presses on, picking up the silk scarf she left that morning from the end of the bed and twisting it between her fingers. 'I stopped eating for a while when I was your age – maybe a bit older – and had to go to hospital. I was put on a programme too.'

I'm so floored by this information I can't even speak.

'It was very difficult,' she continues, and lets out a long exhale, seemingly struggling to find words too. 'So, I do understand . . . I understand something of what you're going through,' she tails off quietly.

I cannot discern which emotion pulsing through me is the strongest. Shock. Relief. Compassion. Gratitude. Rage. Curiosity. Confusion. Betrayal. Everything at once. She sits there on the edge of the bed, seemingly lost in a moment of faraway contemplation, and I want to grip her shoulder and shake her, to look her in the eye and ask why she didn't tell me this before. Why hadn't she *said* she understood? Why has she pitted herself as my eating disorder's most prodigious enemy all these months, when it had once been a friend to her, a friend she knew all too well? But she hasn't offered to save me from this prison – it's too late to be friends now, and she doesn't deserve my forgiveness. I can tell my silence will be the most punishing, so I turn back on my side, facing away from her.

'You don't,' I reply, concluding the conversation. She remains quiet for a while after that, still lost in contemplation, the muffled beeping of machines and the murmurs of other patients' mothers the only sounds permeating the silence. With an effort, she tries to start the conversation again, asking what clothes or books or posters I'd like from home, but I ignore all her attempts. She stays another ten minutes or so, sitting silently by the bed, and then just after 9pm she stands up, quietly tidies away my new treasures into the corners of my nightstand, and starts to gather her own belongings.

'I'll be in tomorrow after school,' she tells the back of my head.

Silence.

'It will get easier,' she tells me, uselessly. 'It's just a couple weeks, and then you'll be back home.' She waits for a response, but I do not relent. 'OK,' she exhales, giving up. She bends over, plants a kiss on my head and makes to leave, but then hesitates another moment. 'Will I leave this here?' she asks.

My curiosity gets the better of me and I turn my head fractionally to see her holding the silk scarf and looking at me enquiringly. She wears an expression of mingled guilt and sadness, and I want to nod my head, the tiniest possible gesture I can offer, the flimsiest nourishment of the heartstrings connecting us, but then she'll think she's won, she'll go home with a lighter heart and I'll be the only one suffering in the dark, so instead I turn on my side and make no reply.

'I'll take it, so,' she says sadly, and this time she does leave, the sound of her heels echoing along the empty corridor. No sooner has she passed through the doorframe of the ward than my facade seems to crack, tears streaming down my face, and I turn back to look for her through the glass window that looks on to the hallway corridor. I want the scarf back. I want a hug. I want to cry out and plead with her to stay, but she's already gone, and it feels as though my heart has vacated my body, abandoning me too, following her out along the corridor, down in the lift and out into the night. *Come back*, it begs. *Save me.*

My hunger strike continued for two bitter days. I terrorised the entire ward. I gave up the silent rebellion quickly, deciding instead to make my presence loud, nerve-shattering and utterly wearisome – a body of pain casting the ward in a cloud of darkness. And I made my protest efforts known in other ways, refusing to shower, change out of my pyjamas or let them change the bed. 'What is the point of getting dressed,' I snarl at the nurses as they rap the bedframe and try to chivvy me out of bed, 'when you won't even let me walk down the stairs!' A normally quiet and watchful person, this ruthless compression of me and my disorder had wrenched forth a vicious, foul-mouthed, vengeful protectress, an uncharacteristic, no-fucks-given, ferocious bitch. I only left my bed to use the bathroom, jumping up abruptly and stalking quickly down the corridor away from Miriam, trying in vain to shake her off, and then subjecting her to a steady stream of insults from the toilet seat, telling her what a disgusting pervert she was for watching me piss. Miriam and I were united only in our utter disdain for each other, and, I think, in firmly believing that there was nothing seriously the matter with me. She showed zero compassion for my predicament and seemed to regard me as nothing more than a spoiled and entitled brat.

I rejected every meal, shoving the plastic trays forcefully back across the table, ignoring Miriam's tutting and the pleas and guilt-trips of everyone else – my mum, Dinner Lady, Áine, the eavesdropping parents of other children – glowering hatefully back at them all. And even though I was starving, my stomach making odd squiggly noises and pronounced groans through the long hours of the night as I lay there clenching and unclenching my muscles in covert attempts to burn calories, I was tormented by the awful, stifling, inescapable feeling that I was getting fat. It's a unique form of agony, known intimately by anyone who's struggled with anorexia: a terrifying, smothering sensation; the keen sense that you can actually *feel* the fat cells creeping their way under your skin. It's an unbearable, claustrophobic feeling, and the only way to dispel it is to jump up and frantically move your body: to sprint so fast up a hill that your lungs burn and stitches pierce your sides, to do so many jumping jacks that your limbs shake and your vision starts to blur, to run and run just up to the point where you feel like you might collapse. In desperation, I tried to sneak in bursts of exercise at night after Miriam had gone, when I was permitted to draw the curtain around my bed for a few minutes under the pretext of changing my pyjamas. I'd hit the floor and quickly crank out fifty sit-ups, careful to make my breathing noiseless, but once I'd discovered this trick, I couldn't stop testing the limits of how much I could get away with, silently drawing the curtain several times throughout the night to crank out intermittent bursts of cardio. That had always been the problem, knowing when to stop, chasing that entirely elusive feeling of having done enough. Whether it was fifty sit-ups or five thousand, I continued to lie there wondering should I, could I, have done more? At what point did I deserve to sleep? I quickly stretched the limits too far, a nurse catching sight of my feet below the curtain with a sharp exclamation of 'Hey!' and after that I was banned from closing the curtain and one of the night nurses stationed herself by my bed with a large stack of trashy magazines. With each passing hour, it became more and more unbearable. One day since I'd done any physical exercise; two days; three. It felt like being slowly smothered to death. They'd taken away all my things, all my methods of self-soothing, the only ways I knew how to cope with the abject, agonising torment of feeling fat, and the only choice I had left was to sit there and feel it. I wept and wept, my knees gathered to my chest, my face buried in the crooks of my arms, wishing I could just step out of my body and be anything else.

'Would you ever stop that carry-on?' Miriam tells me coldly on Tuesday afternoon, as I sob into the bedcovers. 'You're disturbing all the children,' she adds furiously, seemingly of the opinion that I am more demon than child.

'Then just send me *home*,' I plead through my tears, my pride and sass eroded by my misery, ready to beg and bargain for my freedom with anyone, even this crotchety old toad.

By the third morning, I am spent and severely depressed. I've never gone this long without eating. Despite how much the gnawing feeling of hunger comforts me, I've always eaten something and never gotten as far as total food deprivation. My head pounds painfully as I look at the cover of the magazine that Miriam is reading contentedly. *Stars and their Body Issues!* jeers one headline, underneath which a dozen female celebrities have been candidly photographed at unflattering angles in varying states of undress, and are being ruthlessly body-shamed for being either shockingly skinny or riddled with cellulite. Gazing at a photo of a famous actress frolicking on a beach and counting the vertebrae of her knobby spine, I wonder what I've done to deserve this. Nothing is fair about this. I haven't hurt anyone or committed a crime or asked for any special attention. I've never done drugs or shoplifted; I've never even skipped a day of homework. I just want to diet and exercise and be left alone. I'd had everything under control until they all interfered.

I am lying quietly on the bed, truly wondering which will come first, starvation or my parents losing their resolve and deciding to discharge me from the hospital, when the two of them enter the ward, followed by Dr Nolan. The expressions on my parents' faces are grim and distressed as they peer anxiously at me. Dr Nolan, on the other hand, wears a hardened expression today that shows he means business. Any trace of compassion he'd displayed at our first meeting has been wiped clean away by cold impatience.

'Right, let's head next door,' he says brusquely, by way of greeting, his mouth an unsmiling line.

Having virtually no energy and no reason to object, I slide my legs off the bed and traipse after Dr Nolan, not stopping to greet my parents. I've cried so much I have that strange sense of disembodiment and lightness that comes after a considerable emotional upheaval, like I am half of this world, half lost in another dimension, and someone else is deftly manning the controls of my body, robotically lifting one foot after the other. We file into the empty room and I sit on the edge of the bed, where not two days ago I'd perched, full of Rice Krispies and a naive hope that I'd be home by afternoon. I sidle up to the top of the bed, away from my parents, cast my eyes down and wait for the verdict. Dr Nolan sits on the edge of the bed opposite and clasps his hands together. He is actually quite a tiny man himself, the fabric of his green corduroy trousers tenting over two sharp kneecaps and not much else. He crosses his legs and sighs heavily, letting the silence settle a moment.

'This is not going as we had hoped,' he begins, pulling no punches. 'I know you're finding this difficult, but the way you're acting, it's about to get a whole lot harder for you.'

I look up at these words, meeting his disconcertingly abstract gaze, staring hard into his sharp-jawed face. How much worse it could get, I cannot fathom.

'We had hoped you'd adjust and cooperate, and that you'd work with us in a collaborative way to recover your health. Unfortunately, you've done everything to resist our efforts and to make it impossible for the nursing staff to treat you.'

Good of you to notice, I think, drily, hating this cold, bloodless little man, who is talking to me like I'm a war criminal.

'What you need to understand is we have ways of making you better even if you refuse to cooperate with the programme, and under our care, you will not be permitted to deteriorate like this. If you continue to work against us, we will have no choice but to implement a more direct, hands-on method to help you gain weight.' His tone remains measured and maddeningly conversational, but there is no mistaking the blatancy of his unveiled threat.

'What does he mean?' I ask, turning to my right, dagger-like eyes raking my parents' faces. I have nothing to say to Dr Nolan anymore, and if he is going to treat me like some kind of subhuman medical experiment, I am going to do one better and ignore his entire existence. My mum and dad exchange a glance and my mum reaches for my hand, but I snatch it back swiftly, glaring fiercely at the two of them.

'You're going to have to start eating, pet,' Mum says gently, her voice full of pity. 'Otherwise, they're going to start tube-feeding you.'

A chill grips me at these words. Tube-feeding. I've heard only vague allusions to this practice, this unthinkable torture. From grey-faced sick people on reality TV with dead eyes and reddened, crusted nostrils from which a thin plastic tube hangs ominously. From my mum, her voice high and breaking, at the height of an argument when she would loudly exclaim that she'd given up, she couldn't help me, that she would have to hand me over to the doctors, who would strap me to a bed and tube-feed me. I've read nightmarish stories in gossip magazines from hollow-cheeked, large-toothed, emaciated forty-year-old anorexics, in which they describe the process of force-feeding, of being subjected to the stomach-churning reality of having a plastic tube rammed up their nasal cavity, down their throat, reaching all the way to their stomach, through which was pumped a steady stream of liquid fat. The very thought of it makes me want to gag, makes me clasp my own throat defensively. There can be nothing worse than getting steadily fatter even as you refuse to eat a bite.

'They can't do that,' I protest, my voice rising as I feel the panic mount inside me. 'That's not fair. They can't just decide to make me fat without my permission.' And then, with desperation gripping me, my breathing becomes shallow, and it feels like the walls of the room are closing in. I grab my mum's hand and plead: 'You won't let them do that. You won't let them. You'll take me home. Why won't you just take me home?'

Dr Nolan clears his throat pointlessly and recrosses his legs, evidently only slightly perturbed by my hysteria. My mum looks like she is about to say something, staring back at me with a conflicted expression but it's my dad who speaks next.

'We can't do that,' he says emphatically. 'We can't discharge you. If we took you out of hospital now and you got worse, you'd be sectioned by social services and then we wouldn't be able to see you anymore. And we wouldn't have a say in your treatment at all.'

My mum is still wearing that curious hesitant look, like she is paralysed by indecision, like she is not sure of anything anymore and is thinking through the logistics of simply seizing my hand and calmly leading me out of the ward, into the car and driving us away from this precise point of pain. But she doesn't say or do anything, she just sits there holding my hand too tightly and searching my eyes, so a moment later I retract my hand again and stare at the floor.

I am not going to cooperate. I am not going to meet their target weight. I am not going to sit in a bed and passively be pumped full of fat. I am going to fight every step of the way, I know that. I am going to kick and scream and fight through every bitter attempt. I am going to claw through their plastic tubes and cough up their poisons. I will bite their fingers off if I have to. I will not consent to their unjust takeover of my body. If they want to tube-feed me, day in, day out, until I reach a set target weight, they will have to knock me out.

'Look,' says my mum, her forced calm betrayed by an undeniable note of desperation. 'We understand you don't want to be here. We know that. So, we've been speaking to Dr Nolan and we've discussed something of a compromise.'

I let my eyes close at her words, tired, just tired of the hope-lessly transparent pretence of a democratic process in treating my eating disorder. Tired of the ceaseless negotiations that aren't really negotiations, that are just decrees made in my presence but in spite of my feelings. Apparently, this is the level of sophistication of the so-called 'programme' Dr Nolan spoke of. Apparently, the methods for overcoming anorexia in the medical field comprise nothing more complex than a delicate combination of blackmail and bribery.

'We know how much you're looking forward to the new *Harry Potter* book,' she continues, calling me sharply back into the present moment.

With a screaming sense of dread, I suddenly know exactly where this is heading.

'And we know how much you want to be able to get it in person at the bookshop . . .'

My eyes are swimming with tears now. They are taking too much from me. The book release is three weeks away, and it is the only thing left that I am looking forward to. They can't possibly take this from me, this humble, innocent, simple wish to go to a shop and buy a book. Whoever managed to bring their BMI down a few notches by buying a book?!

'No, you can't take that away,' I say aloud, the tears spilling down my face. 'I've already ordered my copy . . .' I tell them, weakly. I ordered it months ago, even braving an encounter with a stranger on the telephone to ask that two copies be set aside, one for me and one for my sister Emily. Emily liked the books too, but was accompanying me more for the novelty of sitting on an empty street before the crack of dawn with an assortment of the town's most eccentric nerds as they salivated at the tantalising proximity of a new *Harry Potter* book, than for the fervent fangirl pride of being the first person to lay hands on a copy. I know they won't keep the actual book from me; I know I'll get it eventually, probably passed to me unceremoniously in a rumpled plastic bag by a harried nurse, as if it is of no more significance than a hastily packed change of underwear or a forgotten sandwich, a mere afterthought. And though it really shouldn't matter how or where or from whom I get the book, though the story will be untarnished and perfect no matter what time of the day I read it, it does matter. It matters so much. And in taking that away, they are robbing me of the strong sense of destiny surrounding this moment, this moment I've visualised and planned for months. It matters so much that there is a book out there with my name on it, and that I have to go to the shop, pick up the book in my own hands and take it home. There just aren't that many things that give me such a sense of purpose anymore. Exercising gives me a sense of purpose. Stepping on a scale and seeing my weight reach a new low gives me a sense of purpose. Throwing food in the bin as my stomach protests in hunger gives me a sense of purpose. And the thought of going to the bookshop on 21 June – that also gives me this elusive sense of purpose.

'We're not trying to take that away,' my mum reasons. 'We know how much that means to you. But you're going to have to cooperate with this programme. And the doctor has agreed that if you hit your target weight, you'll be able to get out of hospital and get the book.'

It is a meagre proposition. I had not realised, a few days previous as I sat in the car on the way to the hospital, gazing out the window and thinking fondly of the goats with only a small twinge of regret, that there was a world in which I would not be a free citizen on 21 June, free to wander in and out of bookshops at my leisure. They are only offering me something I hadn't realised was in jeopardy.

But suddenly there is this pressing urgency to claw back this dream, this precious dream. I look over at Dr Nolan again, scanning for a shred of mercy, a thread of connection, but he just stares back, his stony green eyes completely inscrutable. He might well be part-amphibian. His face betrays no emotion and no hint of remorse, but it is abundantly clear in that moment, looking at him, that I am not getting out of that building without gaining a considerable amount of weight. Whether through bullying or bribery, they are going to force me through this programme. *The carrot or the stick*, they seem to be saying, their palms open, their expressions expectant. *You decide.*

And that is how my hunger strike ended. Not to be completely short-changed, some other compromises were negotiated. I was to have a say in which foods went on my diet plan. A vegetarian by now, it was agreed I would complete my programme on a vegetarian diet. Natasha was to be consulted and treated as a part of my team. I was to be allowed to do twenty minutes of yoga by my bedside every morning. And, to absolutely nobody's disappointment, least of all hers, Miriam was to be disposed of and I was to regain the vastly underrated privilege of peeing in private. Thus, my life in the corner bed on the children's ward on the fifth floor in St Kevin's Hospital commenced, and, grudgingly, I got on with it.

It wasn't all bad all the time. People were very nice to me. I got so much attention that summer, not to mention loot. Cards from distant cousins I hadn't heard of in New Zealand and America telling me what a 'great girl' I was. A series of Mass cards from my dad's side of the family and assurances that I was being prayed for. My more exciting, sophisticated Dublin cousins arrived one weekend with

CDs and obscure fantasy books, and my glamorous cousin Amy gave me a beautifully wrapped, intricately packed box of beads and craft materials that I would open and gaze at in the evenings with a sense of wonder and excitement that I couldn't quite explain. My aunt Teri went out of her way to cheer me up too, visiting every weekend with funky clothes from her uber funky daughter, and she even wrote and illustrated a magical-realism hospital saga in which a bad-tempered, though well-intentioned little hedgehog-man named the Grumpet stole into the children's ward and set about executing an elaborate but woefully clumsy mission to break me out of there. Each weekend, she brought a new instalment chronicling our increasingly far-fetched escapades to outsmart the nursing staff, but each week a nurse would show up at the pivotal moment of our near-escape, startling the nervy Grumpet, who had a profound phobia of doctors that I could entirely relate to. He would disappear into thin air with a small *pop!*, leaving me to explain to a stern-faced nurse how I'd managed to daisy-chain several metres of cannula tubing, and what exactly I was planning to do with them. Mum continued to bring me treasures every few days – teen magazines, Harry Potter trivia books, shiny packets of Pokémon cards, pearly lip glosses and lurid nail-art transfers – and I did, I really did like the treasures.

Natasha also visited, sweeping on to the ward in flowing, gauzy fabrics, turning heads and beaming warmly at all the sleepy, drugged-up children and their dowdy parents, her elegance and poise the like of which had never been sighted in this dreary, disease-ridden place where everyone was either coughing up phlegm or trying not to pass out from the exhaustion of a gruelling night shift. My heart soared every time she showed up, this beacon of light and love and beauty, and I would scramble out of bed to dust crumbs and stray bits of lint off the chair next to it, embarrassed by my cheap cotton pyjamas and the ugly place I'd dragged her to. Nurses and nosy children would drift past us, curious, tell-tale eyes darting to our corner as we conferred about angels and fairies and Natasha shared insights on notes she'd made in my diary. Natasha made no secret of the fact that she disapproved of the hospital's approach to treatment, that she felt there was no significant healing being done here, loudly declaring it daft and unhealthy that I couldn't even leave the bed to go for a walk, unbothered by who might be eavesdropping. She encouraged me to keep writing in my diary, to just get through the programme and focus on getting out.

'You just get through it, honey,' she told me bracingly. 'Get through this shitty bit and get them off your back, and then we'll get back to work.'

School finished a couple of weeks after I was admitted to hospital, and friends came to visit me, bearing greetings cards and helium balloons and teddies – so many teddies. They eyed me nervously at first, possibly only vaguely aware of what was wrong with me, and I didn't volunteer the information, opting instead for idle chit-chat about summer plans and boy bands and all the episodes of *Pokémon* I'd missed. It was too painful to breathe the words 'eating disorder' aloud. Any time I heard the word anorexia mentioned in passing by nurses swapping shifts or my mum and dad chatting amiably with new parents on the ward, I'd feel a deep, cloying humiliation set in, a desperate urge to move, a panicky need to quickly talk about something else. Not because I was ashamed of my eating disorder, though – quite the opposite. I was ashamed of 'getting better'. How could I talk to people about my serious eating disorder as I sat there getting fat? It was too surreal, too absurd. I felt like a fraud; I felt like a waste of space; I felt like I was betraying the most precious part of myself.

Soon the numbers on the scale started to turn, the weight creeping back on. Weigh-in days were never good days – there was just no possible positive outcome, torn as I was between my fear of fat and my desperation to put it on and get my life back. Áine had quickly become my favourite nurse, her laid-back breeziness and undimmable humour the energy I needed to distract my mind from the mounting horror I felt each day at my own body, so I asked that she be the one to weigh me, so that this private, horrible trauma could at least be shared with someone kind. I would press the heels of my hands into my eye sockets, every muscle in my body tensed, as I stepped on to the cold rubber of the scale and listened to her adjusting the dials carefully, never knowing which outcome would feel worse.

'Good girl,' she would say brightly, as I stepped off the scale, trembling, and then a terrible feeling of hollowness would follow me out of that tiny room and pervade the day as I speared potatoes and veggie burgers and shovelled them into my mouth, sometimes stiffly, robotically, and other times choking them down through waves of tears. Other days, I stepped off the scale and Áine didn't say anything, and as I looked over to see her make a small note on my chart, an expression of grim disappointment on her face, a burst of energy and happiness surged through me that I knew was stupid, and that ultimately, I would pay for.

But for the most part, my weight continued to climb, and I did everything I could to avoid thinking about it. I read voraciously, through hysterical children's wails and chattery nurses gossiping about their favourite soap. I reread all my *Harry Potters*, tore through *A Series of Unfortunate Events*, Jerry Spinelli's *Stargirl*, and virtually anything else I could get my hands on. I started making cards again, with beaded creatures on the front, replying to all the distant cousins and Mass-goers, telling them I was fine and expected to be home very soon. I set up a nail-art station at my hospital table, painting dozens and dozens of tiny daisies on all the tired mums' neglected fingernails. Áine patronised my nail-art station any time she had a date, sneaking over to my corner when the ward was quiet and leafing through the nail-art booklet to choose the flower that spoke to her that day. As my talent for nail art progressed from hearts and polka dots to spirals and paisley print, we chose riskier and riskier designs to catch the eye of her suitor of the week. One evening, I branched out into false nails, sending her out into the night with a set of undeniably whorish American-flag print acrylics that even Áine looked dubious about, which somewhat damaged the reputation of the nail-art salon – after that, it went back to being a humble hobby. But as the weeks wore on, there was really no getting away from the agonising mundanity of lying on a bed all day, and many a wistful hour was spent staring at the ceiling listening to Christina Aguilera's 'Stripped' on repeat, a little blue-and-silver CD Walkman whirring rhythmically beside me. '*You are beautifuuuuul*', she crooned in her distinctive throaty warble. '*In every single wayyyy!*'

Hmmm, I thought contemplatively, not buying a word of it.

Fortunately, 21 June was looming ever closer, and that vision of lying in the sun reading my very own copy of *Order of the Phoenix* was becoming clearer. *Un*fortunately, my weight was not progressing on such a steady upwards incline. Though I was still gaining weight, I was not meeting the agreed-upon targets each week, and the actual reality of being checked out of hospital and regaining my freedom one of these days was only getting foggier. I could see my fate changing in the tense smiles my mum gave when I talked about the logistics of camping out all night for the book, and in the way my parents had pivoted from cheerfully indulging conversations about late summer plans to vaguely asserting we'd 'talk about that another day'. I could feel all my hopes and dreams unravelling, being tugged away behind my back, like a beloved knitted jumper rapidly unspooling thanks to a rogue thread. I could sense conversations happening out of my earshot, powerful people discussing my body as I lay on my bed, trying bitterly to eat my way out of that building.

And I was so bored, just so bored. The novelty of being the centre of attention, an object of curiosity and recipient of treasures, was wearing off as the summer went on and people started visiting less frequently. I was looking healthier, too, which tormented me. Though I tried to avoid it, looking anywhere but at the mirror in the bathroom and shutting my eyes tightly whenever I showered, I could feel my body changing. 'You're looking well!' oblivious friends and relatives told me brightly each time they visited, and I tried to smile, tried not to flinch, tried hard to believe that they weren't really saying: 'You're looking like a lazy, fat bitch!'

'I have to get out of here,' I whine to my mum a few days before the book release, as she bites her lip, looking worried. 'I'm trying so hard. I'm eating everything! I don't know what I'll do if I can't get my book!'

'I know,' she says, her tone serious. 'We're going to do what we can. Dad's going to have a word with Dr Nolan.'

'Urrghhhhh,' I reply, grabbing fistfuls of my own hair and pulling. It would be too soon if I never heard his name spoken again.

By Thursday, I am designing my own Grumpet-inspired escape

route, making mental maps of all the possible exits and the hours of day when the store cupboard containing the cannula tubing and various other useful tools is unmanned. Grumpet or no Grumpet, I am breaking out of this building and buying my damn book.

It doesn't come to that, however, as by Friday afternoon another compromise has been negotiated. I am not getting out of hospital to continue my recovery at home, and I am not allowed to camp outside the bookshop throughout the night. I will, however, be permitted to leave the hospital for one hour on Saturday morning to go and pick up the book, and then return to the hospital to read and continue the programme uninterrupted. My dad delivers the news with an air of triumph that suggests he has personally arranged a second Christmas. Apparently, it took much cajoling of the medical team and many phone calls with the management of Eason's bookshop to carefully plan and secure this excursion. It is not the dream I've longed for for so many months, but by this point I am desperate for any crumb of hope, and the news of one precious, sacred hour of freedom comes as a relief. The nail-art station is re-erected that evening, and with the utmost care I paint my nails in electric blue, decorating them with an alternating pattern of tiny golden snitches and the letters 'HP' as I jabber away happily to my dad about my predictions for Harry and his friends now Voldemort has risen again.

'Seven am sharp,' I tell my dad as he makes to leave, and I lay out a pale blue Harry Potter T-shirt. 'Seven am, seven am! Don't be late, OK? Don't be late!'

The next morning, my parents arrive on the ward at 7.04am to find me pacing frantically despite the nurses' protestations. I have gone all out this morning, full maniacal fangirl, scrawling 'I ♥ HARRY POTTER' in black face paint down each arm, circling my eyes in two messily drawn rings, purportedly to replicate Harry's glasses, and baptising myself with a post-box red squiggle on my forehead to represent Harry's scar (you can look up this precise unfortunate ensemble on Google by the way: just type in 'Order of the Phoenix book release Drogheda', and there's my toothy grin and shoddily drawn glasses, described by the reporter as 'very authentic indeed', which can only be read as snide sarcasm).

'You ready?' Dad asks me brightly, excitement colouring his tone.

'Ready!' I tell him, grabbing my backpack and heading for the door, my heart featherlight and beating fast.

It is so odd to simply walk out the door for the first time in a month and realise that the world outside the hospital's entrance is as peaceful and calm as it has ever been, that there is no indication of the consternation raging in a corner of that building, which has seemed to swallow me up for weeks on end with no reprieve. The brisk morning air is so cool, so fresh, and people are just strolling calmly down the street, walking their dogs and picking up poop. In the car on the way to the bookshop, my eyes rove over every shop-front, every open space, every bright-eyed face, seeing all the details anew. I can't stop staring at the people, sweat-drenched bald men in luminous running gear puffing their way uphill, and old women with crumpled faces and identical perms inching slowly along the footpaths, all of them completely lost in their own worlds. How curiously oblivious they are to the marvellous joy of freedom. *Look at all your freedom!* I wanted to yell to a scowling teen as she nudges a chunky baby strapped into a buggy down a narrow garden path. *Look at the world and its infinite possibilities. Look at the day and all you can choose to do with it.*

Ten minutes later, we've parked the car and are making our

way to the bookshop. Outside the bookshop, a small, quiet group of people are lined up waiting, all decked out in similar regalia to mine. There are Harry Potter-printed tote bags and T-shirts, and a few are wearing genuine spectacles. Dad raps his knuckles on the glass door of the newsagent department of the shop, just one door up from the line of Potter fans, and moments later, a tall, smiling, bespectacled man appears and unlocks the door, beckoning us inside. I feel very bad for the twenty or so Potter fans watching us through their owlish lenses. Imagine queueing up and spending the entire night on the cold, hard concrete in a valiant effort to make history as one of the first people to swipe a copy of *Order of the Phoenix*, only for some stupid sick child to shuffle on in under your nose and steal that honour from you! I'd have been warlike! I assume a hunched posture, cast my eyes down and fix a pained grimace on my face, trying my very best to look terminally ill.

Inside the shop, I am treated like a VIP. The two shop managers, John and Mary, welcome me warmly and shake my hand enthusiastically. It's smiles all around, everyone just keeps beaming at each other, delighted either to be out of hospital or doing their bit for sick children first thing on a Saturday morning. I feel a rush of affection towards tall, lanky John and kind-faced Mary as they politely ask me about my plans for reading the book, these lovely people who deal in fantasy books and back-to-school stationery. They're the first adults I've seen in weeks who aren't waving calorie-dense foodstuff in my direction or threatening me with feeding tubes. I could just about stay here forever. In between the chit-chat I keep checking my watch as the minute hand ticks towards seven-thirty, but suddenly, at seven-twenty-one, John hands me a rectangular paper bag printed with the cover of *Harry Potter and the Order of the Phoenix*, and I reach out a trembling hand to take it. My heart is pounding as I lift the massive book out of the bag and stare, entranced, at the vibrant yellow, red and blue cover, where a magnificent phoenix displays his majestic wingspan. Here it was at last, this precious world, contained in a simple book, these words so new and alive. The book seemed to buzz with energy.

'Open the cover,' John prompts eagerly, nodding at the book. It seems a tad antisocial to me, to crack open *HP5* in the middle of this shopfloor and start reading amid the hubbub, but John is so insistent, and, needless to say, I am quite eager by now to find out how Harry spends his fifteenth birthday, so obligingly, I open the book.

For a moment, I just blink in stunned disbelief at the Bloomsbury sticker pressed on to the first blank page of the book, on which an all-too-familiar signature reads 'J. K. Rowling'.

'Wow,' I breathe, my hands shaking as they grip this priceless treasure. 'H-how did you get this?' I ask John, unwilling to tear my eyes away from the loopy signature lest it might vanish. Beaming, he tells me they got it from the publishers, and that it was 'meant' for me. I can't help but think guiltily about #1 HP fan, still shivering outside in the brisk morning air at the top of the queue. (I really hope that gal never tracks me down . . .) But it's mine now! It feels like some kind of transcendent moment as I gaze at the signature of the woman from whose mind and pen this magical world has spilled, and who, for a few moments, had trained that same mind and pen on writing her name on this page, the same page that was now in my trembling hands. It is a tangible connection to something distant, something impossible, someone I hadn't quite believed was real.

In a blink, the hour is up and we're on our way back to the hospital, but I'm not paying attention, not gazing longingly out the window at dog-walkers. I'm deeply immersed in the magical world, drinking in each word thirstily. 'OK, bye, see you later!' I call cheerfully to my parents, barely looking up, after they've returned me to my hospital corner with my book. I spend the rest of the day hunched over the book, monosyllabically deflecting nurses and visitors who amble over to make inane chit-chat.

'Oh, did it come out already?'

'Yep!' I answer definitively, making a point of loudly flicking the page over and staring even more intently at my book.

'You must have been one of the first to get it, so?' a nosy parent, not taking the hint, presses on.

'Yep.'

'Is it good then?'

'Yes,' I breathe, looking them meaningfully in the eye, chasing them back to their side of the ward. I read all day long. The nurses eye me warily, probably wondering at what point this marathon reading session might count as physical exertion. At lunchtime, an argument breaks out when I try to continue reading on my hospital table as I shovel pasta bake into the side of my mouth. A sharp-featured nurse with a close-cropped haircut and an air of brisk efficiency threatens to confiscate the book if I don't put it down during mealtimes. Glowering, I stash it protectively under my pillow and bolt down the food like I'm in a national pie-eating contest, and I am back with my book in five minutes. At dinner I do the same.

'Jesus,' says Áine, watching in awe, as I gulp down a cheese sandwich in three bites. 'It's a shame she couldn't write more of those books.'

I love it. I love it all. I love the fierce, rebellious spirit of the secret Order of the Phoenix. I love Mrs Figg being so much more than a batty cat lady. I love Sirius's messed up childhood home and the pure disdain he shows it. I love Tonks and her ever-changing hair colours. I love angry, hormonal Harry letting everyone have it.

And then Luna Lovegood shows up in chapter ten, and I am not prepared for her. I am instantly entranced by the girl with the straggly, waist-length, dirty-blond hair and aura of distinct dottiness. At first, she just seems funny, and extremely odd, laughing too long and positing bizarre conspiracy theories. She's the weird girl at school, pulling focus from all the other anxiety-riddled misfits, who breathe a sigh of relief and unite to ridicule her in the hope that, amid a crowd, nobody will see the bits of them that stick out too. She's the comic relief, the mad girl, the butt of people's jokes, the one who it's easy to deride and scrutinise, sparing us from scrutinising ourselves. She's that silly, strange girl who hums in class and loiters awkwardly on the edges of society, her presence too prominent to ever fit in. And yet, she is more than that. The more I read, the more I search for her, flipping pages ahead to find her name, wondering when she'll show up again, hoping for her to make an appearance, looking for that wonderfully elusive feeling of, I think, relief. Lightness. I can't understand why, but every time she shows up, something deep within me seems to sigh. She makes my mind still. She makes me laugh, she makes me curious. She hooks me in the present moment. In her presence, anxiety, fear and shame seem to dissolve. My *self* seems to dissolve. She makes everything seem less important, less serious: the teenage drama whirling around Hogwarts, Voldemort's return, Harry's increased potential of being murdered in his sleep, and my nonstop obsessive thoughts of food and calories and fat. Here is somebody who will not judge me, because here is somebody, no matter the persecution and prejudice she faces, no matter how many times she embarrasses and makes a public spectacle of herself, here is somebody who will not judge herself. She is not silly, it turns out. She is not ditzy or oblivious. She is deep and wise. Inalterable. She possesses this rare, wonderful and yet simple quality of total self-acceptance. With this foundation of complete ease and comfort within herself, she is able to fully immerse herself in the world around her, to look deeply and unselfconsciously into another person's eyes, to love things without needing to understand them, to listen to other people talk and not worry about how to respond. She is deeply curious about everything around her, absolutely still and attentive at the same time, drinking in every detail and citing aloud her startlingly insightful observations on them. Her body isn't a protective cage from every being around her; it is a springboard from which she can dive deeper into her surroundings, to explore, to understand. Hers is a gaze unclouded by biases or judgements or insecurities: it is a clear gaze, a gaze of compassion, curiosity and appreciation. With every short encounter with Luna, I find myself laughing, and longing to be in her presence. I want to feel what it's like to be around that. I want to be like that. I want to *be* that.

'OK lovie, it's really time to put the book away now.' Áine places a glass of water on my nightstand and reaches out her hand for the book. 'You have all day tomorrow to read it.'

'OK,' I acquiesce, oddly quiet. I feel strangely unsettled, discombobulated. I hand her the book and she tucks it into a drawer under my nightstand, then flicks the light switch above my bed and leaves me in peace. Though I am exhausted, my eyes itchy and sore, my limbs weary, I can't sleep. Something has deeply disturbed me. I sit there in bed, arms crossed, propped up on the pillows leaning against the bed frame, staring into the darkness, mulling. Why does this character fascinate me so? Why does she seem so . . . perfect? She isn't perfect by my usual definition. It has nothing to do with beauty or bones or discipline. She isn't exceptionally talented or super smart or shockingly thin. She is just completely, disarmingly, unabashedly herself, whatever that is. She isn't trying to veil or enhance it. It is that simple and that radical. These thoughts aren't soothing to me, though, as I lie there in the darkness contemplating this unfamiliar new presence in my mind. On the one hand, I want to grab the book, dash into the hallway and enthusiastically shake it at the nurses, to point to it and exclaim: 'Here! Here she is! Here's someone like me! I'm this!' I want to point to her and then point to me. And yet . . . I'm not like her at all. I am diametrically opposed to her in my every behaviour. While she dreams and gazes at the world around her, I snarl and rage at it. Where she looks at people with respect and appreciation, I see only their ugliness and flaws. As she exists and floats along in her body, I shrink from mine in disgust and hatred. As she seems to emanate love and lightness, I stew angrily in the dark. I have only mean thoughts for myself and others, thoughts that won't be quieted until they've whittled me away to nothing and repelled everyone else with their cruelty. How can I identify with her, how can I want to be like her, when I act like I do? When I obsess over something as mundane and shallow as calorie-counting and the circumference of my upper arms? When my closest literary counterpart is . . . Gollum?

Lying there, in the near darkness of the children's ward, I don't actually feel comforted or uplifted by her presence; I feel infuriated by her. I will never be able to just 'be' like her. I will never be able to risk that. I don't know what it is about her that makes her wonderful: it is impossible to pinpoint, and nothing you could capture. It is completely indiscernible, except for the arbitrary and confusing concept of her unvarnished self. But whatever it is, I will never have it. I will always have to strive, to stress, to hurt, to justify the 'being'. The ward is quiet tonight, the bed directly opposite me empty and perfectly made. And as I sit there fuming, frustrated, baffled, I have the sense that this strange girl is sitting on the bed opposite and staring at me, just staring. It's not a critical or provocative gaze; it is completely neutral. She is just looking at me, and I'm looking back at her, and I feel she's trying to tell me something – but for the life of me I don't know what.

It was just for a few moments before I dropped off to sleep and the image disappeared. It was just a childish fantasy, a foolish dream – it might have been nothing more significant. Or it might have been a seed planted . . . There's a practice I like to use in my day-to-day life now, one that helps me, when I'm feeling lost or stuck, to divine what I want, where to go next, what to do. It's a practice called Creative Visualisation, a term coined by author, Shakti Gawain. It's pretty self-explanatory, really. You create something in your imagination, you visualise it clearly with all the details, you let your dreams unfurl and your mind wander into ludicrous, faraway, unknown places your physical body can't bring you to. The result is that you end your visualisation feeling ever so slightly more hopeful or determined, or uplifted. And you have a clear sense of what step you need to take next. When surrounded by an impenetrable darkness, it helps you to see a way through. For me, visualisation was a powerful tool to help me begin to see my way out of my eating disorder. I believe that until you begin to see your way out, physical recovery will never be effective. You have to take a leap of imagination and see something beyond the darkness, and only you can do that. You have to fix your mind's eye on something far above, something distant; you have to throw the dreams out there, hope they'll catch and then pull yourself up to that point. I sometimes recall this time and think getting the role of Luna three years later might have manifested from this very moment, from this visualisation dreamed up in a corner of the children's ward. But, lying there in the hospital ward in the darkness, I was not to know that yet. There was no fairy godmother to descend and grant me my wish; no wide-eyed seer to grasp my shoulder and urgently tell me what awaited me beyond recovery. It was just a simple, quiet wish, a longing of the heart, curiosity plucking the strings of my imagination. But an ocean of painful transformation lay before me between this moment and that. I was not to know what lay beyond the darkness.

Ultimately, I was in hospital for five and a half long weeks. I finished *Order of the Phoenix* in three days and crashed back to my bleak reality in the decidedly non-magical world of the children's ward – and it was only getting tougher. As the summer wore on, friends went away on their holidays and I had fewer and fewer visitors. People had expected me to be better by now, and I looked better too. The drama and excitement of coaxing a malnourished child away from the brink of death had dissipated. I was out of the danger zone and no longer being prayed for. My parents, Teri, and the indefatigable Grumpet soldiered on loyally, but their breezy shorts-and-T-shirt ensembles and the smell of sunscreen lotion rising from their shiny forearms only put me in a bad mood. I was going stir-crazy and was tired of cooperating with this unjust usurpation of my body. I was so fed up with being surrounded by disease and chirping machines and wailing kids and starched sheets and plastic. Little children with gnarly appendicitis scars and putrid breath would waddle up to my bed, asking what was the matter with me.

'Nothing,' I would huff, arms crossed and glaring at the ceiling. 'Nothing.' Children came and went, and with them many tonsils. The ward grew quieter too. People seemed to decide that high summer was not the optimal time for their children to have their tonsils out. The sky beyond the big window was a pure, tantalising cornflower blue, and summer would be over soon, and I sat there wasting hospital time and money and just putting on weight.

The thing about it was that nobody really knew what to do with me in that hospital. It was a children's ward, intended for binding up broken bones and whipping out appendixes, soothing physically ill wee ones with lollipops and helium balloons and then sending them on their merry way. The programme I was on consisted principally of food and bedrest. A couple times a week, a woman in a tweed suit sporting a bowl cut would drop by and ask me to colour in pictures depicting my emotional state, and they called that 'therapy'. The problem was, they were treating a mental condition in the same way they'd approach any other purely physical ailment they saw in other children. Whip out the appendix and watch the child's health restore. Feed the child and watch the eating disorder melt away. Except it wasn't that. It was more like: stuff the eating disorder with food so no one has to see it anymore. But eating disorders are not problems with eating (at least not initially); those are the superficial symptoms that make their way to the surface. Anorexia had been there before anyone could see it. It was an invisible condition and could not be treated by visible means. Dr Nolan and his team hadn't really concerned themselves with why the condition had taken root in the first place, and five weeks in, it was just simmering angrily, invisible once again, beneath all their food. So, was it my fault later on when it came screaming back?

My parents discharged me in early July, against the medical team's wishes. I was still several kilograms off the target weight, but they could see I was struggling mentally, that the continuation of the programme and lack of emotional nourishment it provided had sent me into a deep depression. Ultimately, my mum and dad didn't think it was healthy for me to stay in those circumstances with no physical or social stimulation. I'd proven that I would eat and gain weight and work with them towards recovery, so we agreed I'd continue to manage my problem at home. There was no farewell party from Dr Nolan, which made my release that much sweeter. Just my parents' signatures on some paperwork, a few reproving glances from the nurses and we were out the door! *Those doctors can suck it!* I thought triumphantly as I wheeled my suitcase out of the hospital entrance and breathed in the smell of boundless freedom.

I ate steadily for a while; I was so relieved to have my freedom back. I knew everyone was watching me, and my parents had been spooked by the cautionary words and acrimonious parting with Dr Nolan. They were determined to prove him wrong, to validate the instincts they'd followed against medical advice, and to show that they had been right to place their faith in me. I wanted to prove him wrong just because I thought he was a dickhead. So, I followed the hospital meal plan for a few weeks. My mum made it her mission to fill the remainder of my summer with social outings, trips to the beach, the cinema. Later in the summer, I went to stay with Teri and her family in Dublin and attended a fancy art camp for two weeks. It had been my favourite place for several summers, sitting in little wooden chalets in the Wicklow mountains making clay pots and friendship bracelets. But it felt different this year. I couldn't get lost in the marbled pictures or the papier-mâché monster faces as I used to, because no sooner had I got there and fixed my name tag to my denim jacket than I felt the anxiety of being surrounded by strangers – cool, loud, funny young people – and of wondering where the heck I would fit in. As usual, the loud, confident, attractive kids found each other like magnets, and I drifted over to a shy girl named Fiona with a cloud of frizzy brown hair, who seemed nice and normal – until I discovered her bizarre obsession with rocks.

I tried to get on with things, tried to enjoy the classes and block out the pervasive feeling of worthlessness and oddness that was triggered whenever a confident kid asked me to pass the paints, and I reached in vain for something funny or interesting or smart to say to them, and ended up mumbling and averting my eyes, only alienating myself further from all the people I wanted so badly to get on with. At lunchtimes, Fiona insisted we go walking, away from the little rock pool where all the cool kids clustered, to a secluded patch of the mountains where there was a stream that presented an excellent array of rocks. I sat on this empty mountain, watching Fiona squatting, frog-like, to squint at the rocks, and it really felt at that moment like it didn't matter to anybody, anywhere, whether I existed or not. What was the actual point of my life? What was I doing, sitting on this secluded mountainside, chewing a cheese sandwich and watching this strange girl, who was by now chatting animatedly to a pile of rocks and apparently finding them much more scintillating company? Why was I here? What did it matter? I'd never felt like such a useless blob of a girl. I didn't want to be a blob of a girl, soft and shapeless. I missed my edges. I wanted them back.

I looked down at the lunchbox on my knees and all the fancy artisan foods my aunt had carefully packed for me. These were Dublin snacks for cool, cultured town kids. They didn't come in family packs for €1. Everything, even the snacks, just made me feel so unworthy. I looked at the lunchbox and saw all the love and kindness and effort that everyone was putting into me, all the money being spent to make me happy and healthy, to keep me on the straight and narrow, and I was grateful for it, I really was, and I tried to push down my feelings and eat for everyone else. But by Wednesday, the choice of whether or not to eat was tormenting me hellishly. How could I justify eating all this food? How could I pay for all the space I inhabited? I followed Fiona to her secluded mountain to look at rocks again. Here, where nobody saw me and nothing mattered, who would mind if I surreptitiously rumpled up the top of a muffin and quietly rolled it down the hill? Who would know? A moment later, a crow swooped in and snapped up the muffin in her beak, and I felt a twinkle of delight. This wonderful symbiotic relationship with wildlife that I had so missed! A new order of the food chain had been established: one that suited me.

After that, the thoughts of how much to eat, how much I could get away with, how much I deserved, consumed my mind again and it was a relief to just focus on that. It was thrilling, once again, to see how far I could take it. Every lunchtime thereafter, I fed my lunch to the crows and I felt productive. Worthy. That familiar, lovely, comforting assurance that I was paying for the space I took up. By the end of the two weeks, Fiona had a stunning rock collection, the mountain was covered in crows and I was not eating lunch. I rode the bus home happy, my stomach gurgling loudly, a sense of equilibrium finally restored.

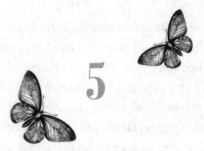

5

A choking, phlegmy, gagging noise rends the silence. *Yuck*, says my subconscious, and a deep, primal knowing jerks me fully awake. I turn over on my side to the unwelcome but all-too-familiar sight of a stripy-haired, squat nurse in a navy cardigan, sitting by my bed and loudly hacking up a lung. Miriam. She finishes choking on her own noxious insides and looks back at me from those pouchy, sullen eyes, bloodshot and watery from her coughing fit, as she dabs at the corners of her mouth with a hankie.

'Fuck's *sake*!' I hiss loudly to the heavens.

'Nice to see you again, too,' Miriam replies smartly. She could always dish it out as well as she could take it.

January 2004. It had taken me six months to lose all the weight I'd gained back in the hospital, and then some. It wasn't deliberate, a vindictive operation to thwart the loving efforts of my parents and everyone who'd invested their energy in my recovery. It was just the only way I knew to get by in life by now, the tools I'd picked up to arm myself against the inevitable pain of existing, because

164

nobody had managed to teach me an alternative. I thought I could do it quietly, without provoking the worries and offence of all the people who'd tried to help me, covering myself in baggy jumpers and loose T-shirts, playing at recovery and pretending to enjoy the food my mum presented me while stealing to the side of the school building at lunchtime and hurriedly emptying the contents of my lunchbox down a ditch, a sense of euphoria and relief coursing through me. I made concerted efforts to appear more normal and be more sociable, scrounging for invites from my friends to trips to town or their siblings' parties, anything to be out of the house and away from the intently watchful gaze of my mother. But everyone was on high alert now. It was not the unspoken battle being waged secretly beneath a facade of politeness and civility that it had been before hospital, before my coping mechanisms had been outed as a disorder. It was everyone vs anorexia, and now that it bore the name and all the baggage that came with it, all the havoc it could wreak, suddenly I was expected to collude against it too, to recognise it as the enemy. And yet, day after day, in the moments of silence away from the noise and peer pressure, I returned to the one unassailable truth; that it was the one thing that comforted me above all else, the one thing I could rely on, that it was my truest friend.

It didn't take long for my mum to identify me as my anorexia's ally again, to sniff me out as a traitor to the recovery efforts and to monitor my every movement with studious watchfulness. I did not want to be at war with her but the more she scrutinised me, trying to catch the anorexia, the more I dug my heels in and vigorously protected it. She was much less easily outsmarted now, an uncharacteristic suspicion clouding her expression every time I announced I was going to a friend's house or made towards the back door after dinner. She was ready to pounce at any moment at the first sign of anorexia getting the upper hand, and I would catch her secretly checking the bottom of my schoolbag in the darkness of the hallway, or the pockets of my jackets hanging in the cloakroom. She even started tailing me after mealtimes, and I would meet her loitering anxiously outside the bathroom, a fierce, accusatory expression on her face. The admission that she suspected me of being bulimic startled and amused me in equal measure. For me, anorexia manifested itself as an all-consuming phobia of fat, and for that reason, consuming any more foods than I absolutely had to only to vomit them up was unthinkable. These accusations of purging only served to flatter me and strengthened my unwavering commitment to starvation. *I am stronger than everyone else*, I thought, smugly satisfied, as I made my way back to my bedroom to do sit-ups, the rumblings of hunger lovingly caressing my insides. But it wasn't all paranoia, as my mum well knew, and she quickly established herself as a worthy adversary. The more I fought to disguise and protect the anorexia, the more she devised ways to expose it.

We were never closer, nor was our relationship ever more fraught than it was during this time. The days began in tense negotiations over the precise measurements of porridge oats at breakfast and escalated into high-pitched shrieks at dinnertime when I would catch her trying to hide lumps of butter in my rice, but they always ended quietly, tearfully, when I'd creep into her bedroom in the evenings and curl up beside her as she read books about teenage psychology and eating disorders. I'd lie there, still, silently contemplating the swirly patterns of the paisley wallpaper. I was twelve years old by now, but I did not feel like a child. I'd become adultlike – driven, industrious, productive, humourless, with no time for play or creativity, silliness or idle chatter – and I didn't relate to other children anymore. But when I finally stopped at the end of the day, conceding to the undeniable exhaustion and letting it weaken my defences, I felt lost and vulnerable. She'd stroke my hair and I'd feel a keen longing to be as small, helpless and dependent as I'd once been, to crawl back inside her and be engulfed in darkness.

Soon we were back to discussions with Dr Nolan and the Irish Health Board, and weekly visits with Deirdre. She and I were equally displeased at seeing each other again, and there was an impatience and sharpness to her attitude towards me now, which I matched with a snarky, uncooperative impudence. A see-saw battle of wills commenced. One week, my weight would drop a few notches on the scale, and Deirdre would insist I gain one kilogram back, threatening hospitalisation, her expression severe as she made adjustments to my diet plan with firm strokes of her pen. But the next week, with the scrutiny and pressure from all angles to quickly gain weight, I would end up gaining more than a kilogram, triggering a catatonic meltdown, feral screams emanating from Deirdre's office, and the evening spent sobbing, railing about how fat and disgusting I was, screaming at my mum that I'd betrayed myself, that she had forced me to betray myself. We'd negotiate a new deal where I could lose some weight and get back to the originally agreed target, but in my vigour and terror of the weight that had stealthily crept on to my body without my knowing, I would end up losing another two kilograms. I'd return home ecstatic, relieved, while my mum and dad devolved into panic, shutting the kitchen door and whispering to each other, an anxious undertone to their murmurs.

Natasha seemed to be the last person left who had not grown weary of me and my problem, and she continued to offer the one sacred space where I could share my honest thoughts, feelings, dreams, and remember who I was away from my disorder. However, more often than not, we did not get to the feelings and dreams, because we were forever putting out the fires started by the bombshells of my weekly weight gains and losses. It became Natasha's first job to pick up the pieces of the previous day's meltdown in Deirdre's office, whether that involved repairing frayed relations between my mum and me, or slowly guiding me away from self-destructive reflexes.

But Natasha was not one to pass time fruitlessly, and spoke up against the hospital's intense scrutiny on weight, which she saw as interfering with my recovery. We could not do the work we needed to do, she insisted, if we were always in crisis-control mode. 'How on earth do they ever expect her to recover and move on with her life,' Natasha reasoned with my mum one evening as we sat in her living room, me sniffling into a pile of tissues because I'd gained two pounds, 'when they are keeping an even closer eye on her weight than she is?'

Natasha didn't do a whole lot to endear herself to the men in white coats, however. Hers was an intuition-led, faith-based approach. She believed in the universe, in a higher power and in the journey of the soul. She regarded anorexia not as this dark, parasitic force that needed to be chased away with food and threats, but as the shadow self making itself known, delivering a message that needed to be heard and heeded. She saw anorexia as a difficult path, but one that the soul had chosen to embark on nonetheless, and one with a purpose. The medical board, on the other hand, followed what Natasha has since described to me as 'a purely allopathic approach' to treatment, concentrating solely on the symptoms of anorexia. She also described their methods, a note of distaste in her voice, as 'fear-based'. Their differences were starkly delineated in one particular case review that put the nail in the coffin of their collaborative efforts. My parents and

Natasha were fighting for me to continue my recovery at home under Natasha's care, while Dr Nolan's team were advocating immediate medical intervention. I wasn't privy to these meetings, apparently too young and unwise to have a say in my own future, but my mum recalls a pivotal moment of the case review vividly, where Dr Nolan posited a scenario in which I might be struck down with a sudden unprecedented bout of flu and not have the immunity to fight it off.

'Pah!' my mum recalls Natasha bursting out in undisguised hilarity. 'She's not going to catch the flu, for God's sake! These girls never do.' She was referring to the collective of spirited young women she treated who struggled with various forms of mental illness, whom she firmly believed had predestined missions on earth, and who would not be taken down by something as meagre and ineffectual as a cold. But it was the wrong thing to say to a statistic-reliant man such as Dr Nolan.

'You don't know that,' he told her coldly, and after that, the medical board regarded Natasha through a fog of mistrust and wanted nothing more to do with her.

'I know what she meant,' my mum groaned later that evening, her head in her hands, looking utterly worn out, 'but now I'm just going to have Dr Nolan breathing down my back each day.' She paused to knead her brow. 'And I am sick of that wiry little man lecturing me on the dangers of malnutrition,' she burst out spontaneously, 'when I could already write a book on the subject. He looks like he hasn't seen a square meal himself in years.' I suppressed a snigger, smiling in spite of my mum's despair. I thoroughly enjoyed the moments when she joined in on doctor-bashing with me. It gave a fleeting but thrilling sense of camaraderie that most often eluded us.

There was something else significant that occurred in this six-month period. One day, in a moment of desperation, or maybe just taken by a whim of pure, childish fantasy, I went to my room, pulled out my stationery set and wrote a letter to J. K. Rowling. I just wanted to thank her. I wanted to tell her how much I loved her books and her stories and her characters, and how reading her books was the only thing that took my mind off the series of lists I was constantly making in my head. I told her about my eating disorder: I even admitted it was a problem, and that some days I imagined being free of it, but I couldn't really imagine a way out. I told her I felt utterly, utterly trapped, except for the moments when I opened her books. And I told her how much Luna meant to me, and how it rattled and mystified me that she was so odd and yet so perfect, exactly as she was. I told her everything. I didn't overthink it; I just wrote what I felt, and then stuck it in an envelope addressed to her publisher and asked my mum to post it. I didn't stop to think of the repercussions of sharing my most private thoughts, my pathetic problems with the person I looked up to the most in the world. I didn't really believe she existed in a humble human form anyway. It was just nice to imagine she did and that she might care.

So it was unexpected, to say the least, when one day out of the blue, a simple cream-coloured envelope with an embossment on the back reading 'By Owl Post' arrived through our letterbox. As it transpired, J. K. Rowling had written back. It was that sudden, that spontaneous, that – dare I say it – magical. I read the letter with trembling hands and watery eyes, my heart hammering. Here was the hand and mind that had spun the stories of the magical world I loved so much; here they were, addressing me directly, with such kindness and compassion. Here was her penmanship, writing, I saw with a jolt of embarrassment, about my problem, sympathising with me, telling me she'd known people who'd struggled with it and understood how difficult it was to come out of it. She was so kind. She told me she knew I could get over my disorder and go after my dreams, but that I would need to be fit and healthy to pursue them. She was as witty and wise and interesting as you would expect the woman who created Albus Dumbledore to be. I finished the letter and handed it wordlessly to my mum, who'd been standing there pestering me to know what it said. Her face worked curiously as her eyes darted back and forth across the page. I couldn't tell what it was; confusion, hurt, discomfort, embarrassment. I hadn't told her what was in my letter, and perhaps she thought my confessions too frank. But when she looked up at me, she appeared emotional and strangely serious, fixing me with an intense stare as she held the letter up.

'You have to take this as a sign,' she said, firmly. 'You have to take this seriously.' Her hand grasped the precious letter rather tighter than I would like. 'She's gone out of her way to write to you and encourage you, so you have to take this as a sign to commit to your recovery.' Her eyes bored into me as she shook the letter. It was like she was trying to wring a promise from me before giving the letter back.

'Yes,' I told her, reaching up and delicately plucking the letter from her, smoothing it protectively against my chest. 'Yes, I will.'

I took the letter everywhere with me. On cycles, to Natasha's, to bed. I even took it to school, wedged neatly between my textbooks, though I never showed it to anyone else. It was too personal. I read it over and over, drinking in each word, imprinting each line on the inside of my mind, laughing heartily at her clever witticisms long after they'd ceased actually making me laugh. And some days, the letter really did fill me with vim and determination to make her proud. I'd eat my dinner without complaint (though not without guilt) and remind myself that I was doing this for her. But just a few hours later, the guilt had already bested me, and I would shove the letter in a drawer, resolving to do 1,000 sit-ups to try and cancel out the fact that I had eaten a full meal, chastising myself for being so silly as to think that J. K. Rowling really cared, or that her kindness could do anything to change how worthless I was. *How easy it must be*, I thought as I sweated through my sit-ups, *to accept yourself just as you are when you're as talented and brilliant as J. K. Rowling*. I was conversing with a near-deity. It was foolish and idiotic to take tips from this innately superior being. And Luna Lovegood, one of my primary inspirations for recovery, was a fucking fictional character. Oh, to be a formless fictional character and not a pathetic girl caged in flesh and quietly expiring in a wretched human body. My naivety disgusted me, and I resolved to stop entertaining fantasies as I gritted my teeth through the discomfort in my abs.

J. K. Rowling and I continued to write to each other every few weeks. We actually became pen-pals, and I came to know her as 'Jo'. I'll never know what possessed her to keep up a steady correspondence with a desperate, depressive twelve-year-old, but I'll always be grateful that she did, because her letters meant the world to me during the darkest times. They hinted at magic and miracles and dreams that I'd almost entirely given up on. But they did not mean recovery to me, and that is a crucial point to establish here. I've told the story of our pen-friendship to journalists and presenters many times, and it has always been simplified and trivialised to a neat, inspiring, bite-sized narrative: that I wrote to J. K. Rowling, that she told me I needed to recover to be in a *Harry Potter* film, and that I went right ahead and got on with that. It's a romantic notion. It's nice to think you can sweet-talk someone into conquering their demons, but I'm sorry to say it does not do justice to the ugly process of recovery from anorexia. I am sorry to dispel the delightful fantasy, but I feel I must, lest someone else grappling with this same darkness is waiting for their own J. K. Rowling to rock up on a fire-breathing dragon and seduce them into recovery with a fabulous alternative life as an actress in a world-renowned film series. J. K. Rowling is not coming to rescue you! She doesn't have a dragon and the *Harry Potter* movies are already over! What I mean to say here is you cannot incentivise recovery. You don't get better to please anybody else, be they your parents, your partner or J. K. Rowling. None of those people, no matter how wonderful they are, can take away the pain that caused you to reach for your disorder in the first place. You only begin to let go of your eating disorder when you find something worth living for. The letters gave me great comfort, warmth and inspiration. Her words resonated and seemed to create an echo somewhere deep within my soul, but I did not buy it when she told me life would get better when I overcame anorexia. I believed in her characters, in her castle of witchcraft and wizardry, I even believed that she supposed that what she was saying to me was true, but somehow, I could not be convinced when she told me to believe in myself. So, while I wanted to be able to write to her and tell her emphatically that I was on the road to recovery, I did not want to actually recover. She would be just one more person I had to lie to.

So, recovery didn't happen just like that. I continued hiding food and over-exercising and setting myself lower target weights, even as I wrote to Jo claiming to be trying really hard and telling her that I dreamed of playing her most fey, carefree and egoless character, while in my real life I was about as far as anyone could get from Luna Lovegood. I was lying to everyone around me, about what I ate, where I went, how I felt. Everyone except Natasha, but when I made it to hers for my one hour of honesty per week, the emotions were just spilling out of me, and I would spend most of the time crying and putting myself back together in time to go out in the world again and continue self-anaesthetising. She tried to ground me and help me to keep it together enough to stay away from Dr Nolan and the hospital, but I was obsessed, and they were obsessed, and I couldn't stop thinking about my weight, and the only way to keep my head above water was to just zone in on losing it. '*I am so tired of everything*,' reads the final line in a journal entry on 10 January, 2004 – and the journal ends there, because two days later, my parents brought me back to the children's ward of St Kevin's Hospital, where once again I fell on to a bed and into a deep slumber, only to be rudely awoken by the thoroughly unpleasant sounds of Miriam gasping for oxygen through dense globs of her own mucus.

'Urrghhhhh,' I groan in reply to Miriam's sass, a heavy weight of despair pressing down on me as I blink back at the fluorescent yellow lights and the beeping machines of this sterile, medical world that I had only escaped, it seemed, mere moments ago.

The mood in hospital is different this time: sombre, and lacking hope. The skies are grey and dark outside the window of the ward, and fewer people come to visit me. There are no more Mass cards or poorly teddy bears. I have essentially nullified everyone's efforts over the summer. Their kindness hasn't made me better, and I have given no substantial commitment to recovery. It feels good to invest in a loved one's recovery when it seems to be helping them, when your time and efforts are progressively making them better. It feels like you're doing something altruistic, something productive, and who wouldn't want to commit themselves to such an endeavour? But when that person is privately conspiring to dismantle these efforts, people grow exasperated and hopeless. Everyone feels sorry for sick people. Illness prompts a wave of sympathy and calls forth humanity's most superior instinct: that of compassion, to nurture and protect the vulnerable. But that sympathy quickly turns to frustration when people realise that you are the one keeping you sick, that you are the sickness. People feel disrespected. They feel like their love has been thrown back in their faces. I understand their frustration, but I do not feel remorse when a nurse scolds me for 'landing myself' back in their care.

'I didn't ask to be back here,' I snap at her venomously. 'I didn't miss you either.'

She shoots me a filthy look and goes to coo over some poor little baba struggling to slurp soup through a straw. I don't care that I am insulting people or that they are all giving up on me, one by one. *Go ahead and give up on me*, I think, *I'm doing fine without you*. Friends get on with their lives and I am happy for them to do so, because all the attention and concern has been an inconvenient burden. I just want to be left alone, to keep my head down and get out of here as quickly as possible, for everyone to give up harassing me and leave me be. But my parents don't give up. They are tired, frustrated, exasperated, stressed, sad, furious, full of despair and pain, and sometimes they threaten to give up, but they never actually do. The evenings in hospital are quiet and uneventful, so different from my first hospital stint in the summer. Dad reads the paper as I work on a cross-stitch pattern or weave a friendship bracelet for him to take home to Mum. But it's quiet because it is temporary. Everyone knows this treatment isn't working, and conversations are being had behind the scenes between my parents and the powers that be about a transfer to somewhere 'specialised'.

As I remember it, I was lured into going to Peaceful Pastures Clinic with the promise of horse-riding. My mother arrives one afternoon at my bedside with a thick pamphlet. She reads out the details of this specialised eating disorder rehabilitation centre as I flip through my teen magazines, making a deliberate show of my thorough lack of interest. In a bracingly cheerful voice, she reads aloud that the clinic in north London is 'more like a home than a hospital', that I wouldn't have to sit on a bed all day and could attend school and other classes. I'll be with 'other young people' who are battling the same problems as I am, not snotty-faced children with contagious diseases. I'll have to gain weight, but I can do it while completing schoolwork and playing games, and even doing 'gentle exercise' like yoga and 'outdoor walks'. I exhale in response to her, fuming as I glower back at the bony models on the pages of my magazines, dolled up to the nines and prancing across poppy-speckled country estates, while I go slowly insane on bedrest.

'And there are lots of great activities you can do,' my mum presses on insistently, 'like dancing and acting – and they even have horse-riding.'

That gets my attention. 'Did you say . . . horse-riding?' I search her face for the lie.

'Yes, look!' she exclaims enthusiastically, gesturing to the pamphlet, realising that she has piqued my curiosity. 'It says that patients will have the opportunity to participate in a range of activities as they progress through the programme, including yoga, dance, trips to the city centre, and yes, absolutely – horse-riding!'

Hmmm, I think, scanning the page and seeing that she is in fact telling the truth. Horse-riding . . . I love horses. Countless are the times my sisters and I have begged our parents for a pony, pledging our humble service to them for life and promising never to take drugs or alcohol in exchange for said pony. Sitting in the hospital bed and gazing out at the impenetrably grey sky, I picture myself cantering gracefully across an open plain, a powerful, pristine white horse bearing me away from all my troubles, including Dr Nolan as he shakes his fist at me from the receding horizon. I long to be outdoors, trying adventurous new hobbies and living my life. It does sound better than where I am now, day in, day out, eating veggie burgers and Petits Filous, abstractly hoping to gain enough weight to get out of hospital and have my life back. And the clinic is in London. Legend has it Daniel Radcliffe lives in London! Might a treatment centre in London not be glamorous, might it not be interesting? It torments me to think about gaining weight, but if I can do it while dancing and socialising and horse-riding, wouldn't that be not altogether odious?

Eventually, I agree to go to London. To satisfy my parents, to get away from the Irish Health Board, to get my life back, potentially to stalk Daniel Radcliffe . . . But mostly for the horse-riding.

The taxi pulls up to the kerbside of a deserted road on the outskirts of World's End in north London and I get my first glimpse of the huge, blocky, yellow-brick building of Peaceful Pastures Clinic, or, as it was irreverently referred to by its inhabitants, 'The Farm'. Driving down the winding road to the clinic you might almost miss the imposing, ugly house tucked away down a long driveway, just visible over a tall, sturdy wooden fence. But as I step out of the taxi and look up, this vast building fills my vision and for a moment, as the taxi driver hoists our suitcases out of the car and plonks them down on the footpath, I wonder at what experiences await me inside those brick walls. I do not know yet that I am going to spend the next few weeks gazing out of windows and fantasising, with an increasingly fervent longing, about what it would feel like to be standing once more on this side of the fence.

The very first thing I notice about Peaceful Pastures is the girls' eyes. Dark, angry, haunted eyes, with purple shadows, leap out of pale, wan faces as a cluster of teenage girls flit through the hallway, quickly disappearing through various doorways, but not before they casually rake me with their scary eyes, a cursory head-to-toe scan that communicates instant animosity. The eyes are circled in crumbly kohl liner and they seem to bore into me hatefully or hungrily, I'm not sure which. They wear long, shapeless hoodies in shades of black and near black, and expressions of contempt and bitterness framed by long, lank curtains of poker-straight hair. I, meanwhile, have dressed up for rehab, wearing a flowy, rustic, pink floral kaftan, greenish denim jeans with lacing down the side seams, and a cream crocheted hat to top it off. Under their contemptuous glares I feel foolish, excessively bright and girly in contrast to the shadowy aura of darkness that emanates from these angry youths as they sweep swiftly through the hallway. I fix my hat self-consciously and shrink closer to my parents.

'The new girl's here,' I hear one of the girls mumble indifferently from a room on the right, and a moment later a short, flame-haired lady with broad shoulders and flushed cheeks emerges and strides towards us.

'Oh, hello,' she greets us, in a cheery Cockney twang. 'I'm Jen, the head nurse here. You must be the Irish people.' She doesn't look like any nurse I've ever seen. She's wearing a ridiculously juvenile white T-shirt with a cartoon unicorn prancing across a lurid rainbow, paired with plain blue jeans and trainers. She just looks like someone's mum, albeit one who refuses to dress in an age-appropriate manner. I'm used to nurses in stripy blue-and-white uniforms with tightly secured ponytails and fastidious nail-hygiene routines. I don't yet know if I trust this loud woman in a too-small My Little Pony T-shirt to regulate my vitals, but she certainly offers a stark alternative to Dr Nolan, so I decide to reserve judgement for now. I see my dad subtly bristle at being addressed directly as 'the Irish people' by an English person. A passionate history teacher, he is naturally inclined towards an initial mistrust of English people, and I see a small frown crease his forehead before my mum jumps in, answering politely:

'Yes, hello, we're the Lynches. Nice to meet you.' She introduces herself and my dad, and exchanges idle pleasantries about the weather as I cast my eyes about, taking in every detail of my surroundings. I am conscious of frantic mutterings coming from the room to the right where all the teenagers disappeared to, but I can't make out what they're saying. A moment later a very short, hollow-cheeked boy, no older than nine or ten, wearing a long Nirvana hoodie, sidesteps from the doorframe and stares openly at me. He has the same haunted, intense gaze as the girls, but instead of glaring angrily, he smirks at me a moment before sidling back into the other room to rejoin the whisperers. The excitement and curiosity I'd felt that morning at 6am on the children's ward as I squashed my last few belongings into a bulging suitcase and zipped it up is rapidly evaporating, and I grasp my mum's warm wrist as she chit-chats aimlessly to Jen about the plane journey here.

'And this is Evanna,' my mum says, adding me to the conversation as she clasps my left hand in both of hers. Jen leans down, perching her hands on her knees and addressing me brightly, as you might a fluffy little bunny rabbit cowering in the corner of a cardboard box.

'Hello, darling! Nice to meet you. Oh, it's not so bad here,' she tells me, conspiratorially, as I grip my mum's wrist tighter, though none of us had made any derogatory remarks about this place. 'You'll feel right at home in no time.'

I do not yet know how I feel about my new surroundings, but I know 'home' is not a place with brusque London accents and cruel-eyed youths.

'The other girls are really lovely. You'll make lots of friends here.'

A short, sharp cackle bursts from the room to the right.

'Dr Grimm will be doing your admission walk-through, so we'll head to the therapy hut in the garden,' Jen tells us, and I lean down to grasp the handle of my suitcase. 'Oh no, darling,' she stops me. 'You just leave your bags here; we'll take care of them.'

'No, thank you, I'd like to take them with me,' I answer, politely.

'Sorry, lovely, we have to take your bags. We have to search them for any sharp objects.' At that moment, a dreadful suspicion occurs to me: that I probably should have read the glossy pamphlet my mum had been perusing by my hospital bedside, particularly the ten pages of information about this rehabilitation programme that had preceded any mention of horse-riding.

'But . . . why?' I ask blankly, genuinely baffled, thinking only of my expensive craft scissors nestled neatly in my beading box.

'Just so's you don't do anything silly,' Jen answers brightly. 'Don't worry, lovely, you'll get your things back eventually.' There's a foreboding use of the word 'eventually' if ever I've heard one. I shoot a panicked look at my mum, who smiles briefly back, but doesn't quite mask the guilt that has crept into her eyes.

We follow Jen out into the back garden, and down a narrow, paved path to a small wooden chalet. I don't look back, but I sense those eyes watching me from every angle, and I don't let go of my mum's hand for an instant. The door of the wooden chalet snaps open, and a spiky, grey-haired lady swathed in layers of thick, black knitted fabrics steps out to greet us. Her forehead lines are crosshatched in near geometric precision. She looks like a feminist writer or a sculptor who makes expensive, angular modern art pieces that populate the desks of lawyers and Ivy League professors. Jen returns to the house as my mum, dad and I step into the airless hut and settle on the small sofa that Dr Grimm gestures towards. She leaves momentarily to root around in a set of drawers in a second room marked 'Office'. My parents tweak their hair and fidget nervously with their coats.

'Great name,' my dad says under his breath, jerking his chin to the room beyond, where Dr Grimm is rifling through papers. 'Suits her face,' he adds, with an impish grin as my mum shushes him, and they seem to relax a tad, sitting back into the sofa cushions and waiting patiently. But I am not relaxed, sitting between my parents on the very edge of the couch. Something in my gut tells me to be on high alert, that it is important from this point on that I listen critically and with sharp attentiveness, the way adults do. Something tells me that my parents are not paying heed to the subtle hints of danger, and that I'm going to have to be the one who protects me from whatever is about to happen. I've already decided that I'm not going to stay here long, if at all, and I know it is crucial that I conduct myself like a mature, emotionally stable young adult and not betray the terrified, frantic voice inside that is screaming at me to get up and run as fast as I can away from this place.

Dr Grimm returns from her office, her swathes of shapeless woollen fabric shifting like tectonic plates with her movements. She settles herself in a creaky bamboo chair across from us and offers a perfunctory smile as she hands my mum three identical pamphlets titled 'Peaceful Pastures Clinic – Patient Welcome Pack'. Mum distributes them between us.

The adults begin making pleasantries again, incessant pleasantries, but I'm already flicking through the welcome booklet and trying to still my trembling hands as I skim-read the blocks of text in front of me. *Twelve-week minimum stay.* That's the first thing I see. No matter how much weight the patient has to gain. *Patients will work towards their target weight by gaining a minimum of 1kg per week.* I do a double-take, my heart rate increasing as a keen awareness grows that I have walked directly into the enemy's lair. *Each patient will start the programme under Total Supervision by one of our nurses as you adjust to your new routine. Once we are satisfied that you are not a danger to yourself, you will earn more freedom and privileges back and you will be able to sleep, shower and partake in activities privately.* Did they actually say I had to earn the privilege of showering in private?! Yes – it turns out, as I read the sentence three more times – they did. *There will be no access to phones or internet, except for two phone calls per week, providing you are meeting your target line and cooperating with the programme.* My grip on my mum's hand tightens again, my palms sweaty by now. *Failure to meet your weekly targets will result in higher calories, privileges being revoked, and your discharge date being postponed by an extra week. You may also need to be put back under Total Supervision. Exercising in secret is strictly forbidden and, if caught, will result in you being put back on Total Supervision immediately. We expect patients to look out for each other and confide in a nurse if you suspect a fellow patient of breaking these rules.* I try to steady my breathing as all of my muscles clench involuntarily. *No dietary preferences will be catered for, unless in the case of allergies. Each patient can have three dislikes, but no more. As an anorexic, you may struggle with your fear of high-calorie, high-fat foods, otherwise known as 'fear foods'. You must face and conquer all of your fear foods in order to complete the programme.*

What absolute bullshit, I think indignantly, stifling the urge to scoff at these extreme rules. I've always been a fussy eater. I don't even like most vegetables, which has nothing to do with fat or calories. I'm not *afraid* of tomatoes; they're just inarguably unappetising. I read on.

Weight is calculated according to your BMI. You will be expected to reach a mid-range BMI of what is considered healthy for your age. Your discharge date will be calculated depending on how many kilograms you are required to gain.

No, no, no, I think, flatly, firmly. A healthy BMI is just so far out of the question. I've always been on the small side; I don't think I've ever reached the median weight for my age. I'm certainly not about to cross that threshold now.

I read ahead to the list of activities on offer, that are available only as a patient succeeds in meeting their gradually increasing target weights. The low-calorie-burning activities, like drama and yin yoga, are available after a few weeks of steady weight gain, while the higher-burning cardio activities, like dancing and swimming, are earned much later in a patient's stay. As for the horse-riding, that doesn't come until a patient has reached ninety-nine per cent of their target weight, somewhere around the final month of their stay. I shut the booklet. I've read enough.

Dr Grimm is describing the logistics of the latter part of the programme, when the patient is sent home for the weekend as a test to see how they fare with the freedoms and pressures of adapting to the family environment and my parents are nodding along calmly as though this is all fine, as though it's perfectly acceptable that I won't see my home for three months, as though they are considering actually putting me through this regime.

'No,' I pipe up abruptly, silencing Dr Grimm, and all eyes swivel to rest on me. I squeeze my mum's hand tighter and summon a knot of courage from deep within, collecting myself to address Dr Grimm directly. 'Sorry,' I tell her calmly. 'I mean that I don't think this programme is right for me. My problem is actually not that bad, see. I'm not as bad as the other patients here. I don't need to be force-fed and I think it would be better if I continue my recovery –' I borrow a word I don't believe in, purely to humour them, to speak to them in their language '– back at the hospital in Ireland. I can see now that I would do better on *that* programme,' I tell her peaceably, smiling to show my commendable maturity and willingness to find a reasonable compromise. 'But thank you for seeing us, Doctor,' I add, with a small, respectful inclination of my head.

Silence.

'I'm afraid,' Dr Grimm responds in a deep, throaty voice, looking completely unafraid and unconcerned as she regards me from grey, heavy-lidded eyes, 'that option is no longer available to you. The choice of where and how you are treated is not yours to make. You have not been cooperating with your doctors in Ireland and they have conceded that they are unable to treat you. That's why you are here.'

'No, but I will!' I tell her enthusiastically, my eyes widening emphatically, my composure slipping ever so slightly. 'I can see now that that programme was much better for me. So, I'm ready to cooperate with Dr Nolan.'

I hear my mum inhale beside me, her anxiety palpable, but it's OK; I'm the strong one here. I will handle this.

'You have done nothing so far to suggest that your parents, your doctors or I should believe you,' Grimm tells me plainly, placid as an empty lake. 'You're here now of your own doing, and you will complete this programme.' She's different from Dr Nolan. Her eyes are as cold as his, but his had a steely determination and fierce resolve that matched my own. Hers are vacant, empty, lifeless. There is nothing in these eyes I recognise; nothing I can relate to. I can't make this person understand me.

I turn instead to my mum on my right, abandoning my facade of calmness, sensing the mounting urgency of my situation. My mum is the epitome of kindness and understanding. She can't walk by a single beggar on the streets without emptying her purse, even when she's stopped for two others previous. My mum is not cruel. She won't leave me in this wretched place.

'Mam,' I tell her seriously, switching instinctually to the Irish variation of mum. I'd long ago traded in the flat, frog-like croak of the Irish 'Mam' for the neat, purse-lipped chirp of 'Mum' in a purely pretentious bid to sound sophisticated and English. But now in this strange, huge city where people with leather-bound notebooks and crisp, upper class accents are already threatening to take away my freedom, England seems scary and I just want to go home. 'I can't stay here. You know I can't stay here. Please can we just go home? I promise everything will go well at the hospital and I won't ask to get out.' I clutch at her hands, trying desperately to meet an agreement in her eyes, but she won't look at me. Her eyes are darting around the room, to Grimm, to the door, to her hands, to the ceiling. If I can just make her look at me and see the fear, then it will be OK. She will rescue me from it. But still she won't look at me.

'Evanna,' my dad says in his gravest tone. 'We don't have any more options. The health board has paid for our flights and your treatment here. They won't let you come back. We have to go through with this now.'

But he is a man. What would he know? He's strong and sturdy, not soft and vulnerable like I am. He doesn't know the fear and torment of having some external force rule and control your body, so I keep my eyes fixed firmly on my mum, even as I address him.

'I'll talk to Dr Nolan. Just call him up and let me talk to him. I'll make a deal with him. I swear I'll be good. I'll be nice to him!' I insist, believing every word I'm saying, desperate to communicate the truth beneath my words, how much I mean them, how everything will be better now. My mum is stroking my hands softly, over and over, and I know there is no way she will let us be separated, but still she will not look at me. 'Please, don't leave me here,' I whisper to her, and I can't stop the tears jumping to my eyes and falling into my lap. 'Please.'

'OK,' says Grimm in a tone of brusque finality, rising to her feet and making towards the door. 'I think it's time for you both to leave.' She looks at my parents meaningfully.

'No, no, no, no, no, no,' I say to my mum, frantic by now, because it looks like she's thinking of leaving. I follow them back up the garden path to that huge, threatening building. 'No, no, no, no, please, please, you can't leave me here. Don't leave me here.' I am pawing at her coat, her bag, her arms, her fingers, but I cannot get her to stop and look me in the eye and tell me everything will be alright. 'You won't leave me here, will you?' I ask in disbelief. 'You won't leave me!'

We've reached the back door again and my parents are inching down the hallway to the side door we came in through, and I am going back out that door with them, no question. Already, my large suitcase with all my most precious worldly belongings has disappeared, but I don't care. I'll leave it here, if that's what my freedom costs me. Dr Grimm drifts away and I am only abstractly aware of her calling for the nurses because I am clinging to both my parents' wrists and ordering them to take me with them, still unable to believe that they have it in their hearts to walk out that door and leave me behind as I cry for their help.

'I'll eat!' I tell them fiercely. 'I'll eat anything!! I swear! I'll do whatever you want me to! Just don't leave me here.'

Jen, and two other tall women – nurses, evidently – appear in the hallway, their faces set for battle.

'You two need to leave now,' Jen barks at my parents.

But they just stand there and blink back at her, looking clueless, lost, and kind of small.

'Have I no rights?!' I plead, utterly desperate now and clawing at my dad's coat sleeve. 'Have I no rights at all?' I implore because it can't be legal to tear a child from their parents' arms and surely my dad will fight for me, but he just stands rooted to the spot, looking shaken, his mouth pinched tensely into a small line in the centre of his face as he looks down at me from scared eyes.

'Just leave!' Jen insists. 'You have to leave right now. You have to go!'

My parents look at each other, dumbfounded. They are the bunny rabbits now, cowering in the corner of the box, so I decide to take more decisive action.

'No,' I insist, releasing my grip on my dad's sleeve and wrapping both my arms around my mum's waist, my right hand seizing my left wrist, assuming a grip that no one on earth could possibly break. She will either have to stay here or take me with her. 'No, you're not leaving.'

'OK, come on,' Jen commands the nurses, snapping her fingers briskly, and suddenly I feel hands on me from all angles. Clammy, alien hands fix upon my wrists, my forearms, my shoulders, and yank, pulling me back but not managing to break my hold. My mum is stroking my head and walking backwards at the same time, and I am screaming now. I am screaming and sobbing like a newborn baby, making a holy show of myself, but there is nothing else for it now.

'MAM! MAM! STOP! DON'T LEAVE!'

'It'll be OK, pet,' I hear her say in a strangled voice as she continues inching backwards, and now my dad's hand is on the door handle and a blast of cool air hits my reddened face. 'It'll be OK.'

It's a blatant lie, straight from her lips. She knows it's a lie, for her benefit only, as I wail and beg. It's not just my freedom I'm fighting for now, because I don't know what will happen in this place. I'm fighting for my life. I am still holding on with all my might, but the audacity of her lie weakens me for one moment, and suddenly the nurses have broken my grip and are pulling me backwards, away from her. My hair is flying, my little crochet hat is on the floor being trodden on by the nurses, my pink top is halfway up my torso, exposing my belly, the centre of my shame to everyone, but I don't care. All that matters is that I kick and scream and claw my way back to my mum. And I am still screaming at her at the top of my lungs, begging and pleading and wailing as she follows my dad and steps out the door, and I see it, I see the moment she looks back at me – an expression of fear, panic and confusion frozen on her face. She looks me directly in the eye as I flail and sob and beg, and then I see her turn her back and walk away.

If you've ever been held down by hands that didn't care for you as you fought, tooth and nail, for your life, then maybe you know what this feels like. Maybe you understand this kind of defeat. Not before and not since that moment have I ever kicked, clawed, bit, thrashed, screamed and fought so hard for anything in my life. I don't know if I even have that in me anymore. I think, until that moment, I actually believed I could do anything. I think I thought I was sort of invincible.

'You're being a baby!' spits one nurse from behind. She struggles to hold my upper arms to my sides as I continue to squirm and thrash. 'I've never seen anyone make such a fuss!'

'MAAAAAAM!' I yell at the top of my lungs, tears streaming down my face, my eyes still fixed on the door handle, willing her to come back. 'Come back, Mam! Please come back! MAM! Mam! Mam . . .' I don't know how long I fight the nurses off, bellowing for my mum to come back – five minutes or fifteen – as they drag me from the hall into a small, stuffy room with a sofa. My breathing is coming in gasps now, and it doesn't look like my parents are coming back. I feel winded by their betrayal, but I am still trying to fight my way to the door. Finally, after all three nurses are out of breath and covered in bite marks, Jen threatens to administer me with a sedative by needle, all bright cheeriness gone from her voice as it becomes abundantly clear why she's the head nurse of this brutal place, and I wilt on to the sofa, my head pounding painfully, snot, tears and drool pooling on to the cushions as I lay my head down and weep.

I stay in that spot for several hours, soaking the cushions through, crooning softly for my mum to come back. It feels as though my life has reached an abrupt dead end. There is nothing for it now but to stay here and wither in this windowless room. But that is not my choice either.

'Right,' says Jen sharply, some time later, clapping her hands together. 'Up you get. It's dinnertime. Time to pull yourself together.'

I am exhausted, sore, defeated. I can barely imagine standing, let alone swallowing down some cheesy, fatty, carb-laden dinner, so I keep my cheek pressed into the couch cushion and refuse to look at this obnoxious, bossy woman.

'I want my mam,' I tell Jen in a croaky whisper.

'You can talk to her on Thursday,' she replies officiously. 'Come on, now. Time for dinner.' It was only Monday afternoon. Thursday was a lifetime away.

'I'm not hungry,' I mumble. 'Just leave me alone.'

Jen guffaws loudly. 'Do you think I haven't heard that one before? Come on, I'm not about to carry you.'

'No,' I tell her bluntly.

Jen crosses her arms and glowers down at me. 'Well, I'll just go and get the feeding tube then, shall I?' she smirks. 'That's no problem for me. I'll go get the feeding tube and make you up a nice milkshake with full-fat cream and butter and mayonnaise, and you can just skip your dinner. How does that sound?'

Sniffling and trembling, I follow Jen to the kitchen.

I take my place at the long, brown table, where an offensively colourful collage card displays my name. They are already claiming ownership of me in deviously cheerful cut-out lettering. It looks like it's been cut, pasted and sprinkled with glitter by a child – but not one of the other children sitting at this table look like they have the corresponding emotional state to produce such a saccharine piece of art. Across the table and to my left and right, I am framed by two rows of stormy-faced, angular-shouldered teenagers, some of them crying quietly into the sleeves of their jumpers, while others glower stonily at the placemats in front of them. A fair-haired, wide-eyed girl with a heavy fringe and a look of sincere emotional trauma rocks very slowly back and forth as she gazes vacantly into the distance. On my right, the small, scathing boy who had eyeballed me in the hallway has lost all his swagger: his elbows on the table and his head clasped in his hands as one of his feet tap out a frenetic pattern beneath his chair.

Welcome to the Brown Kitchen! The Brown Kitchen is where every patient admitted to Peaceful Pastures starts. You do not come to the Brown Kitchen to eat dinner; you come to the Brown Kitchen to be *bullied* into dinner. It's where the newest recruits, the most severely underweight and notoriously non-compliant patients must eat all their meals and snacks for the day, presided over by two eagle-eyed nurses who prowl up and down the table and seem to harbour a fetish for watching every single piece of crockery being licked clean by protesting adolescent mouths. They bark orders like prison wardens as bony-fingered, trembling teens choke down buttery breakfast muffins through their tears. So, in the Brown Kitchen, even if you have a rare impulse to sit and actually enjoy your dinner, you can't.

'Jumpers off,' commands Jen suddenly, and all around me the other kids wriggle out of jumpers and shrug off hoodies, sighing sulkily and cursing under their breath. The traumatised-looking girl with the fair hair reveals pale arms marked all the way from her wrists to her elbows with a series of criss-crossed flesh ridges, like she has been severely burned or tortured, except the lines are satisfyingly neat and symmetrical. The other girls around me hug their elbows and hunch in on themselves, their eyes downcast, in a posture that mirrors mine, the source of the contempt pulsing from their eyes suddenly evident. This is how you hold yourself when you hate the body you're in. This is how you look when you can't bury the burning hatred in your own body anymore and so it pours out your eyes, scorching everyone else.

'You need to tie your hair back,' a nasal voice nags. 'You. New girl.'

I look up to see a small-eyed, sour-faced lady with a long, dull blond ponytail looking at me expectantly. She has a very thin nose, and nostrils that flare expressively with each syllable.

'I . . . I don't have a hair tie,' I reply, in barely a whisper, twisting my fingers around one another.

'Here you go,' says Jen, handing me a black elastic. 'And you need to take your hat off.'

'Why?' I ask her, frustrated by this grating series of commands from people I don't respect.

'Do you talk back to your parents like that?' asks the blonde, squinting at me and flaring her nostrils. For some reason I feel an immediate dislike towards this snide woman, even more pronounced than that I'd felt for the nurses I'd bitten two hours ago.

'You have to take it off so we can see that you eat all your dinner,' answers Jen. 'So we know you're not skanking any food in your hat or hair.'

'In my hair?!' I look at Jen in alarm to be met with an expression of frank sincerity. 'I don't hide food in my hair,' I insist. 'I'd like to keep my hat on, please.'

I'd been up since 6am, flown across the Irish Sea, been wrenched from my mother's arms, had a wrestling match with three fully grown adults and not once had a moment to check my reflection in the mirror. Surely, I could be afforded this small measure of dignity and be allowed to hide the trauma my hair had suffered during today's indiscretions under my hat.

'Take off your hat,' Jen casually orders, proffering her out-stretched hand.

'Oh, just let her keep her hat, Jen,' a sullen, freckled teen from the end of the bench pipes up in my defence. Her rainbow name card reveals her name as Rose. 'It's her first meal, for God's sake.'

'No,' says Jen firmly. 'She'll be treated the same as everyone else. Give me the hat.'

With all eyes in the Brown Kitchen on me now, I reach up and slide the cream cap from my hair, passing it to Jen in wordless defeat. I feel totally humiliated, as my greasy, unkempt roots are revealed, and I sense all these cruel strangers' eyes studying my exposed, reddening face, and I burst into tears again, grasping my elbows and keeping my gaze fixed determinedly on my knees.

Shall I tell you the origin of my intensely personal vendetta against tomatoes? Yes, I shall. I have never liked tomatoes; not in a sandwich, not on a pizza, and not mashed up deviously in tomato ketchup. Cold, slimy, evil bastards. I just didn't like them; it was a simple sensory fact. But after my first meal at Peaceful Pastures Clinic, my aversion to tomatoes became suddenly, and forevermore, an intensely personal affair.

'Aw, no – tomato pasta bake!' complains a sharp-elbowed, sandy-haired boy loudly from the very end of the bench. 'We just had pasta yesterday! You said we wouldn't have it again 'til the weekend!'

'It's your own fault, George,' fires back a brassy-haired girl with racoon-ish eyeliner and chipped black nail polish. 'If you hadn't complained about it so much, they wouldn't know it's your fear food. Maybe if you'd shut up, we'd get some healthy dinners.'

'Shush, you two,' Jen reprimands them. 'It's nobody's fault, I just changed my mind about the menu. I'm allowed to do that. And all foods are healthy foods for you lot.'

I gaze at the meal in front of me. By anyone's standards, this is a generous helping of tomato pasta bake. I've not eaten a generous portion of anything in . . . I don't know how long. A huge mound of fusilli pasta, doused in thick tomato sauce and topped off with handfuls of crusted, browned mozzarella cheese, cheese that seems to touch every piece of pasta. And then, worst of all, there are those plump, shiny, seedy segments of tomato, glistening nastily from amid the cheese and tomato sauce. Oh God, it's just so much food! I gaze at it in horror and take a shuddering breath as everyone around me starts to pick up their utensils and grudgingly spear pasta on to their forks. I'm still weeping as I regard this metaphorical and literal mountain I have to overcome. My throat is constricted and unwilling. The very last thing I want to do right now is eat. I look out the darkened kitchen window, yearning to see my mother's face, but still she does not come back.

'Come on, Evanna,' chivvies Jen. 'You have to get started. Otherwise we're going to be here all night.'

I take another deep breath, pick up my fork and begin to eat.

'Eat with your knife and fork,' barks Sue, the blonde, almost immediately, and I look round at her quizzically. 'Don't look at me like that, you know exactly what you're doing.'

'I'm just trying to eat!' I splutter back in disbelief.

'Eat with your knife and fork,' she repeats, her eyes narrowing, deeming any further explanation unnecessary.

So even though I've never actually eaten with a knife and fork – it's always just been one of my quirks to slice everything with the side of a fork – I clumsily pick up the knife in my left hand and try to tip the slimy pasta shells into my mouth with the knife tip. I get shouted at for that too. It seems no matter what I do, as I gulp my way through the pasta bake like Bruce Bogtrotter with his chocolate cake, I can't get them to stop yelling commands and criticisms at me.

'Eat faster! Eat more! Don't tank your water like that! Don't forget that blob of sauce, I can still see that saaaauce!'

It wasn't good enough to just get the food down your throat. Here, you had to eat like a 'normal person', and any behaviours deviating from The Farm's very narrow definition of 'normal' dinner table etiquette was not tolerated. In their opinion, they were quashing all anorexic tendencies from us with an iron fist. 'Eat with your knife and fork,' they shouted. 'Stop eating from around the edges! Drink some water. Now you're tanking. You need to hurry up! Stop skanking, stop skanking! I want to see you take your next bite with pasta, tomato and cheese in one go.'

Many were the times I wondered bitterly if the nurses were deriving some kind of sick sexual gratification from watching us eat.

At Peaceful Pastures, they were always looking for the anorexia. Everything you did was viewed through the lens of your anorexia, especially at mealtimes. So, it was easy for them to give orders and ignore our protests, because they justified their dominion over us by only hearing the anorexia speaking any time we opened our mouths. They looked so intently for the anorexia that they didn't really see *us*. In the eyes of the Peaceful Pastures staff, we looked like anorexics, we spoke like anorexics, we acted like anorexics. To them, we were anorexics. This might be a helpful tactic when you're a nurse trying to make sure your charges eat every last scrap of food, so you won't be blamed for any unprecedented weight-loss, but it is not good when you're the young girl trying to find herself amid her anorexia. In that environment, it's almost too easy to lose her.

'For fuck's sake,' bursts out the brassy-haired blonde, who I'll come to know as Lexi. 'I can't eat with her whining like that! Make her shut up!'

Glancing up, I see that her angry, black-rimmed eyes are fixed on me.

'Well, then, just let me go home,' I mumble into my meal, which I've reduced to a smaller mound now. 'I don't want to be here.'

'Do you think *I* want to be here?' Lexi snaps furiously, standing up abruptly, her fork clattering down on to the table as she channels her terrible rage directly at me. 'Do you think it was *my* idea to get this fucking fat?' She spits the last word in passionate disgust. I think she's the most terrifying person I've ever encountered, her big, scary, sooty eyes boring into me. She's not fat by any means, but she does look almost normal, like she might be able to hide her problem in society, if it weren't for her murderous eyes.

'Alexis, sit down and watch your language! You just focus on your own dinner.'

Lexi sits back down, fuming, and gets on with her pasta.

After a few minutes, I am the only one still gulping down tomato pasta bake. The rule in the Brown Kitchen is that everyone must finish their meal completely before anyone else can leave the table. I have no intention of attracting more attention to myself – I don't want all those eyes staring at me again – but there is so much food and I hate tomatoes. Eventually, it's just me and the eyes and five cherry tomatoes glistening evilly up at me.

'Some of us have lives, you know,' drawls a bored-looking brunette sarcastically. She's sitting on Lexi's right. 'My TV programme starts in five minutes. I'd really like not to miss it.'

Their taunts only serve to make me cry harder, though, as I spear a tomato with a trembling fist and force it towards my mouth.

'You're so lucky it's just pasta bake,' sighs a dark-eyed girl across the table as she surveys my tomatoes. 'My first meal was a cheeseburger!'

It felt like they despised me, but this was the standard initiation process for the new girl joining the unit. They'd all been through this particular trauma of the first meal before, had all had their spirits broken, their resistance crushed, so it was painful to see someone skinnier come along who hadn't given up yet. The innocent, wide-eyed ingenue whimpering piteously reminded them of the harsh fact that they had given in to this regime, they had stopped fighting, so they felt no qualms in punishing her for it. I, too, would come to hate the new girl, to roll my eyes as she wailed for her parents from the kitchen floor, but on that first day, they just seemed unconscionably cruel.

'Come on, they're only tomatoes, they won't kill you,' Jen urges.

'But I hate tomatoes,' I wail.

'No, you don't,' replies Jen automatically. 'That's just your disease speaking. Anorexia is telling you not to finish your dinner . . . try and fight it,' she adds, lazily.

'No, I *hate* tomatoes. Please, I can't eat them. Please don't make me.' I look out the window, praying for a reprieve, a glimmer of hope, a shred of mercy.

'OK, look,' says Jen finally. 'Will you eat something else? Just because it's your first meal. You won't get this special treatment again, OK? Will you eat a digestive biscuit instead of the tomatoes?'

I am silent a moment, sniffling and contemplating the slimy red pustules on my plate, and then I nod. Fine.

'Are you insane?!' exclaims Lexi, sounding half-delighted. 'Biscuits have way more calories than tomatoes!'

'Shut up, Lexi!' replies Jess, the dark-haired girl on her right. 'Let her eat it and then we can go.'

I chomp my way through the dry biscuit slowly, grimacing as I swallow. It's actually very difficult to cry and swallow food at the same time. Jen insists I open my mouth afterwards, to prove I've eaten the whole biscuit. I tilt my head back and show her the back of my throat as tears leak into the corners of my mouth, and I wonder where my mum and dad are. Why have they left me here? Where are they in this big, alien city? Maybe out to dinner or at a movie, in some fabulous part of London, clearly far away from me and my pain. Tomorrow morning, they'll get the plane back to Dublin, and then there'll be nobody left in this city who cares about me.

'OK,' asserts Jen, straightening up again. 'You can all go.'

The other kids bolt.

To this day, I regard tomatoes as my mortal enemy, sneaking their way succulently into innocuous falafel wraps, ruining the one vegan option on so many menus with their obnoxious, tangy slime leaking its way across an entire lettuce leaf. Foul. No matter how long I live, how many hours of therapy I have, how much distance I put between that first meal and this moment, on principle and out of loyalty to my poor, defenceless twelve-year-old self, I will never – never – forgive tomatoes.

After dinner, I was introduced to another nurse, Pat, a butch, gum-chewing, stripy-haired nurse with a beak-like nose, who informed me I was on Total Supervision, or 'TSV'. This meant that I was to drift around the house in a dark cloud of the most depressed, most catatonic, most-likely-to-do-themselves-bodily-harm patients on the unit, while Pat surveyed us impassively and took notes. There were four other girls on TSV my first night at the Farm. Lexi, who was sixteen, and who I learned was a repeat offender, yo-yoing in and out of inpatient treatment every few months because she kept brazenly flouting the rule of losing more than two kilograms of her target weight, and her parents kept bringing her back. This was why she looked healthier than everyone else, and why she openly despised all the skinny new admissions around her. The only person she liked on the ward was her cynical, sarcastic brunette counterpart, Jess, who'd also done several stints at the Farm, but who had a cooler temperament and avoided staying on TSV by blithely cooperating with the nurses every time she was frog-marched back into the Brown Kitchen. There was Naomi, thirteen, who barely said a word as she balled herself up into a corner of an armchair, keeping her face hidden behind the chewed-up cuffs of her oversized cardigan and two long, black curtains of straggly hair. Nobody really knew how long Naomi had been there; her admission predated every other patient's, and every return admission patient was on familiar terms with her, though I rarely saw her speak to anyone. Then there was Ruby. She had the most impressively prominent clavicles I'd ever seen, stylishly layered strawberry-blond hair tucked neatly behind her ears, and, unlike the other girls, she sat up poker-straight, her shoulders thrown back proudly, though her erect posture could sooner be attributed to her compulsive devotion to burning calories than to a healthy sense of self-esteem. Ruby was an intriguing presence from the get-go. She was prim and tidy but had a fiercely defiant glint in her eyes, and possessed an aura of spiky power.

Ruby perches herself on the very edge of the couch cushions and starts up a curious behaviour I've never seen before, tapping the balls of her feet up and down in an energetic seated running motion.

'Stop jigging! Stop it!' Pat insists sharply.

Ruby shoots her with a look that could pierce armour and stills her feet, but she maintains her unnaturally upright posture, refusing to relax.

Meanwhile, I retreat into a corner of the living room, press my face into the walls and cry. This first day at the Farm was then, and still remains, hands-down, the worst day of my life. I've never been in so much intense emotional pain. I've never felt so heartbroken, abandoned and hopeless. And I have the unbearable, unfamiliar feeling of fullness too: no pangs of hunger to console me and tell me I am doing something right. Instead, my belly growls and squawks under the strain of digesting such a large amount of food. The sensation of fullness, and of fat creeping on to your bones as you sit there doing nothing about it, is just the most agonising feeling when you're in the throes of anorexia. It's so intense that you find yourself grasping for anything that will save you from the feeling. I keep fantasising about running out in front of a speeding bus or throwing myself from a top-floor window, but the side door is locked, the key nowhere in sight, and the members of the TSV cloud are confined to the downstairs living room. It is suddenly abundantly clear why the first thing they do at Peaceful Pastures is confiscate your pointy objects.

'My God, do you ever shut up?' erupts Lexi furiously, and Pat doesn't tell her off. The rest of them are trying to watch a *I'm a Celebrity . . . Get Me Out of Here!* and block out their respective traumas while I loudly and unceasingly give voice to mine. I am being insufferable, a real brat, and further destroying any chance I have of making any friends here, but I am hundreds of miles away from my home, my bed, my cats, and I am determined not to stay here anyway, so I just keep crying.

201

'I don't want to be here,' I whinge into the wall, my hands pressed into my eye sockets.

'Well, neither do any of us!' Lexi spits back. 'Not one of us wanted to come here!'

'My mam will come and get me,' I say petulantly. 'She won't leave me in this place.'

'Ha, ha,' laughs Lexi, hollowly. 'Suuuuure.' A mean smile creeps into her voice. 'Your mum will come and get you.'

At 9pm, a very overweight, cropped-haired nurse with an air of profound indifference named Janet appears in the living room doorway and addresses me bluntly.

'Come for your supervised shower.'

Cradling my elbows, I follow her out through the hallway, into a second kitchen, known as the Blue Kitchen, where patients in the latter half of their programmes were trusted to eat away from the surveillance of the nurses, and then into a second hallway with stairs leading up to the bedrooms. I climb the stairs wearily, and then look up ahead of me as two enormous, trembling buttocks – a butt almost the width of the stairs – fill my vision and I see . . . my future. Janet shows me to a bathroom off a bedroom with six other beds and wedges the door open as she sits on the edge of a bed and tells me to start showering. I stand under the stream of water and scrub myself frantically, trying to get it over with as quickly as possible, but Janet trudges in and out every minute or so to check I haven't done anything sinister. I cower against the wall, shielding myself every time I hear her footsteps, hating that someone else is privy to my naked shame. And then I catch a glimpse of myself in the reflective surface of the tap and I recoil, because I can see – plain as day, and nobody can tell me any different, even though I've just been admitted to an anorexia treatment programme, even though I'm as thin as I've ever been – I can see that I am still fat.

The other girls shower one after the other as I sit on the edge of a bed, combing my hair and sniffling quietly. At 10pm, the lights are turned off and I sink weepily into a bed. Pat stations herself on a chair by the door, reading a gossip magazine by the light of the hallway. As I lie there, my eyes feeling raw, itchy and tired, I hear other lonesome sniffles permeating the silence. I cannot allow myself to sleep. It's been a whole day and I haven't done any exercise and I've eaten a huge meal laden with fat and calories. I can't just let them take my thinness away. I've worked too hard for it. Under the thick duvet, I tense the muscles of my abdomen tightly and then squeeze every muscle in my body that's covered, being very careful to keep my face blank. If I just keep doing this for the next few hours, I should be able to burn off most of the dinner. If I just keep—

'Stop tensing! I can feel you tensing!'

My eyes snap open and I look over to see Pat eyeballing me warningly. Everyone is so damn scary in this place!

'Stop it!' she barks, and reluctantly, I unclench.

I am not on the children's ward anymore, where at 2am I could noiselessly draw a curtain around my bed and knock out a hundred sit-ups. Here at Peaceful Pastures Clinic, they know their shit.

6

'Phoebe was like you!' exclaims Jen from the top of the table in the Brown Kitchen the next morning at breakfast, as once again I am the last one chewing my way through a huge bowl of fruit and nut muesli and a butter-soaked muffin while everyone else waits impatiently. 'Now look at her, look how happy she is!'

Standing by the kitchen counter, a rosy-cheeked, tan-limbed girl meets my eyes and smiles sweetly. Like me, Phoebe is twelve years old, but unlike me, Phoebe has almost completed her stint at the Farm and is being discharged today. This morning, she's finished her breakfast in the Blue Kitchen quickly and is saying her goodbyes to the residents of the Brown Kitchen as she prepares for her parents to pick her up and take her home for good.

'Give us your leaving book,' Jess calls to Phoebe from across the table. 'I think we're going to be here a while,' she says, jerking her head in my direction and reaching a hand towards Phoebe, who passes her a colourful notebook emblazoned with jovial cut-out lettering that reads: *Phoebe's Leaving Book!*

'Yeah, don't hurry up for our benefit,' Lexi adds, her chin resting on the palm of her hand as she surveys me through freshly made-up panda eyes. 'If you keep going at this pace, we might all get a day off school.'

I ignore their remarks, my head bent over the giant bowl of cereal, which doesn't seem to be shrinking no matter how many nutty clusters I shovel into my mouth.

'Take a bite of your muffin,' orders a young auburn-haired nurse with braces, her arms crossed as she watches me choke down another large mouthful of Jordan's Fruit & Nut with orange juice. 'Don't forget to wipe up that melted butter with your muffin. Don't think I can't see that.'

Seriously, Bruce Bogtrotter and the Trunchbull. Every freaking meal gave me flashbacks.

The leaving book was a tradition at Peaceful Pastures. Towards the end of their stay, patients would buy a notebook, decorate it with a collage of stickers and pictures, and then the other girls and boys would write parting messages of support and encouragement. Close friends would put hours of work into their leaving messages, asking for the book a week in advance and spending several days writing thoughtful, loving words surrounded by beautifully illustrated flowers and stars and photos of the two of them mounted on brightly coloured card. They clipped motivational words and slogans out of magazines, reading 'BEAUTIFUL!' 'STRONG!' 'YOU BABE!' They also cut and pasted photos of fatty foods with little notes reminding them of the most traumatising meals they'd endured in the Farm. 'Remember the day you vomited your dinner into a plant pot, and we all had to watch you drink this 1,000-calorie milkshake?! DON'T COME BACK, BABE!'

Less familiar friends would just scrawl curt, somewhat begrudging well wishes and words of warning. 'Well done on getting out of here. You look good at target. Hope I don't see you back here.'

'I'm really gonna miss you all,' says Phoebe fondly, beaming round at the residents of the Brown Kitchen.

'No, you're not,' says Lexi, a hint of bitterness in her voice as Jess slides her the book and she uncaps a pen to start her own message. 'You've got too much going for you. You're going to move on and you're not going to come back here.'

I look at Lexi's sullen face a moment, unable to tell if she means to compliment or insult Phoebe. At face value, it sounds like encouragement, but I can't help but detect an almost indiscernible note of smugness, and wonder, secretly, if she judges and pities Phoebe for reaching a healthy target weight.

It takes me forty minutes to get through breakfast. I slurp down the last droplets of full-fat milk and lower my head in defeat as the other patients leap to their feet and skitter off to brush their teeth and collect their schoolbooks. I follow the TSV cloud out of the kitchen, down a narrow hallway and into a large, L-shaped room set up like a classroom with desks in the centre and lockers lining the walls. The other patients set themselves up at the desks, laying their books around them, their faces quickly sliding into study mode, like this is all so normal, like it isn't a gross injustice that we are all being kept here against our will, like the day hasn't just started with two fully grown adults screaming us through our breakfasts. I loiter awkwardly by the wall for a minute, but everyone seems consumed in their own work, as if they've suddenly forgotten I'm there, so I slide quietly into an empty seat at a desk, fold my arms in front of me and bury my head in the crooks of my arms, so there is only blackness and I can block this all out for a while. But a moment later, a hand taps me on the shoulder and Jen is in my face again.

'We have to do your assessment. Come with me to the weighing room.'

Zombie-like, I follow her into a small room just off the classroom. Another nurse, Angela, sits by a small table next to a large weighing scale. Angela sports a mullet, a deep husky voice and the musculature of a rugby player. Her eyes flick up and down the length of my body without saying a word.

'Why didn't you weigh her yesterday?' she demands of Jen in an accusatory tone.

'We couldn't,' Jen responds. 'She was being a *very bad girl*.' She shoots me a facetiously stern look.

Why do they all talk to us like we are naughty children having a strop? Do they think anorexia is a mere childish bid for attention?

They argue back and forth for a bit about the weight being inaccurate due to me already having eaten breakfast, but Jen insists it will make little difference, and instructs me to go to the loo next door before being weighed.

'I'll be right outside,' she tells me. 'So, if you vomit, I'll hear you, and you'll have to drink a whole milkshake.' These nurses, I will learn, are always full of great ideas.

Thoroughly discomfited, I head to the toilet next door and pee as quietly as possible, picturing Jen's flushed cheek pressed creepily against the door. Back in the weighing room, she measures my height and calls it out to Angela, who notes it down. Then she tells me to strip down to my underwear to be weighed.

'Just your bra and pants, please.'

'I don't wear a bra,' I stutter, mortified, colour rushing to my cheeks. *I am twelve,* I feel like reminding her.

'Fine, keep your T-shirt on for now,' she allows. 'But you need to tell your mum to get you some little bras or crop tops so we can weigh you properly.'

I feel a stab of pain at the casual mention of my mum, who is still out there somewhere in this city, but not for much longer. Shaking, I step on the scale and see a number that gives me a happy, swooping feeling inside even as I stand there in my underwear flanked by nurses. It turns out all that crying and struggling has been extremely productive. I step off the scale, feeling very slightly better, calmer. At least one thing in my life is OK.

'You can put your clothes back on,' Jen tells me, as Angela fills in a box on the form in front of her.

'Take a seat, please,' Angela insists, and I sit in the cold plastic chair by the desk, an illicit sense of pride rippling through me, the number on the scale flashing across my mind. I feel thrilled, purposeful, strong. That glorious feeling of empowerment, that I am worth more than nothing, that I have managed to do something difficult and set myself apart, that I can do other difficult things too. I don't feel like I'm suffocating anymore, and with that elusive sense of equilibrium restored, I feel capable of civility towards these nurses and this system – at least while I strategise my way out. As long as I can get out of here soon and stay at this pleasing weight forever, everything will be alright again. I can forgive these nurses and my parents the trauma of the past twenty-four hours – no hard feelings.

'OK,' sighs Angela, flipping the page and conjuring a new chart, filled with figures. She references my chart with her pen and then slides her hand across to the other chart, and colours in a little box with a number I can't make out. 'So, your discharge date will be the tenth of May,' she says carelessly, almost lazily. 'You've got twelve weeks to gain the weight and two weeks to maintain.'

There is silence as I blink between the two nurses, confused.

'No,' I say simply. *14 weeks?!* This must all be a misunderstanding.

'Yes,' she answers plainly. 'That's the programme. Everyone does twelve weeks minimum, and then additional weeks depending on how much they need to gain to reach a healthy weight.'

'No, I can't be here for . . . fourteen weeks. I'm . . . I'm fine!'

Jen and Angela exchange a look of pure sardonicism.

I lean over to scrutinise the chart in front of me and the little box Angela has coloured in, this horrifying number that feels like a death sentence. The target weight has been calculated at ninety-five per cent of the national average of other children of the same height and age. It is that precise and uniform. Nothing else has been taken into account; not my genetics, not my build, and certainly not my preference. I gaze down at a number that seems unfathomable, absurd, ridiculous – a number my parents and Dr Nolan have never even whispered – and I feel panic rise inside me. Fourteen weeks in this hellish place, being bullied into eating my way to the national average weight. If there was one word I detested more than any other in the English language, it was *average*.

'No,' I tell them firmly. 'I've never been that weight. I'm not meant to be that size. Ask my mam.'

'Sorry,' answers Angela bluntly, snapping her folder shut and binding it. 'That's not your mum's decision. That's a healthy weight for you. Same as everyone else your age.'

So, I throw another tantrum, screaming and scratching at them, scrabbling for the door handle as they strain to keep me pinned to the chair. One thing I want to make abundantly clear to everyone in this godforsaken building, no matter how much power they wield, no matter that they have trapped me here, aided by my own flesh and blood, no matter that they have a rigorous, carefully designed plan to keep me here for fourteen weeks, from which I have no apparent escape – I will not go quietly. A puffy-haired, stormy-faced teacher barges into the weighing room at one point to chastise the nurses for the almighty ruckus I'm causing, which is rendering study impossible.

'I won't be quiet 'til you let me out of here!' I snarl through gritted teeth, chasing the teacher out of the room with my rage as I try to wriggle underneath Angela's meaty forearms.

'Right, I'm going to get a sedative,' Jen affirms crossly, marching towards the door with intent.

'No!' I exclaim, and Jen stops in her tracks, glaring at me challengingly.

'Are you going to behave then? Are you going to sit quietly like a good girl?'

I hold her gaze defiantly for a moment, my eyes brimming with tears, wishing I could laser this cruel woman with my hatred. I *hate* her. I hate this place. Most of all, I hate my parents. I hold her gaze a moment longer, searching for a hint of compassion, a tiny shred of kindness, but there is none forthcoming, so again I wilt, defeated, sliding on to the floor to lay my head on the seat of the chair, and I cry. I stay there for a while, hopeless and homesick. Angela files out, muttering about what a brattish nightmare I am as Jen tells me to pull myself together so I can re-join the classroom, but I ignore her and continue sobbing into my elbows.

All I want is to get far away from this place, to walk out that door with simple self-autonomy and sit quietly on a footpath with my freedom. I think of all the neglected, starving children that teachers and parents taunt *their* children with, in geography lessons or over unappetising bowls of lumpy potatoes, and I feel zero sympathy for their plight, as they pick their way through dumpsters and wander aimlessly through a world that is loveless and harsh, but free, totally free! I am the opposite of a neglected child, pinioned to this chair by threats of further control and intrusion into this body I cannot bear. I am cornered and watched from every angle so I can't struggle, can't run, can't walk away, can't slice the pain I'm feeling out of my skin. I can only sit here and let it leak out of my eyes.

A while later, Jen gets to her feet, claps her hands together and insists I stop being a baby and go to do some schoolwork, but I have no intention of cooperating, so I sit there stubbornly and refuse to budge. She grabs me under the armpits and drags me out the door of the weighing room – the eyes of every classroom occupant following us – and plonks me back into an empty seat at a desk, whereupon I fold my arms in front of me, tent my cardigan over my head and bury my face in the darkness, sniffling quietly.

Some time later, I feel a light touch on one of my shoulder blades, a touch so distinct in its gentleness that it makes me start. I peek out from the edge of my cardigan fortress to see the freckle-faced girl who'd defended me at dinner. She has blue-green, clear eyes and a halo of flyaway hairs poking out of a messy ponytail. She's one of the older girls on the unit, sixteen at least, and relatively healthy-looking, though she's wearing the customary shapeless, oversized hoodie down to her knees, so it's hard to tell how close she is to target. She folds her arms in front of her and rests her head on her forearms to meet mine.

'Hi, I'm Rose,' she tells me. 'I thought you could use some company.' Her speech reveals a slight, endearing lisp.

I look back at her for a second, seeing the kindness, the sympathy I've been craving since I got here, but I don't know what to say, and I'm not ready to give up resisting this place, so I bury my face in my arms again and give a loud sniff in response.

'I know it's awful here,' Rose continues, and her tone is not simpering or patronising like that of the nurses; it is just kind. 'I know how angry and upset you must be feeling . . . I hate it here too,' she tells me, through my cardigan barrier. 'But it will get easier.' Somehow, her kindness isn't making me feel better. It's making me feel like I'm breaking. It's seeping under my heavy cardigan, permeating my steely anger and pooling in the tender cracks of my heartache, making it sting painfully. I just want my mam. I just want it to be her gentle touch and her kind voice soothing my pain and telling me life won't always be this awful.

'No, it won't,' I tell Rose, through bitter tears. 'It won't get easier. I don't want to be here. I hate it here.'

'Why do you hate it here?' she asks, patiently.

'. . . because everyone is so mean . . . and they're trying to make me fat. I can't get fat. I can't be fat.' I can feel the panic rising again as I chant this.

'They won't make you fat,' Rose says reassuringly. She is so patient and sweet. I hear other girls scoffing and tutting around me as I whine, but Rose remains neutral, trying her best to reach me and offer comfort despite the venom I'm spewing. 'They'll make you get to a healthier weight, but they're not going to make you fat. I promise you, nobody leaves here fat.'

But everything she says just makes me cry harder. I don't want to surrender. I don't want to accept that things will get better and that I will eventually feel OK here. I am bent on resistance, and that means clinging fiercely to my pain and rage. As much as I crave a hug and her sympathy, I also want to wear her down, to quash her positivity and make her give up too.

'I don't want to be here,' I say again. 'I don't like English people.'

This was a lie. I was practically an anglophile. Growing up, I'd always idolised the sophistication and cosmopolitan glamour of the English. I cringed at the bumbling awkwardness of my fellow Irish natives, who seemed so uncivilised in comparison to the self-possessed, confident English. Mam became Mum, as I already mentioned and I worked carefully to cultivate an ambiguously neutral accent and often complained at home about the tediousness of learning a practically defunct language. *Harry Potter* sealed the deal for me. I watched with longing as glossy-haired, upper-class, drama-school Brits graced magazine covers and went off to Hogwarts, while I sat at home conjugating verbs and learning the rosary in Irish. As far as I could tell, Irish people didn't get to go to Hogwarts. But the thing about anorexia – or maybe it's just self-loathing in general – is that it likes to push people away. It bites and spits and lashes out until, eventually, the other person gives up their kindness, stalks away in disgust, and you sit back, perversely satisfied that they, too, have recognised your worthlessness. It gives a strange sense of power and safety when you keep love out. And there was something about the events of the past twenty-four hours that had awoken the long-dormant Irish nationalist in me, so I summoned all the pain and spite from my ancient ancestral wounds and directed it at the well-meaning, kind-hearted Rose.

'What do you mean you don't like English people?' she asks, scepticism creeping into her voice.

'You took away our language and culture! Now you're taking away my thinness!'

'I don't think that's anything to do with politics,' Rose reasons, lifting her head and pulling away from me.

'Yes, it is. You English people like to dominate us! You're trying to dominate me!' My history lessons were finally coming in handy. 'I don't like the English,' I add, sulkily.

'Well, that's actually kind of *racist*,' Rose snaps, her patience finally crumbling, and she gets up and stalks to the other side of the classroom. I sniff, feeling a small twinge of regret as the lovely wave of warmth and compassion she'd created dissolves, and I'm left alone again. *Let them all leave*, I think as I bury my face once more in the darkness. *Let every last person give up on me and leave me alone with my thinness*.

At ten-thirty, a nurse calls down the corridor that it is 'snack time', and all the patients get reluctantly to their feet and slope to the Blue and Brown Kitchens. An array of horrors meets my eyes on the table of the Brown Kitchen. *Chocolate bars*. Terrifying words like 'king-size', 'chunky' and, worst of all, 'man-size' glint jeeringly from shiny blue and purple wrappers. These chocolate bars always seemed to brag nonchalantly about their nauseatingly dense calorie count and the gross indulgence they represent, which is precisely why I have been avoiding them for years. It's not like I haven't tasted any chocolate for two years, but it's only ever been from under shy, demure wrappers that apologise profusely for their sinful existence, showing an appropriate level of shame under self-flagellatory marketing terms like 'low-sugar', 'no-sugar' or 'skinny', and even those have always been followed by a frenzied bout of cardio, expelling their corruption immediately from my body.

And now here they sit, on white paper plates with names written on the top and their calorie count beneath. *Allison, 180 cals. Nina, 210, cals. Lara, 185 cals.* Weekly calories, I will learn, are calculated according to how close to the weekly one-kilogram target weight-gain each patient's weight had settled at their last weigh-in. Weigh-ins take place on Monday and Thursday mornings. The Thursday weigh-ins spell out the specifics of your weekend privileges, while the Monday weigh-ins monitor how consistently you are moving towards the target line, and indicate which calorie adjustments need to be made, or privileges revoked. Patients whose weight is floundering below their weekly target are subject to a significant calorie increase, a chocolate bar here, an extra chunk of cheese there, while patients who gain more than their weekly target enjoy a calorie cut and the least scary of the chocolate bars.

'Yes!' says Lara triumphantly as she grabs the plate with her name and a Crunchie bar listed as 185 calories. Other girls eye her enviously as they slink off to their seats with 250-calorie Mars bars and Snickers. By far the most feared chocolate bar, though, is the brutishly named 'Boost', coming in at a dreaded 265 calories. Lexi swipes her Boost angrily from the table and stations herself at the very end of the bench, propping her elbows on the table to glare at the offending chocolate bar. There is one more Boost on the table, sitting, predictably, between 'Evanna' and '265 calories'.

There was no respite from eating at Peaceful Pastures, not for anyone, under any condition. It didn't matter how young or sick or traumatised you were, or how much you were suffering, there was never a break from eating. Every single calorie from every meal or snack went in at the Farm, either between screams or through mute, tensely held jaws. It felt like the entire purpose of our lives was eating. No sooner had your belly stopped hurting and whining from the last ambush, than another meal or snack time was launched. And as you sat there, chewing your way through hunks of chocolate and caramel, you couldn't help but frantically calculate the river of calories consumed, especially compared to the meagre amount that had previously sustained you.

Chocolate was everyone's fear food, because it was unanimously acknowledged as a treat rather than a necessity – and what was the point of food, other than to get fatter, if it wasn't *necessary* for survival? So even as I ground my way slowly through the dense chocolate caramel bar, and some muted, distant part of my brain danced and relished the sweet chocolatey deliciousness, I felt, with each swallow, like I was ingesting poison.

No sooner has the final crumb been licked clean again than everyone leaps to their feet, disposing of the plates and wrappers in the bin, and hurries out of the Brown Kitchen. The TSV cloud is last to trudge out, impeded by a heavy veil of depression, inertia and the most uncooperative personalities on the unit. Just as I'm about to slink back into the hallway, Jen calls me back and tells the TSV nurse she'll see me to the classroom. She presents me with a small plastic Woolworth's bag.

'Your parents came by to deliver this,' she tells me casually.

I snatch the bag off her, but keep my eyes fixed hungrily on her face. 'My parents are here?' I demand. 'Where are they? Let me see them.'

'They're gone already. They're gone back home. You can talk to them on Thursday.'

'Please, please, *please* can I see them? Just for a minute. I won't try and run away.' My lip trembles as I look at her and implore her to understand. It is so important in this moment that she understands that I need my parents. I feel as though I can sense them moving further away from me. Soon they will be at the airport, buying bottled water and hard-boiled sweets, choosing fridge magnets for my siblings, and they will board a plane without me, return home and get on with their lives. There is something irretrievable about that, like something precious is leaving with them – a last chance, hope, a piece of me I won't get back. So, I look this woman in the eyes and plead from my soul. But she is blank and business-like. It's just a job to her, boxes she needs to tick to fulfil her role. She's trained not to notice the soul crying out for help.

'You can speak to them on Thursday. These are the rules. You don't need to talk to them now.'

'Is there . . . is there no way I can talk to them?' I ask desperately, my eyes darting to all of the windows, still nursing that feeble, faint hope that my mum's face might appear at one of them.

'You can write them a letter,' Jen offers, shrugging. 'But it won't get to Ireland before Thursday.' She escorts me back down the hallway to the classroom, where everyone is glumly resuming their seats. I station myself at my desk again, avoiding the eyes of anyone around me, and with trembling fingers I pull out a thick envelope bearing my name in my mum's writing. Tiny inked flowers and vines curled elegantly around the letters. Inside the bag are more treasures:

an *Art Attack*, a *Mizz* magazine, bright socks with sunflowers and butterflies, and a *Harry Potter* bookmark. Tearing the seal of the envelope, I pull out a cluster of cards with cats on them, round-blue-eyed calendar cats with coiffed tails set against dreamy cloudscapes. Opening the cards, reams of my mum's curly, feminine script meet my eyes, and a few lines of my dad's loopy, stylised penmanship down the bottom of the last card. Tears blur my vision again as my eyes flick back and forth over the lines on the page and I think I might dissolve with sadness. They are sorry. They love me. They didn't realise it would be so harsh. They wish they could take me home. They'll come visit me. They'll call every day. They'll think of me. They'll look after my cats. And then at the very end, framed by a hectic smattering of 'x's and 'o's, my mum's slightly shaky pen has written: '*PS It will get easier.*' A thousand tangled feelings pulse through me as I sit there, looking at the cards in front of me. Relief. Gratitude. Love. Hope. Warmth. Hurt. Sadness. Fury. Fear. Despair. Abandonment. Disbelief. Longing. Loss. All of it swirls around inside me as I read and reread the cards and try to make sense of the fact that, despite all the loving, lovely words on these pages, all the assertions that they wish they could help me and will be there for me, somehow, they have still walked away from this place – not once, but twice – and left me in it. The more I read, sitting there trying to still my breathing, the more my emotions settle and the presiding feeling I'm left with is rage.

'It will get easier' is probably the most offensive thing you can say to someone in the grip of pain. You are borrowing from a future that isn't promised, a future that depends entirely on their endurance of the pain. You are taking for granted a well of strength within them that they may not possess, fast-forwarding through the ugly bits that you don't want to watch but they must live through, nonetheless. 'It will get easier' is not a helpful thing to say to someone for whom only the present moment can exist, so vivid, so intense that it's not possible to imagine a moment beyond it. The future doesn't matter to someone enduring an unimaginable pain, so let's not entertain that childish fantasy. All that matters is the pain that is consuming you in this moment, that you grit your teeth and try to survive it. You invalidate the pain and the damage it inflicts when you hasten to skip past it to a brighter tomorrow. Sometimes things are just unremittingly shit and the only respectful thing to do is to stand next to the person going through it and scream along with them.

I close the cards and look back at the beauty pageant kittens and their shiny marble eyes. Words. That's all they are. Useless, empty, ineffectual words. And these cats, they are not *my* cats. My cats in Ireland have lean, velvety bodies, wild green eyes and stripy coats matted with their own fur and sticky green balls from the tall weeds they prowl through at night as they hunt. I do not know these stupid, fluffy, doll-like show cats. I do not love these vacant-eyed distortions of nature. I do not need empty words and frilly socks and frivolous *shit*. I need my freedom.

I storm across the classroom and ask a tall, grey-haired, woolly-jumpered man – Nigel, the headteacher – for a pen and some paper. He looks hesitant for a moment, as if about to venture some verbs that need conjugating, but seems to sense the simmering rage I'm barely containing and quietly acquiesces with my demand. I storm back to my seat, lay the paper out in front of me, and proceed to write a letter to my parents. '*Dear Mam and Dad*,' I begin, scratching furiously. '*It will not get easier . . .*'

I spend the next few days writing letters. It's the only way I cope. Meals keep coming around far too often, meals upon meals upon meals, each one presenting fresh horrors I'm not prepared for. It is physically uncomfortable and emotionally torturous to be eating so much food. I cry and cry. I wait at windows in case my parents come back. I sit and stare vacantly into the distance, lined up on a couch with all the other dead-eyed girls on TSV. My eyes linger on kitchen knives, pointy edges and steep drops from bedroom windows, fantasising about a way out. It would be nice to just be dead. I shower for a different nurse each night, the taps cruelly taunting me with my bloated body. I can't read *Harry Potter*, because everyone suddenly has bossy English accents and in my nightmares Professor Dumbledore screams at me to lick steak and kidney pie off the Great Hall floor while the students – even the Gryffindors – jeer from the four house tables. Everyone in the Brown Kitchen despises me for my incessant hysterics and for the way I keep making them miss the start of *I'm a Celebrity . . .Get Me Out of Here!* It's the season where Katie Price and Peter Andre meet and fill the Australian jungle with their knuckle-biting sexual tension, so their frustration with me is understandable. The only kind person at the Farm now thinks I'm a xenophobe and carefully avoids me. The days are lonely, loveless and calorific. And it is so unfair that my parents are at home, away from all this, with my cats and their lives and their other children, and that they're still pretending that they love and care about me. It is not fair that they get to avoid all this and simply imagine that things will get easier, so I use the only tool still available to me and I punish them with my words. I tell them how much I hate them.

I tell them I don't forgive them. That I want to die. That they will regret this. That I *can't* do this. That soon I will find a way to actually kill myself and it will be their fault and here's the written proof. Oh, I go *in* with these letters! I even borrow some colouring pencils from the school store cupboards and take to illustrating the corners of the letters with increasingly graphic pictures of my death. I draw me in a hospital bed with lacerated forearms. I draw me hanging from a shower curtain. I draw me as a sad ghost. *Lots of love, your erstwhile daughter*, I sign the letter, sealing it up, addressing it to my mum and plopping it in the clinic's post box, which sits on a windowsill on the way to the Brown Kitchen.

I write other people letters too. This whole experience has radically shifted my opinion of Dr Nolan, who I think of with a soft fondness now, his small-boned, puffy-haired form angelically backlit in my imagination. I seriously consider sending him a Valentine's card. *How I miss you, Fergal! We had a good thing going! Please can we give it another try?* I write long, melancholy epistles to my friends at school, full of profound wisdom and ominous warnings. *Don't do what I've done. Live your lives, children! Be grateful for every moment!* I am a poet possessed of an otherworldly sagacity that only comes from deep suffering! I work carefully to give an impression of steadily declining sanity in my letters, becoming increasingly more cryptic and incoherent, planning to eventually devolve into pure nonsense. I want everyone to think I'm dying, tragically expiring in a brutal institution, my spirit sadly fading! Yes, I am a seriously dramatic individual, and some of expressing myself this way is therapeutic, but it all still hurts keenly and, behind my quest for vengeance and attention, I want someone to recognise just how much it hurts. I want them to help me. I want them to care. The letters to my mum become darker still, with specific dates for my intended departure from this world, and instructions for my funeral and who will inherit which cat. I finish one particularly awful letter with a Tim Burton-esque illustration of my tombstone and my tortured mother weeping beside it. *This is what the future holds!* I rail at her. *This is all your fault!*

Looking back on those first few days at the Farm, I am struck by the intensity of my rage towards my mother. Why was it she who felt the brunt of all my anger, when my dad had been there too? He was equally guilty of abandoning me in that shadowy hallway and turning his back as he walked away. So why did I not blame him with the same furious passion? Why did I hate her so much for something that was not her doing alone? It's hard to see a clear rationale for all this maternally aimed rage. It could be a number of things. Maybe it was because there is a deep-rooted strand of misogyny to anorexia that loathes and fears the female form, and so it is natural to direct this ire towards the mother. Maybe it's because she was my original caregiver, had grown me deep in her being, protecting me from the elements with her own body, and so on a primitive level, I just expected she always would. Maybe it was more of an existential agony, that she had spit me out of her womb, the one safe place on earth, and life had only gotten progressively harder ever since. Maybe it was because she also hated herself and as a part of her I was bound to self-hate too. Or maybe I hated her for how she had made me – normal, flawed, human – and how nobody would ever love me like she did, and for the way her love doomed me to walk the earth, hollow, and searching for it elsewhere.

Needless to say, daily life at the Farm in those first few weeks was entirely grim. A large part of that could be attributed to the undeniably twisted dynamic that existed between the staff and patients: an atmosphere of constant conflict and antagonism, and a relationship that can only be likened to one of Prisoner vs Captor. Today, I often refer to the Farm as 'Anorexic Prison Camp'. That's just what it felt like. The nurses treated us like criminals, being punished over and over for the crime of trying to be thin. There was no kindness or sympathy on offer for anyone showing resistance to the programme or inclinations towards thinness. Even the smallest transgressions – standing up for too long in the classroom, or sectioning your dinner into different food categories before eating it – would earn you admonishment, a series of threats levelled loudly in your direction. The nurses were always hunting for signs of our deviousness, bursting through closed doors to check nobody was secretly doing sit-ups in the corner, and routinely searching our possessions in the bedrooms for sharp items, or plastic bottles that might be used to 'tank' water the night before a weigh-in. Our shoes were all confiscated too, locked up in a cupboard in the hallway, to discourage us from making a run for it should we manage to get out the back door.

Their suspicions weren't always unfounded, of course; more often than not we *were* all frantically scheming for ways to burn extra calories, skank foods and tank liquids, but the problem with them only seeing us as naughty, devious anorexics was that it created an atmosphere of silent warfare. The thing about declaring war on someone is that either you crush them, or you create a warrior. And when you declare war on anorexia in a ward full of furious teenagers, you inevitably create an army of anorexic warriors. The schism this environment established between staff and patients was profound and only helped foster a spirit of bitter resistance. It became personal very quickly, the patients focusing their hatred narrowly on the nurses, and they'd cluster together in the evenings after mealtimes and bitch with savage ferocity about every detail of their captors; their hair, their husbands, their style choices, most certainly their weight. But the nurses always got their revenge at mealtimes, their tone coming across snidely pleased as they reminded us of the sickening mixture of liquid fat that would be pumped into our stomachs via a nasogastric tube if we failed to finish our grilled cheese sandwiches. All of the nurses – as long as I was a patient there – were female, and I was grateful for that, especially during supervised showers, but sometimes I do look back and wonder was the atmosphere missing a much-needed strand of masculine evenness to balance all that fiery-tempered girl-on-girl hatred. Certainly, in my experience, female captors could be just as cruel as men, though their punishments weren't dealt through their fists; their cruelty was psychological, subtle, insidious. Perhaps not everyone on the staff was a bully but any softer, gentler personalities were usually drowned out by the loud-mouthed, harsh disciplinarians and so they are the ones I remember most clearly. Patients' programmes were enforced by a regime of fear and punishment, at least in the early part of their stay when they were refusing to cooperate, and I think that environment hardened many of the staff members and honestly, the power often went to the nurses's heads. Certain nurses and patients developed more personal, pointed animosities, singling each other out to taunt and deride a disproportionate amount, their personalities clashing explosively. Sue, the mean blond nurse I'd encountered at my memorable first meal, became *my* arch-nemesis. Whatever the hell her unresolved issues were, she seemed to relish taking them all out on me at mealtimes.

❧

'You just think the world revolves around you, don't you?' Sue says to me, a smug smile pinching her features as I gag at a chicken Kiev oozing greasily on my plate. (Vegetarianism is regarded as a symptom of eating disorders at the Farm, an ally of thinness, and is forbidden on the programme. It is not respected on ethical grounds, and any claim to care about the welfare and rights of animals is explained back to us as anorexia in an artful new guise.)

'You think you should get to have everything your way.' Sue leans down on her elbows across the counter and squints at me through small, rectangular glasses.

'No, I don't,' I sob, my hands shielding my eyes from the breaded carcass in front of me. 'I just don't want to eat a dead chicken.'

I ate the dead chicken. I ate everything. You always did in the end. That was the worst thing about the war between the nurses and the patients; they held all the power over us, and our resistance, however fiercely and bravely we wielded it, was ultimately futile. They won every battle. And there was something really soul-crushing about that.

Much like prison making masterminds out of petty criminals, the Farm made everyone better at anorexia. The average age of the patients on the ward was fifteen to sixteen, and they were mostly girls (though there was always at least one boy there during my stint) who had been grappling with anorexia for years by now. One key thing about anorexia is that the longer you have it, the more your life deteriorates and the better you become at maintaining your disorder, until the *only* thing you're maintaining is your disorder. Some of the girls were practically professionals at anorexia, having spent most of their adolescence bouncing in and out of various treatment centres and fighting bitterly to hold on to their eating disorders, biding their time until they reached the mythical age of eighteen, when their lives would be theirs alone and nobody could force them into recovery. So, they knew *all* the tricks and were happy to brag about their extensive knowledge of overcoming hunger cravings, optimal fat-burning activities and their most impressive escapades in outsmarting the scales. In the evenings after dinner, when group morale was at its lowest, the savvy older patients would hold court by listing the calorie count of obscure foods from memory, the younger patients gripped and hanging on their every word, absorbing the precious knowledge like wide-eyed children listening to a wizened old bard reciting ancient fairy tales. There was definitely a respect and reverence afforded to the most experienced, hardcore anorexics on the ward. They had submitted further and sacrificed more to anorexia, a social currency that was prized above all else in a house of anorexia devotees. And though all the patients were sympathetic to the mutual pain and inevitability of each of us gaining weight, no matter how 'bad' we started, there was an unspoken hierarchy of thinness. Extreme thinness won you envy, respect and vigorous scrutiny. This accounted for the way the girls flitted through the hallway when a new admission appeared, their eyes roving over her fleshless thighs and spiky hip bones.

'She's so thin!' they'd whisper to each other in the living room, a note of awe and excitement in their voices. 'I don't know how they let her get so bad!' There was too, that smug satisfaction and a note of haughty dismissal in their voices when the new girl didn't look 'sick enough'.

'She practically looks normal,' someone would scoff. 'I bet she only does twelve weeks.'

Privately, the older girls rolled their eyes at twelve-week stay patients. Twelve weeks was for little girls, amateur anorexics. I grew to be proud of the additional two weeks I'd earned through two extra kilograms lost, which signalled I'd crossed a threshold in thinness that afforded grudging respect and protected me from the unspoken accusation of not having quite got 'sick enough'.

These were the thoughts you picked up around long-term anorexics. Everyone made each other more obsessed. Watching the other patients' behaviours at mealtimes and overhearing snippets of conversations, I learned of new ways to get rid of food, discreet dense objects that could be hidden in your hair, underwear – various orifices, if it came to that – on weigh-in days to trick your parents, and of a habit called 'jigging', that bizarre rapid pattering of the feet I'd seen Ruby do on my first night, a practice which was of course banned at Peaceful Pastures, but which broke out – a wave of bony knees in motion – the moment a nurse turned her back. Above all, I learned that nothing was ever enough when it came to anorexia. That standing burned more calories than sitting, so stand up. That cold temperatures burned more fat, so leave the bedroom windows wide open at night. That you could keep on stretching the limits of how much food you actually needed to survive and how many calories you could burn in a day, and that somebody else had already beat you at these feats without dying, so by all means you should keep going. I learned not to relax or to enjoy a single moment of comfort, because all of it – all of it, no longer just the food and the moments of inactivity – was making me fat. And though it was not possible to put this newfound wisdom into practice and take my anorexia up a notch while in the clinic, I filed each trick and tip carefully away in my mind for when I would get out, and I vowed silently to be better, stronger, thinner.

Of course, regardless of these relentless efforts to burn calories, each patient consistently gained weight, and there was just no getting around that. Everyone, at whatever stage in their programme, was scheduled to gain one kilogram per week. The atmosphere on weigh-in mornings was that of a courtroom just before they announce the verdict of a murder trial – impossibly tense and strained, the silence only broken by the occasional muffled sob. We all sat hunched against the wall or – for those desperately afraid of seeing the numbers on the scale go up – stood, jigging from foot to foot, still trying to burn calories even as the line in front of us dwindled and the weighing room loomed, mere moments away.

There was never really a positive outcome to those weigh-ins; either you didn't gain the requisite kilogram and would be subject to higher calories, fewer freedoms and possibly TSV, or you did meet your 'line', which earned you fresh privileges and got you one week closer to total freedom, but also meant you had to grapple with the distressing, undeniable fact that you had put on weight. However, everyone tended to have a preference for which direction they wanted their weight to drift. Patients in the latter half of their programmes tended to be calmer, having grudgingly accepted their fate, their eyes trained fixedly on their target and discharge date that finally seemed within reach. But the new admissions, return patients and the ones who just flatly refused to submit to the idea of recovery, no matter how long they remained on the unit, struggled bitterly with the idea of any weight gain and were usually the ones sobbing into their elbows on weigh days.

On my first weigh-in day, I sit shivering in the corridor in a thin nightdress, hands wrapped around my ribcage as I stare at my knees. It is all so horrible. The regime. The food. The rules. The toxic bitchiness. Over and over, my lack of control and freedom gut me. And the only method I know for riding waves of pain and periods of intense stress is unravelling rapidly beneath my fingertips. As I sit there, grinding my teeth and dreading the scale, I can't help but run my hands all over the familiar bony bits of my body, grasping for angular edges and sharpened points as if urging them to stay, stay, and don't you dare change.

'NaaaaaaAAAAAAAOOOOOOOO!!!' a primal wail erupts from the weighing room, and a moment later the door smacks open and Kayla, a bobbed-haired, brown-eyed sixteen-year-old with a catlike face, is striding down the hallway, with eyes blazing, a terrifying rage pulsing from her like bolts of electricity. The rest of us cower against the wall away from her, clutching our nightdresses and robes around us as she storms past. In front of me, Lara, a shy, dark-eyed girl, starts to cry.

We find out later that Kayla has been tanking for a couple of weeks, carefully calculating what time in the evening to stop peeing and holding an alarming volume of water in her bladder for the whole night before the weigh-in. However, on this particular morning, she'd been unable to hold the massive quantity of water she'd tanked, had fatally gone to the toilet, and now apparently has lost 1.2kg of weight, though in actuality, she just hasn't been gaining. She is put back on supervision so they can watch her beadily and deduce her methods of subversion. She is also told she will not be allowed to see her boyfriend at the weekend as planned. She cries all day, pleading with the nurses, fretting about the fact that her boyfriend has already paid for his train journey and that he will probably break up with her soon, and then how will she cope, but they show no mercy. It's one kilogram or bust. As for me, by Thursday I've gained almost half a kilo, and am allowed my first phone call home.

Communication with the outside world is strictly limited for all patients at the Farm. Mobile phones were forbidden, though in 2004 that isn't a particularly extreme measure. The classroom contains a few enormous, wheezy computers allowing access to emails at lunch-time, but again, 2004 – most of us don't have email addresses. Our principal method of communication with the outside world comes in the shape of biweekly telephone call slots on Monday and Thursday evenings. That first Thursday, the TSV cloud are all scheduled to have our telephone calls at the same time, so we trudge to a brightly lit, starkly furnished room with a telephone at each seat around a large table. I watch as everyone picks up a corded telephone in the crook of their elbow and retreats to various corners of the room, where they curl up, gathering their knees to their chests and wait, with varying expressions of anticipation, anger, and hope for their loved ones to ring. I pick up the telephone that Janet indicates is for me, and carry it over to a bare stretch of wall to huddle and wait, as she seats herself unconcernedly at the table with a stack of magazines. My phone rings at 8.32pm, and I snatch it up on the first ring.

'Hi, pet,' my mum's warm, familiar tone greets me.

As it turned out, my parents had *not* spent their evening in London at the theatre or a Michelin-starred restaurant enjoying an artisan cheese board. Later, I learned that they had staggered out the door of Peaceful Pastures and wandered away, feeling lost and shaken. Just a hundred yards up the road, they had stumbled upon a Catholic church and a convent of nuns and, like any frightened Irish person who finds themselves shuffling around the mean streets of a vast foreign city, their heart crying out for the smell of homemade stew and overly familiar neighbours, had been irresistibly drawn inside the house of God. They had knocked on the door to the convent, two desperate strangers from the street, unheralded and empty-handed, and were immediately escorted to the parlour, whereupon they were met by the Mother Superior, Sister Paula, a cheerful, practical Donegal woman, who sat them down and listened quietly as they recounted the day's events, punctuating their tale of woe with murmurs of empathy and understanding. When my dad finished speaking, she nodded, posed no questions and simply said: 'We can help you. But first, will you have something to eat?'

Later on, Sister Paula had shown my parents to accommodation in the grounds of the convent. She gave them keys to the building and said they could stay there as often as they needed to, so they forewent their booking at a nearby hotel and spent the night – and every other visit to London after that – tucked up cosily amid the Sisters of Charity. Years on, both parents still talk of the Sisters with misty-eyed appreciation. 'Say what you will about the Catholic church,' my mum – an occasional verbal correspondent of God, but not an especially religious person – says anytime the church comes under fire '. . . but those nuns were real-life angels to us during that time.'

Unbeknownst to me, my mum has been calling the clinic several times a day to ask for me, but at this point all I know is that she has abandoned me so I keep my lips pressed together tightly and try to meet her cheerful greeting with icy, unyielding silence, but then she asks me how I'm doing and something in my chest seems to unknot as tears spill freely down my face. For a while, I just weep down the phone and my parents make soothing, sympathetic noises and commiserate with their own series of grievances. They admit the programme is far harsher and more rigid than they'd been expecting. They agree the nurses are cold and impersonal. They balk at the idea of fourteen weeks. I feel a little better to know my family are still on my side. But then I ask them when they are coming to get me out, and am met with a tense, protracted silence. They say we have to give this programme a try. They remind me that the methods of treatment at the hospital have not been working. They tell me that, naturally, this 'period of adjustment' is difficult, but I have to try and 'be strong', 'fight the illness' and tough out these first few weeks.

With a feeling of growing unease, I recognise the terminology they are using as the language from the admission pamphlet used to explain away a patient's cries for help as puerile hysterics and the swan song of anorexia. They have put me and my feelings into a neat little box labelled 'The Anorexia' and sealed it shut to shout itself hoarse and wear itself out. My sense of dread and alarm mounting, I realise my parents are being trained not to hear me, in the same way the nurses don't. They are being brainwashed. So, once again, a calm, reasonable demeanour is dropped, and I resort to begging, blaming and threatening them.

All around me, other conversations are escalating into high-pitched shrieks, frantic pleas and furious swearing.

'I FUCKING HATE YOU!!!' screams Naomi, the quiet girl with the dark curtains of hair covering her face, and slams down the phone with startlingly violent force. A moment later, her phone rings again and she yanks the cord out of the wall, silencing it, and goes back to crying quietly behind her hair.

Ruby, meanwhile, is giving her parents the silent treatment, sitting in her rigidly upright position, her face blank and impassive as she holds the receiver to her ear. Her rage is palpable only through her tightly crossed limbs and the way her jaw keeps clenching and unclenching, but she remains calculated and controlled as she gives only the most terse, monosyllabic replies to their series of enquiries, responses that communicate nothing but her utter disdain for her parents. After a few minutes, they give up trying to coax conversation out of her and she replaces the phone coolly and resumes jigging before Janet casually admonishes her without looking up.

Eventually, it is only me left on the phone to my parents, whining pathetically as I scramble for some sort of compromise, a plan, a foothold of hope so I can survive another few days of this hell until they come and get me. Janet rises from her chair and hovers above me, her hand outstretched for the phone as I frantically ply my parents for a verbal agreement. But they will only tell me that they can do nothing, that it's out of their hands now, that the Irish Health Board would see it as a child abuse if they discharge me from the care of Peaceful Pastures and would set social services on them.

But it is like trying to explain to a sad-eyed puppy that, though you're going away for a week and not taking them with you, you will be back soon, and everything will be as it was. Logically, I can understand that there are complications and restrictions in place that prevent them from intervening, but in my heart, I can't understand why they simply aren't here. In my heart, I can't reconcile the fact that they will not physically elbow their way through the front door and protect me from this pain, as they always have done before. And, right now, I really, truly don't see myself making it through the programme, which just feels unendingly bleak. I *need* them to come and take me home. I don't see any other way out of this place, as I continue to tell them with increasing urgency.

I hear my mum hesitate and take in an anxious breath, unsure of how to answer my discomfiting threats and pleas. She, too, is grappling for footholds, for methods of coping, and she finds them in flimsy, illusory words of hope. The vision of a brighter future is what she sees as the solution to this traumatic situation, even as I scream for her to take action.

'It really will get better,' she offers, in a tentatively optimistic tone. Anger surges through me as I hear her take comfort from her own futile words. Two stone and no moment of respite from eating is not something to sneeze at for a young person in the grip of anorexia. It fills me with panic and despair each time someone assumes this merciless, unrelenting struggle is something I can endure. And it is so much more acute when that person is my mother, when the person I rely on most to protect me can just hang up the phone and imagine that everything will soon get better. By now, Janet is gesticulating impatiently for me to hand over the phone. It is 9.03pm, and everyone is waiting for me to wrap up. Sucking in air through my gritted teeth, I decide that I'm not going to leave my mum clinging on to this offensively happy thought of a brighter tomorrow.

'It won't get better!' I shout at her. 'I'm not OK here! I'm telling you it's not OK! It's not OK and it won't get better!

GoodNIGHT.' I slam down the phone in fury, breathing hard through my tears.

Nobody was listening to my cries for help. I felt like all the little bubbles of hope quietly orbiting my heart were being dashed out. Every day just seemed to get darker and sadder and harder to get through, and something about the repeated refusal to acknowledge the full extent of my pain really played at the edges of my sanity. I don't know what point I'm trying to make here, politically, morally or otherwise. Perhaps I'm just ranting. But to me, there is something deeply unethical about a scared twelve-year-old begging for help and crying 'I can't do this,' only to be met with a blank chorus of 'Sure you can.' You know the end of this story already; I got out of there, and ultimately everything *did* get better, but, when someone is in such a fragile state of mental health and finding no source of comfort, I don't know that it always would get better. Personally, when it comes to anorexia recovery, I don't approve of solely treating the body and turning a deaf ear to the soul crying out for help. A soul can still drown in a healthy body.

A week goes by, and I meet my first weekly target. A few days later, I am taken off TSV and assigned a new bedroom. There is some debate among the nurses and patients over who will have to room with me. 'I don't want to room with a hysterical twelve-year-old!' I hear Lexi shriek to Pat in the hallway outside my new bedroom, as I hang my clothes in the empty half of the wardrobe next to Lexi's row of black shrouds. 'She's unbearable! Make her get out of there!'

After some jostling and bargain-striking, in which Lexi barters her Thursday evening booking with the unit masseuse for an older, more even-tempered roommate, Ruby, freshly off supervision too, agrees to share a room with me temporarily. Scowling, Lexi tears into the room without making eye contact, yanking her clothes from the wardrobe and stalking out clutching a messy pile of her possessions, while Ruby calmly takes to folding her T-shirts and jeans into neat little bundles with retail-assistant precision, and stacking them tidily in corners of the chest of drawers. We ignore each other as we work, her turning the labels of her nail polish bottles to face the front of the dressing table as I pin some photos of my cats and a dreamy picture of Daniel Radcliffe to the corkboard over my bed. I reach over to the window to let some air in, but a series of chains tauten stiffly, stopping the window from opening more than a couple of inches. I fiddle with the chains and try to wrench the window forwards with some more force, as the sense of being literally trapped in this building heightens my frustration and panic.

'*Why* are there chains on this thing?' I burst out angrily to the room, smacking my hand against the double-glazed window aggressively, my blood pumping with the incredible injustice of it all, at the unbearable reality of being imprisoned in a building, a room, a body with no way of escape.

'It's so that we don't jump out,' Ruby answers me flatly, as she regards me through her defiant, kohl-rimmed eyes. For a moment, we just look at each other, a kind of mutual understanding passing between us, an acknowledgment of our shared bitter reality, and the fact that, in private moments, both of us had looked down at the concrete from this third-storey window, and wondered would a drop like that kill or just seriously injure. I can't help wondering about the previous residents of this room, and whether their actions had warranted the chains.

For the next few weeks, I remain unpopular and largely ignored. I focus my energies on my letter-writing endeavours and campaign to get back to St Kevin's Hospital, continuing to pummel my parents with rage, blame and suicide threats. Several members of the Blue Kitchen reach their target weight and are discharged, including Rose, who I am both sorry and relieved to see leave. I am ashamed of my behaviour in the face of her unprecedented kindness. I always think of her when I think back to that dreadful first week: how her presence was the only glint of light on the darkest day. I wish I could thank her; it was rare moments of kindness and understanding like that, that sustained me when there were no reasons to be hopeful. (I also wish I could tell her I'm not a secret xenophobe; it was just convenient to invoke my ancestral trauma and blame the English.)

Lexi and Jess, that terrible twosome, graduate finally to the Blue Kitchen, and mealtimes became considerably less fractious and pressurised for me. I put tomatoes firmly at the top of my dislikes list and never have to suffer another. I also put sweet and sour curry down — a flavour combination that still makes me taste bile, and made for another memorably traumatic dinner – and, finally, peanuts. Although each patient is allowed three dislikes on their menu, you can't list notorious fear foods like chocolate, meat or butter. There are so many foods I find unpleasant, but it gets a bit easier once I've familiarised myself with the menu and can brace myself for the most unpalatable meals, which are usually pre-empted by the anxious whispers of the other patients, who keep meticulous mental records of the rotation of weekly dinners. By far the most feared and dreaded meal – spoken of in panicked whispers as girls compare theories and notes for when it is next due on the menu – was McDonald's. Legend has it the McDonald's experience is sprung on the unit at twelve-week intervals, ensuring that everyone on the programme is subjected to it at least once. The idea is that all 'normal teenagers' eat McDonald's routinely as part of a balanced diet, and therefore we ought to learn to embrace it too. But, rather than cure our fear of fast food, the hype and terror surrounding the mythology of the McDonald's meal only exacerbates our profound belief that McDonald's food is the devil incarnate. It is used as a threat and taunt by the nurses, and as a horror story, told in hushed, fearful tones, by the other patients. 'I know a girl whose first *and* last meal was a McDonald's,' someone would hiss as a collective shiver ran round the table.

I'm not sure if the McDonald's meal is purely a dark myth or if it *is* actually skulking around the corner of my programme – somewhere around week ten or eleven, according to the most scrupulous list-makers and seasoned patients of the ward. So, I try to forget about it and to just get through the food that is put in front of me. For the sake of the other girls – who I've begun to empathise with – I try not to have any more histrionic meltdowns as we all choke down the same gelatinous slop. It certainly gets easier with the knowledge that there are no more tomatoes lurking slyly in the folds of tortilla wraps.

There comes a day, somewhere around week three, where I begin to be accepted into the other patients' social circles – and it is all because of stamps.

'What the hell are you doing?' comes a startled cry from the opposite side of the table one day during school hours. I am calmly sticking a stamp on another suicide letter to my mum. Looking up, I see Lara staring at me, a look of wide-eyed wonder and disbelief frozen on her face. I glance down at the letter, confused, wondering what anorexic secret society rule I've broken now, and who was about to yell at me.

'I'm . . . I'm . . . I'm just writing a letter,' I tell her defensively, pressing the stamp firmly into the top right corner of the letter with the edge of my fist.

'No,' she says, breathily, her tone awed and slightly disturbed. 'You *licked* the stamp . . .'

Around the table, the eyes of other girls snap up and fixate on me, identical expressions of shock and amazement rippling across their faces.

'Yeah,' I tell her, nonplussed, looking back at them all quizzically. 'I licked the stamp . . . so?'

'Stamps,' she tells me, sombrely, hesitantly, as though aware she's breaking some truly terrible news to me, 'have five-point-nine calories each.'

For a moment they all look at me, sincere pity and trepidation in their eyes, anticipating another meltdown over the fact that I have unknowingly consumed almost six evil extra calories. Instead, I burst out laughing. I can't help it. It's just so ridiculous. I am having an out-of-body moment. I may have got down with the jigging, the intentional coldness, and I've even joined in the strange habit of hovering awkwardly around the sitting room couches, rather than sitting on them properly as we watch *I'm A Celebrity*, but the stamps . . . the stamps thing is just a step too far.

'D'you . . . d'you really think that you can get fat from licking stamps?' I quiz Lara, still giggling and looking back and forth between the other girls, who evidently don't find this a laughing matter.

'If you lick enough, of them, yes,' says Lara, seriously, regarding me now as though I might be mentally ill. I laugh them off and continue to lick stamps for my letters, and the next day Lexi approaches me, uncharacteristically polite, and asks me to lick the stamp for her letter to her mum. After that, rumour quickly spreads around the ward that I'll lick any stamp put in front of me, and soon there is a line of patients shuffling meekly up to me with their letters and stamps in hand, and I am so flattered and buoyed by the attention that I fulfil every request, happily demonstrating my amazing capacity to not care about the calorie content of stamps.

It didn't take long for the teachers and nurses to deduce what was happening, however, and I was soon banned from being the unit's official stamp-licker – but by then, I'd started to make friends.

Ruby was one of my first friends there. She was creative and excessively neat, and she spent her free time snipping coloured sheets of card into tiny, perfect little squares, stars, petals and hearts to make the most bright, beautiful, perfectly constructed greetings cards that she would send to her family and friends on national holidays, signed with a few cold, impersonal, but neatly penned words. Encouraged by her example, I got out my bead box and would string together little butterflies as she snipped tiny rose petals on the floor of our bedroom at night, while we talked animatedly about our ideal BMIs and fantasised dreamily about our fabulous skinny futures and celebrating our eighteenth birthdays on lavish weight-loss retreats. Ruby taught me how to jig to maximum fat-burning capacity, and she also taught me how to do it completely noiselessly, feet hovering off the floor and abs tightly engaged, so as not to be detected by nurses prowling the corridor outside our bedroom. Though she complied with the programme, gaining the essential kilogram per week and keeping her head down at mealtimes, she maintained her defiant glint and spirit of resistance, and found many ways to defy her parents and the staff without jeopardising her discharge date. She was furious with her parents, who had fully bought in to the Peaceful Pastures way and heartily endorsed its draconian practices, following the guidelines for parents to the letter, and for the most part she endured their weekend visits and biweekly phone calls in stony silence.

She kept up the same impenetrable wall of silence in her weekly therapy sessions as well. Therapy sessions at the Farm could be described as 'an afterthought'. That's really all they were: a box ticked once a week, without any real evaluation, as far as I could see, of whether or not they were working, so they remained, for the most part, ineffectual. Ruby and I had the same therapist, Dr Jon Walsch, a cheerful, bearded man with a relaxed demeanour. He'd lean back in the creaky bamboo armchair in the therapy hut, his legs crossed, his hands casually tucked into his trouser pockets, and smile lazily. He was, in a word, harmless – which, I think you'll agree, considering the scope of descriptions applied to every other medical professional in this book so far, is actually quite a positive endorsement. He let me spend my sessions talking about *Harry Potter*, and chuckled merrily when I said I intended to get a part in one of those films, but he didn't shoot down my dreams. Ruby, on the other hand, had zero time or words to spare on Dr Walsch. She described him as 'a bumbling fool' and spent their hour a week glaring at him in silence.

'You mean you haven't spoken a word to him at all, in any of your sessions?' I asked her one afternoon in wonder, awed by her rebellious nature and unwavering commitment to insubordination.

'Nope,' she affirmed proudly, deftly snipping a yellow daffodil shape for a Mother's Day card, a vengeful grin creeping on to her face. 'I just stare back at him and keep jigging.'

I also befriended Ava, a shy Turkish girl, who was fifteen and had an edgy, artistic style, with paperclips in her ear lobes and a different slogan T-shirt for every day of the week. She was sweet and funny and good company. Since coming to England for treatment, she'd discovered a missing piece of her heart in the shape of the boy band Westlife, and would pore over their album inserts in the evenings, her command of the English language vastly improving thanks to her careful study of their song lyrics.

There was Mona, a tall, incredibly gentle, soft-spoken girl with a kindly demeanour. She was intensely studious, working quietly at all hours towards her dream of being a doctor. She didn't come across like a teenager: more like a sweet old lady accidentally reincarnated in a teenager's body. And she didn't seem to possess the same meanness as many of the other patients – that caustic, spiky streak of cruelty that personifies anorexia – and yet its presence could be glimpsed in the drab grey jumpers and tracksuits under which she hid her body. Her meanness was subtle, secretive, expressed only towards herself, and though she was always so sweet and lovely to everyone, immediately becoming my parents' favourite patient to encounter in the hallways on their weekend visits, I always felt there was something I didn't know about her, something that nobody knew. Another new friend came in the shape of Natalie, an attractive blue-eyed, bottle-blond seventeen-year-old, whose shockingly prominent hip bones seemed to reach towards opposite corners of the room. By the time she was shunted through the doorway of the Farm, Natalie hadn't eaten solid foods in weeks. Her body protested vehemently to the onslaught of eating, which seemed to cause physical as well as emotional turmoil, and she'd sit at the table clutching her belly and groaning in agony.

'I haven't had a poo in five days!' she told me, wild-eyed and bent double in the hallway one day after a giant lunch of mushroom risotto. The nurses were merciless though, not letting her skip a single meal, and instead just started traded her morning orange juice for a sickly-sweet prune juice. Her body eventually adjusted, her joyful whoops sounding from the bathroom during school hours a couple of days later, and she got on with the programme. I enjoyed her hilarious frankness and apparent lack of inhibitions, and she took to me with a sort of maternal fondness, cuddling me to her bony frame and calling me 'cute'.

Lexi and Jess never really forgave me for my hellish antics in the first week, and they maintained a cool distance. Though everyone had a strongly honed inner bitch, Lexi and Jess were definitely the mean girls of the ward, virtually inseparable, always huddled together at the corner table of the classroom, their angry eyes darting about the room at everyone, possibly plotting a murder. They tended to attract the darker souls to their little bubble, too; Lauren, a tomboy with tightly braided curly red hair and mistrustful eyes, who loved running, and who routinely made bids for freedom, waiting in the shadows of the hall for an opportunity to bolt out the door anytime a visitor passed through it; and Adam, the tiny ten-year-old with the spiky brown hair and baggy Nirvana jumper, whose knowledge of unspeakable sexual acts surpassed his age and level of maturity in quite a sinister manner. He delighted in filling in my very patchy sex education with graphic descriptions of some of the most bizarre sex acts, things I remained convinced he had been lying about until much later misadventures. There was also Tess, who didn't really fit anywhere, but was a cheerful and unmissable presence at the Farm. Tess was an anomaly at the Farm at that time, due to the fact that her struggle was with obesity rather than anorexia. She was also an anomaly because she seemed to enjoy life at the Farm, being regularly readmitted to the clinic for gaining too much weight at home and never seeming even slightly disgruntled to be back. She enjoyed terrorising the anorexic patients with her extra pounds. She was a fairly average weight when she came back to the Farm during my stay, but she had large folds of loose skin from her weight-loss that she would untuck from her waistband in moments of mischief and wobble around, dancing in front of the TV screen crying: 'Mah belly is a bowlful of jellyyyy!!'

'Disgustaaanggggggg,' Lexi would screech, jumping up from the couch and bolting out into the hallway as Tess pursued her, wobbly bits rippling.

'Put your belly away, Tess,' Jen would call from the kitchen. 'Stop frightening the other children!'

There wasn't a whole lot to do at the Farm in the evenings, particularly in the early part of my stay when my activity was extremely restricted and I couldn't take part in the dance, aerobics or yoga sessions that took place in the classroom. There were board games. There was MTV. There was a Playstation2 EyeToy, until the nurses realised how much physical exertion we put into the window-cleaning game, and that too was sanctioned. But the most prevalent pastime (for it could hardly be called a 'hobby') and one over which we all bonded, was flicking through *Heat*, *Closer* and *OK!* magazines to compare and contrast the body-fat percentage of different celebrities. Anorexia was *fashionable* in 2004. It was the era of Lindsay Lohan and Nicole Richie stumbling out of clubs in sequinned sheath dresses that proudly showcased their fleshless chests and ribcages. They were photographed twenty-four-seven, their rapidly diminishing frames chronicled in vivid detail across every gossip magazine cover. *Big Brother* stars who dared put on bikinis were openly mocked and ridiculed for the barest hint of cellulite, while Nicole and Lindsay's figures were 'causing concern' among loved ones. There were no such terms as body-shaming or body positivity in the early nough-ties, and 'mental health' was only mentioned in the same breath as the clinically insane. The magazines we consumed all continued to reinforce the beliefs we already subscribed to: that fat – all of it, any of it – was a shameful, embarrassing thing, whereas extreme thinness got you attention. Together, we fanned the flames of each other's most viciously cruel anorexic thoughts, pointing out 'problem areas' on various supermodels that we all agreed they needed to surgically alter. I learned, through listening to the older girls, who always had the most scathingly creative remarks, that the female body, in all its full-breasted, wide-hipped, soft-bellied glory, was a fate to be dreaded, feared, resisted: that 'normal women' was code for 'weak', and that surrendering to the natural pull of puberty was an outright tragedy.

'Eugh,' Natalie says, pointing with a long-taloned, bony finger to a picture of a beaming bikini-clad reality star with an ample chest.

Natalie, Ava, Ruby and I are sitting at the picnic table in the back garden, the newest editions of all our favourite gossip magazines splayed across the surface of the table. It's our idea of porn.

'Look how big her boobs have got,' Natalie says, wrinkling her nose with distaste.

'Gross,' nods Ruby.

'Fat,' affirms Ava.

I lean over to examine the busty, beaming woman and her offensively large chest. 'But boobs aren't made of fat, are they?' I ask innocently, scanning my twelve-year-old brain for the sparse details I'd collected on the fully blossomed female form. Surely, boobs were made of something functional, innocuous: surely it was something less incriminating than just *fat*. 'They're . . . something else, aren't they?'

Natalie shoots me a penetrating look. 'Boobs are just bags of pure fat hanging off your chest,' she tells me. 'Disgusting,' she adds, lovingly caressing the xylophone shape of her own bony chest.

Disgusting, I think, my thoughts echoing Natalie. I quickly file this information away for a later date. I feel a rush of love towards her, my strong older sister in anorexia, her cheeks hollowing as she sucks on a cigarette and glowers down at yet another picture of Nicole Richie's sizeable thigh gap.

It was strange to be a wide-eyed twelve-year-old amid all this toxic analysis of the female form; I felt relieved to be at the tidier end of the treacherous passage of puberty, watching from afar as the older girls struggled to flatten and deny their newly restored curves, undeniably feminine shapes, but my relief was always underscored by a dulled note of dread, and their reactions to their bodies reinforced my suspicions that womanhood was a grim and pitiable existence. (To be clear, anorexia is not solely a crusade on the female body. It's a crusade on all fat – plain, simple, genderless fat – but because the female body generally has a higher percentage of body fat – wider hips, meatier thighs, fat deposits in all sorts of unbecoming places – a womanly body was a particular object of fear and loathing among the Peaceful Pastures inhabitants.)

One aspect of the mature female body that all the girls anticipated longingly, however, was menstruation. This was not out of any well-adjusted desire for restored bodily health or a sign of anorexia retreating in favour of a fecund, flourishing body. It was purely because menstruation was the single, solitary reason a patient's target weight would be dropped at Peaceful Pastures. Target weight was calculated according to two methods only. Either, as I explained before, at ninety-five per cent of the national average weight of other people of your height and age – *or* the precise weight at which a patient got their period. The period was seen as a clear sign of restored health and an affirmation of a fully functioning body, and could be responsible for shaving several glorious kilograms off the original target weight.

'Yes, yes, YES!!!' a euphoric cry sounds from the bathroom one afternoon during school time. A moment later, Nina, a glossy-haired brunette who still has several weeks to go at the Farm, charges into the corridor, her face shiny with beatific joy. 'I got my period!' she exclaims, prancing towards the Brown Kitchen and hollering for a nurse.

Nigel, the headteacher, clears his throat and furrows his brow as he studies a chart in front of him with greater intent, and the boys in the classroom shift uncomfortably in their seats. The girls, meanwhile, exchange envious scowls and fume silently. For the rest of the afternoon, Nina is put on TSV to ensure she is telling the truth about her period and not simply trying to trick the Farm into dropping her target. She is given a sanitary towel with her initials carefully penned on the underside in permanent marker, because patients have been known to smuggle in previously soiled sanitary towels and try to pass them off as their own. (Yes, reader, just when you think you can't be any more shocked by the lengths anorexia will go to avoid weight gain – *soiled sanitary towels*.) Nina had to provide solid proof of the veracity of her claim as verified by a staff member's naked gaze. By evening, she had backed up her claim and was happily bragging to her friends in the lounge that her target weight had been docked a solid three kilograms.

Most girls did not get their periods back before they reached their target weight. For many of them, it had been years since they'd had a period, and even at target there was no guarantee of a restored regular menstrual cycle, their malnourished bodies refusing to instantaneously snap back into perfect health and fertility. So, most patients were doomed to meet their original target. It was a secret – though commonly held – belief that most people didn't look all that good at target. People tended to look healthy and attractive about a month before reaching their target weight, but after that, the word often used to describe their appearance was . . . puffy. Even the nurses acknowledged it, and reassured girls who were fretting about the notable puffiness around the cheeks and belly that their weight would, a few weeks after discharge, 'redistribute'. The claim was that the unprecedentedly sudden weight gain caused the fat to centre itself around the midsection, and that eventually the body would realise it didn't need to doggedly hold on to these new reserves of fat and could redistribute it elsewhere. Some people did carry off their target weight better than others, the fat settling in more aesthetically pleasing areas, and the common refrain towards anxious girls struggling through the last two weeks of maintaining their target weight was: 'You look so good at target.' But it was something everyone said to each other, regardless of their level of puffiness, a refrain we all knew was hollow and fake, given the viciously spiteful assessments we'd all shared about the barely discernible weight gain of the thinnest celebrities. So, getting one's period and being spared the final few kilograms of weight gain was a joyous occasion, and one the other girls dreamed and prayed for in the final weeks of their stay.

As for me, due to my age, the menstruation factor was pretty much off the table, and I was always fated to meet my original target. But the frenzy and obsession around menstruation wormed its way into my mind, and, watching the older girls, I began to regard menstruation as a symptom of a battle lost, a weak submission to being that most dreaded creature – a normal woman. Despite its association with a reduced target weight at the Farm, I saw it, as it is so often referred to, as a curse. There was no doubt that there was something final about menstruation, a sense of being irredeemably flawed, irrevocably ruined. And though I, too, was putting on weight and creeping towards a healthier body, my anorexic ego was somewhat placated and satisfied by the idea that, as long as I didn't get my period, I would be spared the regrettable fate of being a fully grown, undisputedly normal woman. I was aware that if a woman didn't get her period by the age of eighteen, it was likely she never would, and though she would grow up and older, she'd be spared that final awful initiation into womanhood from which there was no coming back.

'What ages did my sisters get their periods?' I demanded of my mum over the phone one evening.

'Ehhhmmm, maybe around thirteen or fourteen?' she answered me, evidently pleased that for once I didn't want to converse about the process of making a will. I exhaled anxiously, realising that this impending doom was closer than previously anticipated. Privately, I vowed to get out of this place as quickly as possible, to hold fiercely to innocuous girlhood, to never ever surrender to the wicked tragedy of being a normal woman.

The notion of being 'healthy' was a commonly held fear among all the residents on the Farm. To us, words such as 'healthy', 'normal', 'better' were absolutely synonymous with 'fat'. We lit up over words like 'thin', 'shocking', 'sickly' and 'emaciated' – even 'deathly' made us glow with pride.

'I can't stand when people tell me I'm looking "well",' Natalie moaned one evening, gripping her head in her hands as other girls in the circle nodded frantically. I was reminded with a twinge of guilt of my rosy-cheeked, well-intentioned dad at the weekend, clapping Natalie heartily on the back and telling her how well she looked as she responded with a weak smile.

'You have to stop telling everyone they look well, Dad,' I chided him over the phone several days later. 'You're causing a secret exercise epidemic.'

By now, relations with my parents were slightly less volatile. The suicide letters had abated and our phone conversations and their visits to the ward on the weekends, though initially quite harrowing, soon passed in relative calm. They struggled to afford the trips to London, but with the generosity of Sister Paula and the nuns in the form of free accommodation so close to the clinic, one or both parents managed to fly over every weekend of my stay to see me for a few hours. I could see that they were trying their hardest and were struggling with the circumstances themselves, and I'd accepted that they were not the main culprits responsible for locking me up, that the Irish Health Board had terrorised them into submission, and so I'd decided to go above their heads and take matters into my own hands. I wrote Dr Nolan and the Irish Health Board several letters outlining my struggle, my homesickness, my social isolation, and giving them a detailed report of my weight-gain progress so far as proof of my willingness to cooperate with the hospital programme. A week went by, and the letters got progressively more desperate and threatening, insisting to Dr Nolan that my parents' marriage was on the rocks, that my siblings were bereft without me, that my friends at school had entirely forgotten my name, that it was very urgent that I got home and salved all these rifts created by my absence. *Do you really want to be responsible for breaking up a good Catholic couple's marriage, Dr Nolan. Do you?* News reached me that one of my beloved cats had been found dead on the road and I was convinced it was because he'd felt abandoned by me, and driven mad by grief, had deliberately wandered into the path of a speeding car. Dr Nolan got a particularly furious missive after that. But Fergal, my old pal, he ghosted every single letter.

It took another couple weeks of tireless scheming, letter-writing, guilt-tripping and begging, however, for me to finally give up my campaign to win back my freedom and fully surrender to the Farm. This came, about six weeks into my stay, in the shape of a new admission named Hazel. It was always traumatic when a new patient showed up. Inside, when we really paused to think about it, we were all screaming, all day, every day, but now and then the Farm grew quiet and we numbed our pain with MTV and origami, distracting ourselves from the panic alarms sounding within by keeping our hands and minds busy. But every time a new patient showed up in the hallway, bone-thin and shivering, it was like somebody had smashed through glass with their bare fist to sound the alarm again, and a collective cacophony of pain surged through us all, a reminder that everything was terrible and unjust, the pale new waif in the hall showing us who we'd been mere moments ago, and how far we'd all strayed from the feeling of safety since. Hazel was an especially bad case, and so the mutual stress we all felt was at fever pitch. She was severely anorexic of course, her teeny, sparrow-like ankles, just visible below three-quarter-length trousers, seeming to defy the rules of physics in the way they managed to keep her upright. She might have been pretty, except for the fact that when you looked at her face, you couldn't help but notice how easy it was to picture what her skull would look like without skin and eyeballs. She really was skeletal when she arrived, and we all seethed with jealousy from the downstairs lounge.

Hazel isn't just anorexic, though; she has a fancy, add-on problem in the shape of Obsessive Compulsive Disorder (OCD). The skin on her gaunt hands is broken and red-raw from the hundreds of times she insists on washing them each day. Doorknobs send palpable shivers of fear through her body, and she has a habit of circling the lounge and nudging household objects with her long sleeves into neat lines, burning extra calories *and* fixing everything at right angles to each other in one go: two birds, one scone! Her first meal is a particularly lengthy affair for all of us. She arrives just in time for a lunch of cucumber and cream cheese sandwiches, the fatty combination of thickly buttered carbs filled with a cucumber-specked lumpy white cheese concoction making any resident of the Farm, Blue Kitchen or Brown, queasy – and posing a veritable Everest for an unsuspecting new admission. Hazel has a creative new way of trying to skank food. She mushes the cheese of her sandwich into the grooves of her fingerprints and under her nails, and then rubs her fingers on the underside of her hair. Apparently, when push comes to shove, the voice of her anorexia screams louder than that of her OCD. This behaviour does not go unnoticed by the nurses, however, and quickly earns her another quarter of a cheese sandwich, freshly and liberally buttered, just for her.

Swallowing down my own foul cucumber-cheese sandwich with a grimace, I look over at this poor creature sitting across the table, her raw chafed fingers smothered in cottage cheese as dollops of the stuff hang from tendrils of hair, drool and tears pouring down her face as she tries to wail and chew at the same time, her mind screaming at her to spit the food out, while the nurses yell at her to put it back in. *No one is coming to take away your pain*, I think, staring at her forlornly. *This is the place where we do nothing but sit and eat and feel pain*. One thing is abundantly clear to me, as I look at Hazel's wailing mouth, blobs of cheese and spittle dropping back on to her plate, her face a portrait of agony: none of us is getting out of this place skinny.

I become quiet after Hazel's arrival. I am no longer the disruptive one at dinner. I'm not the one drowning and wailing anymore, and I don't want to go back to that place. There is no escape from this hell. The only way out is through. So, each meal, I keep my head down and stuff the food in. They've finally broken my spirit. I've officially given up. But another significant schism has occurred here, one that nobody notices. A schism between my mind and my body. It is too painful to sit there in my body and feel it, to acknowledge her expanding and changing without my consent. She is not mine anymore. She is not someone to be trusted. She is repulsive and only getting bigger. There is everything wrong with her. But I can't fix her anymore. Someone else has taken her over. So, I find somewhere else to hide out. I retreat to the safety of my mind. I become cerebral, reading and writing and reading. I focus on the things around me, anything outside of myself. Like all the more seasoned patients here, I cover her up. She is no longer a part of me that I will acknowledge. I cover her in long cardigans and shapeless dresses that fall to the knees, and try to get on with my life as if she isn't there.

As if I don't live inside her.

As if I could ever get away.

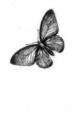

7

'I won't, I won't, I WOOOOOONNNN'T!' Hannah, the newest admission to the Farm, howls to the Brown Kitchen, spraying the table in front of her with clumps of broccoli-and-cheese quiche.

There is a new queen of histrionic meltdowns at Peaceful Pastures, her loud, banshee-like wails echoing through the hallways at all hours of the day. My previous theatrics are quickly forgotten, rapidly erased from everyone's minds by an incessant stream of ear-splitting shrieks as we are all united in contempt for this unwelcome devil-spawn.

It was never really established what was the matter with Hannah, and though it was not for any of her peers to diagnose her condition, it was widely agreed among the other patients that she routinely refused food more out of a stubborn campaign for attention than out of a desperate and secretive compulsion to seize control over her body. Hannah just didn't foster the same idolatry of thinness as the rest of us, and neither did she have the sharp-eyed, coldly calculating discernment of her surroundings of someone with anorexia, looking for means of escape or soft-hearted souls to manipulate. She was never secretive or devious in her conduct at the Farm, and instead wanted all eyes on her at all times, her mouth a gaping, crater-like hole, exposing her tonsils as she wailed her way through every meal-time and screamed, over and over, the one word that we all came to associate entirely with her.

'Won't, won't, WOOOOON'T!!'

Hannah was the first patient I saw being 'tubed'. A casually and frequently wielded threat, the nasogastric tube was actually quite a rarity at the Farm, so terrorised was everyone by the thought of higher calories, prolonged TSV and a thin rubber tube being stuffed up your nose and then threaded all the way down to your stomach. The tube was also not seen as a healthy method of refeeding by the clinic, the idea being that in order to recover and lead normal lives, every patient would have to learn to eat solid foods of their own volition. Having a nurse tail you in order to squeeze fatty liquids into a tube dangling from one of your nostrils at the dinner table is actually very antisocial. Most patients ate the food, despite the difficulty, tears and trauma this involved. Anyone really struggling to consume the meal was given an enormous milkshake with equivalent calories to the meal, and while these were a more common occurrence, we all generally endeavoured to avoid them, because while the calories were matched to the meals, the milkshakes actually contained a higher fat content than the solid foods. It was only after a patient bluntly refused, through tightly pressed lips, to take a sip of milkshake, that the Brown Kitchen was cleared, extra nurses were summoned, and a thin rubber tube was passed through the nostril and taped to the face, at which point a mysterious, creamy liquid concoction was squirted up into the tube and down into the stomach of the loudly protesting patient. Word on the ward was that the liquid was composed of a stomach-churning blend of all the most dreaded fear foods imaginable – mayonnaise, cream, butter and Mars bars. I'm grateful to report that I never had to find out the veracity to these claims, but the horror of the legend alone was enough to keep most of us firmly on the straight-and-narrow terrain of dutifully ingesting solid foods.

And if the threat of the grisly mixture being syringed into the pit of your stomach wasn't enough to put any lingering curiosity about the tube as an alternative to eating to rest, then seeing its effect on Hannah certainly did. It did not do her any aesthetic favours, her belly becoming hugely distended within a matter of days, while her little limbs remained pin-thin. Her cheeks puffed out like those of a guinea pig, her eyes were always bloodshot and watery, and her nostrils quickly became red and inflamed from the number of times the tube was passed in and out of them (the nurses didn't initially leave the tube in in between mealtimes, the idea being that they didn't want to take it for granted that she wouldn't eat her meals and could rely entirely on a nurse painstakingly squirting every calorie up her nose). Sometimes, Hannah coughed and gagged so violently that she actually succeeded in regurgitating the tube, a slimy trail of drool and an unpleasant milky white substance oozing from her moistened lips down the front of her pink velour cardigan. Oh, Hannah did not go gentle into the night, screeching her dissent at all hours, and we all skirted, with knowing looks to one another, away from the rooms she inhabited, her cries penetrating the calm of even the most dull, unflappable teachers. But her abrupt arrival had an upside too, and in addition to the fact that I had officially been dethroned as the unit's most unpopular resident, her unruly antics in the Brown Kitchen stood in sharp contrast to my newly quiet, acquiescent comportment and after a few weeks of enduring

Hannah's disastrous table manners, I caught the attention of the nurses for the right reasons.

'Evanna,' Jen called one evening after dinner, amid the scramble to deposit our plates and cups in the dishwasher.

Instantly riled and ready to defend myself, I turned the insides of my jeans pockets outwards to show her I hadn't squirrelled away any of my crinkle-cut chips, but she cut me off as I opened my mouth to proclaim my indignation.

'No, no, I know you ate all your dinner. What I wanted to say was I think you're ready to move to the Blue Kitchen.'

Finally submitting to the regime at Peaceful Pastures had felt awful, soul-crushing, but it is true to say that life at the Farm became progressively easier the moment I gave up. So while it had robbed me of my remaining shreds of dignity and self-respect, there was a certain measure of relief and calm that came with complying obediently with the programme, and I placated the voice of anorexia that roared ferociously in the background about what a pathetic, fat failure I was by reasoning with it that I had no other way to get out than gaining weight, and privately vowing to it to lose that weight as soon as I was free. It wasn't that gaining weight and having to eat so many calories became an easy daily routine, but it did eventually become, let's say, less torturous. My target weight still loomed horribly in the distance, looking surreal and impossible, but I knew that it meant freedom at last, so begrudgingly, I accepted I would have to reach it. I committed to reaching the minimum one kilogram weight-gain target each week and tried, above all things, to avoid ever catching a glimpse of my body in the mirror.

It helped to be surrounded by other young people whose spirits had been similarly flattened, and whose bodies were not their own.

The Blue Kitchen was populated by other patients whose anorexia had also been beaten into submission, who'd reached that precise point in the programme where they'd given up, and whose eyes were now trained intently on their target weight and ensuing freedom. We were trusted to butter our own muffins and weigh our own muesli at breakfast, and to eat every crumb of each meal without staff members present. There, we bitched about the staff, held serious scholarly discussions about the fat content of different types of nuts, made gagging noises at the tuna pasta bake and prodded the gelatinous slabs of cheesecake with expressions of sincere distaste – all things we would have been sharply reprimanded for in the Brown Kitchen – but still, we ate every crumb. Occasionally someone would slip back, skanking cheese sauce on the inside of their sleeves or shaking the muesli out so there were fewer nut and chocolate chunks, but they would soon be ratted out to the nurses by the other residents of the Blue Kitchen, and nobody had any qualms about doing this. It was too triggering to be around someone who was wilfully trying to subvert the programme and trick the scales – it made you feel terribly guilty for not attempting to lose weight too, and it therefore jeopardised everyone's discharge date – so that person was promptly reported, given a warning and, if they didn't correct their behaviour, demoted to the Brown Kitchen. We still did secret deals with each other – I often traded Lara one-quarter of a cheese sandwich for her blackberry yoghurt at teatime, because cheese freaked me out and Lara was just thrilled by the fact that the sandwich had fewer calories than the yoghurt – but this was done out of camaraderie and a collective effort to get through these trenches together. The freshly emaciated, sobbing teens continued to arrive at fortnightly intervals in the dark hallway, but we in the Blue Kitchen didn't prowl around to study their sharply jutting collar bones, and we didn't dwell on them, because we knew they were doomed too, and it was all ahead of them. None of us envied them the routine bullying, supervised showers and rude awakening.

By now, I'd made several friends on the unit. Tight-knit friendships developed quickly between patients at the Farm, bonded as we were by the uniquely horrible regime we were all living under, and by the isolation we felt from our friends and family back home. I found a sense of belonging and closeness with my fellow inmates that I hadn't had with my friends at school, especially since the eating disorder started. However, I was considerably younger than the majority of the patients there, and there was a gulf between the pre-teens and the older teens that often left me feeling lonely. In general, the older patients tended to have more weight to gain, their stays correspondingly longer, a fact they inevitably all bonded tightly over; it was just harder to empathise with a twelve-week patient when your sentence was twice that. They also tended to be more severely anorexic, because most of them had been battling it longer than the nine-, ten- and eleven-year-olds before they'd been forced into treatment, and this too created more of a distance. The older girls would gather in little circles around the classroom floor in the evenings, as they waited for the yoga instructor to arrive, whispering sombrely with darkened expressions, that would brighten, the conversation abruptly truncated, the moment I entered the room and attached myself to their circle. There was another aspect of age that caused an invisible division. All of us gazed longingly at the mythical wonderful eventuality of being eighteen and having the freedom to discharge yourself and cultivate your anorexia freely: but at twelve years old, eighteen seemed like a virtual fantasy, and the prospect

THE OPPOSITE OF BUTTERFLY HUNTING

of spending six whole years fighting the system and yo-yoing in and out of clinics while your friends in the outside world grew up, got jobs and boyfriends, was unappealing. The prospect of trying to hide your anorexia and deftly dodge treatment for six years ultimately felt like a futile and exhausting mission in comparison to those sixteen-year-olds who only needed to toe the line for a year and a bit before they could turn around and tell Peaceful Pastures, their parents and the authorities to SUCK IT. The older girls also had more pressing health issues to worry about, infertility and osteoporosis posing increasingly more urgent threats, and though they were proud of the lengths to which they had taken their anorexia, secretly gratified by the long-lasting physical damage – distinct evidential markers of the years of self-abuse they'd devoted to thinness – I saw genuine sadness in their eyes when a younger patient was discharged.

'You'll be fine,' they'd say, hugging their friend tight, a faraway expression of mingled bitterness and sorrow playing on their faces. 'You have your whole life ahead of you.'

It was for all these reasons that it was a relief to see another younger girl, a doe-eyed eleven-year-old named Grace, join the Farm, and she and I soon latched on to each other. She was tiny and fragile, of course, but she didn't look like a haunted skeleton. We were somewhat evenly matched in our anorexia, and weren't inclined to corrupt one another further in the way Peaceful Pastures friends often did. On Grace's arrival, Ruby, who was a good friend by now, moved in with Hazel, who was closer to her age, and Grace became my new roommate.

As far as friends not corrupting one other further with their ano-rexic outlook on life, I can't say the same was true for Ruby and Hazel. Hazel had settled in somewhat after a couple weeks; she'd been taken off supervision, had ceased her mealtime meltdowns with the arrival of the new scream queen, Hannah, and her hands were slowly healing as the nurses closely monitored her trips to the bathroom sink and slathered her cuts in ointment. She soon made friends, and after the whining and weeping phase had abated, revealed herself as a force to be reckoned with: a fiery, opinionated girl with a sharp tongue and a sarcastic sense of humour. She and Ruby bonded very quickly, and soon the two of them were sitting side by side on the couches in the lounge like twin Siamese cats, jigging in perfect unison. But finding friends did not mitigate the fact that Hazel was finding life extremely difficult at the Farm, and was furiously resisting the notion of recovery. Ruby was also struggling, her calculating, cool-tempered facade forming cracks as her body was wrested further from her control with each passing week. Dr Walsch was growing irritable with her stubborn silent resistance and obvious lack of respect for him, and now her whole family was being summoned each week to the therapy hut to speak for her and to try and goad her into an outburst. The two girls were both struggling, their discharge dates nowhere in sight, and they could often be glimpsed huddled together after mealtimes in the corner of the classroom or the lounges, identical serious expressions fixed on their faces as they murmured back and forth to each other in an undertone that was drowned out by the din of the TV or the dance class happening in the background. It was very unlike the two of them to miss an evening dance class. That really should have given everyone a clue.

'They've done it!' an excited whisper sounds from the classroom as I wander down the hallway one Saturday afternoon, feeling dispirited and glum after a visit from my parents in which they had revealed that I won't be allowed to fly home for a day to attend my Confirmation with the rest of my class. 'They've got out!'

'No way!' answers Lara. 'How d'you know?'

I hang by the doorway of the classroom. Lara, Ava and Lauren are clustered together by the window with Natalie, watching her with rapt attentiveness.

'Saw them leave!' says Natalie, excitedly, a light in her eyes I haven't seen before. 'They've been gone ten minutes!'

'Who's gone?' I call obliviously from the doorway, stunned by this news.

'Shhhhhhhhh!' The four girls turn and shush me urgently, Ava beckoning for me to join the huddle, so I pad lightly over to them and hunch into the circle.

'Ruby and Hazel escaped a few minutes ago,' Natalie explains to me, grinning broadly and dropping her voice further. 'When the nurses were busy tubing Hannah and the back door was unlocked for your parents. They'd hidden their shoes down the couches a few days ago rather than lock them up in the cupboard after their lunchtime walk. They've been planning this for weeks. They finally did it!'

'You're kidding!' I exclaim, in breathless awe, scanning the eyes of the other girls in the circle. They nod proudly.

'Yes – but you can't say anything to the nurses,' Lara adds quickly, giving me a meaningful look. 'We have to keep quiet to give them a good head start. Apparently they're headed for Brighton.'

It is undoubtedly the most exciting day in all my time at the Farm. News spreads quickly about the escaped convicts via a web of whispers to all the other patients, but nobody breathes a word to staff, and we all keep up a careful show of normality, quietly resuming our activities, but exchanging looks of gleeful knowing as we pass each other wordlessly in the hallways. Nobody resents the girls their transgressions, despite the fact that we would all like to break out and be whisked away from our troubles by a train to Brighton. This is different to sleight of hand in the Blue Kitchen or secret exercise parties at night, which just makes everyone else feel threatened and triggered, because this escape is not about anorexia slithering its way through the slightest opening at any given opportunity. It is about our collective freedom, it is all of us versus the oppressive system we are trapped in. These girls breaking free is like a piercing beam of light cutting through the heavy fog of inertia and despair that pervades at Peaceful Pastures, and it reminds us that one day, we can be free too. Our spirits have been crushed by a series of quietly devastating daily defeats, but now Hazel and Ruby's escape has reignited a small flame in all our hearts, and we are happy for them, proud of them, inspired by them.

By dinner, their absence has been discovered, the nurses tearing anxiously through each room and shouting commands at one another. Each of us feigns wide-eyed disbelief and ignorance, claiming not to have noticed them leave, and denying having overheard any whispers about where they were going. I don't think the nurses believe us, but they are so stricken with fear and panic at the idea of two of their charges – skinny, malnourished, teenage girls without their coats – wandering unsupervised around this vast city that they don't waste much time grilling us. Hazel and Ruby's parents and the authorities are informed, and the police start searching for the duo at once – but even this dramatic turn of events doesn't stop mealtimes from forging ahead as usual at the Farm. The nurses make their thirst for vengeance clear in the massive helpings of creamy carbonara they dole out for dinner, but nothing can dampen our spirits this evening. The mood in the Blue Kitchen is electric, hopeful, euphoric. It feels like a major triumph for all of us, as we cheerfully discuss potential hiding spots in the city, wonder how many calories running away from home burns, and place bets on how long they can evade capture. Lexi and Lara, the two longest-running residents of the Farm, warn that running away is usually not worth the ensuing penalties, and that it is likely, whenever they are found and returned to the Farm, that they will pay for their misdemeanours with a dizzying 4,000-calorie diet. But it doesn't matter that they will be found and punished and made to gain the same amount of weight as before. What matters is that they got out! They've given the middle finger to our parents, the nurses, the doctors – The Man! – everyone who has casually blocked out our cries for help. They've reminded them that we have our own ideas, that we are individuals, that though we might be their children, we are not *theirs*. Ruby and Hazel have broken free, shaken our parents' trust in this institution and reminded the people in power that these are our bodies, our lives.

By morning, the girls still haven't been found, and the nurses are edgy and tense, their tempers snapping easily at members of the Brown Kitchen or a foot absent-mindedly jigging as we watch TV. We are quiet and subdued in the afternoon, the previous day's high-spirited elation slightly wearing off by now as the staff grow more stressed, fielding calls from the girls' terrified parents every hour.

In total, the girls are gone for thirty-six hours before they are discovered by the police in Trafalgar Square. They are shunted back through the side door at Peaceful Pastures sometime in the early hours of Monday morning. They are greeted by two tall, thick milkshakes and then sent straight to bed. By breakfast, the words '4,000 CAL' have been written in stark, angry black letters next to Ruby and Hazel's names on the whiteboard in the Brown Kitchen that records everyone's daily calorie count. Those of us in the Blue Kitchen can hardly believe that even the nurses are capable of such cruelty, 4,000 calories seeming an obscene amount for any human, let alone two scrawny teenagers, and we peek our heads around the door frame to see that the legend is indeed true. They only stay on 4,000 for two days however, and it feels like it is being done not solely to make up for any meals missed, but more as a punishment to the girls, a blow delivered for their impudence via a steady stream of full-fat cream shakes and king-size Mars bars – and also as a cautionary tale to anyone else secretly contemplating a short jaunt to Brighton. They are also immediately put on TSV and stripped of all the privileges their previous good behaviour had earned them. Oh, they pay mightily for their sins, but they do not appear to regret their actions one bit, and instead seem to regard the whole operation as a resounding success.

They have returned from their short sojourn looking physically exhausted, with wan complexions and dark circles under their eyes, but they seem distinctly spiritually reinvigorated, and thoroughly pleased with themselves. They aren't given much opportunity to recount their wild adventures in vivid detail, so heavily supervised are they, but in the classroom they whisper an enthralling account across the desks of how they'd journeyed to Brighton, walked all over the city, miles and miles and miles, eating absolutely nothing, before making their way back to London, where they walked more and took beaming photos of one another in front of the London Eye with a disposable camera. They tell us how they had eventually got tired when they found themselves in Trafalgar Square, settling themselves at the base of the lion statues for a brief nap before they were rudely shaken awake by police officers and driven straight back to the Farm.

'Oh, and look, we got you all gifts,' Ruby says brightly, as she and Hazel reach into the pockets of their hoodies, pulling out handfuls of thick wands of red-and-white rock candy wrapped in plastic. 'The nurses said we could keep them because nobody here will eat them . . . But look, we brought them all the way from Brighton for you!'

We all laugh a lot at the irony of anorexics gifting each other sticks of pure calories, but we accept these offerings happily, passing them around and scrutinising the nutritional content on the labels for the hell of it, admiring our gifts, these symbols of defiance.

After a few days, the excitement faded and life at the Farm returned to its usual rhythm of slowly drawn-out pain, but we weren't the same as before. That determined gleam in Ruby's eyes sparkled much brighter now and had an infectious quality to it. The temerity and daring of the girls had inspired us, had been like a balm to our broken spirits, had reminded us that a fire still burned within us that the nurses couldn't touch. Even now, seventeen years on, whenever I walk past the lion statues in Trafalgar Square, I smile and think of those two skinny teenagers and their lion hearts.

This spirit of rebellion spread quickly throughout the clinic after the breakout, and it was hard for the nurses to quash. Our urge for subversion had been reawakened with the realisation that, though we could not escape these four walls or the authority the staff held over us, we were still free in our own minds. We found ways to remind them of this, to express our dissent and refusal to be dominated. Soon after the breakout, this resistance took shape as a self-harming pandemic. Self-harming had seemed off the table since day one of the programme when the staff searched our luggage and confiscated all pointy objects. There were a few serious cutters on the ward, who bore thick scars all the way up their forearms, but after a few weeks of strict supervision and monitoring by the nurses, their cuts would close, their skin forming an ugly mess of three-dimensional, inflamed ridges, but finally allowed to heal. As for the rest of us, most of us had dabbled in cutting throughout our eating disorders, and it didn't take long for anyone at the Farm to viscerally understand the keen urge to feel a searing pain slice your skin, the perverse satisfaction of seeing beads of your own bright red blood bloom to the surface, the relief of delivering a punishment your body justly deserved and that might for a few moments distract from the insufferable inner torment. But razor blades, nail scissors and craft knives were forbidden, only used under strict supervision by staff or teachers, and anyone caught trying to cut themselves would be put on TSV immediately, so for the most part, self-harming wasn't a thing at the Farm.

That is, until one day shortly after Ruby and Hazel's great escape, when Ava brought self-harming back. Ava was having a hard time at the Farm, deeply submerged in her own self-hate and finding the reality of her body gaining weight utterly intolerable. She saw her family much less frequently than everyone else, given the price of flights from Turkey, and when she wasn't dancing around the lounge joyfully yelling out the lyrics to 'Uptown Girl', she was crying quietly in a corner and refusing to be comforted. One week, her parents cancelled a trip to see her, on the advice of the Farm, after she had somehow managed to lose weight, and that's when she arrived to breakfast the next morning with an angry red patch of cuts stretching from knuckles to wrist on her left hand. Cutting the back of her hand rather than somewhere discreet, like the inside of her upper arm or thigh, meant that the wound was more than just an expression of pain: it was a message of insubordination. It was a message the nurses promptly noticed and punished her for, demoting her to the Brown Kitchen mere days after she'd left it, and putting her on supervision. But somehow, the cutting continued, freshly hewn bloodied scratches showing up every day on the back of her hand, and none of the staff could work out how she was doing it. And now other patients began flaunting angry red incisions in similarly prominent placements along their wrists and forearms, and the Brown Kitchen was quickly becoming overcrowded, the insubordination harder to contain. It turned out that Ava had learned how to cut herself with the small, colourful paper clips she wore as earrings, and she'd passed this skill, along with a couple of stray paperclips, on to her peers. Soon, she had inspired a self-harming revolution.

The trend took off quickly, and it was easy to see why it was enticing. It raised the alarm to our parents, damaging their trust in Peaceful Pastures further. Their children were locked up in a shadowy house in World's End and tearing up their own skin. The spirit of resistance was strong with everyone writing 'fuck you' to the system in their own blood. Those cuts did come from a place of real pain, but it was obvious at the same time that the girls were deriving pleasure from seeing the nurses scramble, from witnessing the chaos they were causing, and they continued to exchange trade secrets on how to create sharp incisions that would draw the most blood. Even after the nurses had twigged about the paperclips and confiscated those, the girls continued, using innocuous objects like thin rulers or broken zips. You had to really hate yourself to draw blood with a broken zip, but some girls managed it. I was tempted by the self-harming craze, and expressed my interest to Ava in a hushed undertone one evening. I was duly slipped a small green paperclip, because it was understood that that kind of pain needed an outlet. I held on to the paperclip, keeping it neatly tucked into the small flat pocket of a pair of jeans that I was rapidly growing too big for, knowing it was a silly, melodramatic and counterproductive gesture, but still fantasising about punishing my parents with a row of deep cuts. Some days at the Farm really were so intensely difficult, your bloated belly straining to digest all that food, and you'd just want to rip your very skin off. I remember, one evening, sitting on the floor of my bedroom waiting for my turn in the shower and looking down at my forearms, which were no longer pleasingly narrow and fleshless, with my paperclip in hand, tracing a white line back and forth. I remember how I looked at my wrists and I couldn't help but see my future. I wanted to hurt, I wanted to bleed. I knew my body was disgusting, shameful and totally unlovable, but somewhere in the very distant future, I dreamed that maybe I could be something more than just thin. I saw myself working and dancing and acting and performing – and I saw myself doing so with pale, unblemished wrists.

Sometimes I think about the word 'recovery' and how apt it is for recovering from an eating disorder – but not for the reasons people think, which are merely the superficial aspects of recovery, such as gaining weight and establishing more consistent, normal eating habits. It's apt because in eating disorder recovery, you're literally trying to recover a whole person, the one who was there before the eating disorder, the one you didn't like and tried to bury, the one who fades into the background and who people stop seeing the more the anorexia intensifies. You're trying to recover this person to the surface, this person who is slipping down and down into ever darker depths, further and further away from the sun. The deeper she slips, the harder the battle will be to recover her. But to recover that person, you have to have a very good reason to pull her back to the surface, because the battle is brutal, and you get so tired of fighting. It is sometimes just easier to give up and let her sink. This, to me, is the most difficult aspect of recovery. People don't develop anorexia without a deep-seated sense that they are inherently worthless. They find solace from their worthlessness in anorexia because it is gruelling and relentless, a punishing way of life that aligns with their opinion of themselves, and then they find that thinness – the sweet bonus of their self-flagellation – is prized and praised by society in an intoxicating manner. This thing they are doing to distract themselves from their own worthlessness just so happens to earn them the attention, affirmation and secure identity they've always craved and could never give themselves. So why would you ever give that up? Why the fuck would you ever choose recovery?

I think this is also the most crucial element of recovery, because until the person finds a reason to exist independent of their eating disorder, it doesn't matter how many times someone fills her with food and sends her on her way again – she will just keep slipping back beneath the surface. But where do you begin to salvage self-worth and recover yourself, when you simply don't have any reasons to like yourself beyond your disorder? How do you choose yourself when everyone around you has forgotten who that is, and when treatment centres like Peaceful Pastures actually reinforce identification with one's eating disorder by fixating entirely on that part? And why would you bother when the eating disorder further embeds your sense of worthlessness as your peers go on to succeed in life, pass exams, go to college, score their dream jobs, and all you are is thin, and there's no hope that you'll ever catch up with them now?

These questions are difficult to answer, but I do have a theory of how one might find the motive and the determination required to begin recovering oneself, whether from an eating disorder or some other seemingly infinite darkness, and I think it starts with nurturing the dreamer. Dreaming is underrated, I think, so often dismissed as a fanciful, childish, passive activity for immature people not rooted in reality. But sometimes, reality is truly unbearable, not worth enduring, and dreaming offers the only way out of it: a light in impenetrable darkness, even if it's an illusory one you conjured by your imagination. And that's the great thing about dreaming; you don't have to have a shred of self-worth to do it, you only have to have imagination. Dreaming makes us better people, because in seeing these wonderful, irresistible, beautiful images of a potential future, we ignite that desire to be around to witness them, to live and become part of the dream. How many times have you fallen in love with a person and put on your best outfit to meet them, pushed yourself beyond your comfort zone without noticing, gone out of your way to do something that makes them smile? You become your best self, regardless of how you felt about yourself when you encountered them, because you are compelled by the dream. Dreaming has a transcendent quality to it, this ability to pull us up and beyond what we saw for ourselves, and while I don't think it's the answer to recovery – because those dreams can crumble and dissipate in a moment, leaving you bereft, alone with yourself again – I believe they can provide a lighted path out of the depths of an eating disorder, and that's where recovering the self begins.

There was one person above all else at the Farm who never stopped seeing the patients as people, and who seemed to make it his singular mission to nurture the dormant dreamers within us: an energetic, quirky and enthusiastic young man named Marcus Freed. Freshly graduated from drama school, Marcus is ebullient, passionate, good-humoured and *crazy* about acting. Marcus found his way to a job at the Farm as the unit's Drama and English teacher, though his enthusiasm for life is such that he dons many other hats, teaching extracurricular sessions that include everything from yoga to religion to meditation – really, whatever he fancies in any given week, according to whatever his latest newfound passion is, of which he has multitudes. Marcus is the kind of person who takes the term multi-hyphenate to medically inadvisable lengths. And he is so different to everyone else at the Farm: a cheerful, bright-eyed young Jewish man who arrives promptly for each lesson clutching the straps of his outdoor sports backpack eagerly, practically quivering with excitement about teaching. Marcus has been teaching at the Farm throughout my entire stay, but somehow doesn't enter my remit until about six weeks in, I think because until this point, we've been operating on completely different energetic frequencies, his cheerful, encouraging tones drowned out by my tormented wailing.

Eventually, though, I calmed down enough for Marcus's relentlessly positive outlook to infect me too.

I think, above all else, what sets Marcus apart from everyone else on the unit is simply that he is a hopeful person. He is brimming with ideas, plans, dreams, and can't help but see potential stories in and devise spectacles out of every mundane moment of life. He is a figure of fascination at the Farm, and of fun, if often at his own expense. He is attractive, but just a little bit too enthusiastic to stoke the flames of dormant teenage sex drive, and the older girls are far too cool for his enthusiasm, so they take to making fun of him. Much hilarity ensues when Lexi and Jess find his actor's website online, complete with a frequently updated blog and a series of moody headshots. They print out several dozen copies of his headshots and, the next morning, stick them up all over the place, so Marcus smoulders out at us from every corner of the classroom and every couple of feet along the hallway, just in time for his arrival during school hours to teach RE. But much as they like to mock him – his sultry headshots, his weekly blog posts, his early experiments into yoga teaching – his pure, positive energy is the direct opposite of that of everyone else stuck in that prison, and we all flock to him like moths to a flame. His undimmable idealism feels like a breath of fresh air in contrast to the stifling atmosphere of cynicism that presides everywhere else in the house. And, contrary to what you may expect of performers, Marcus has very little ego. He is never offended when people fail to show up to his evening drama classes. Instead, he comes parading through the lounges, breaking us out of our TV-induced stupor, hollering for new student recruits.

'Come on, come on, we're unblocking our chakras through our inner animal states this evening! Everyone's invited!'

'Can't you take a hint, Marcus?' Jess grumbles from the sofa. 'We all have better things to do,' she adds, turning her gaze back to *Blind Date*.

But he always finds a few willing participants, me among them. I join first out of vague curiosity, but quickly become a keen and engaged student, with an enthusiasm to match Marcus's – well, almost. Each class, after he's done his rounds, a small group of us traipse after him down the hallway and space ourselves out around the classroom as per his instructions, following him in a warm-up of stretching, sighing, circling the room, growling, squawking – you know, the things you do in acting class. Then we gather in a circle, bellies down on the floor, and with a few prompts from Marcus, share what is on our minds: what is making us sad, furious, frustrated. After this, Marcus springs to his feet, bubbling with inspiration for how we might channel these intense feelings, be it through reciting a melancholy Shakespearean sonnet, becoming wild hyenas chasing each other back and forth across the classroom, playing simple ball-throwing games or even sitting and penning our own monologues.

Invariably, at some point during the class, the older, cooler girls creep into the classroom, keeping to the peripheries of the room, pretending they've forgotten a copybook or that they want to read quietly, even while Marcus and his troupe thunder around in the background as rhinoceroses. Initially, they throw scornful looks in our direction, but over the course of ninety minutes, they are eventually drawn into the circle too, purportedly they claim, because we look like we are burning a lot of calories.

Soon, Marcus's classes become the highlight of my week, and I arrive several minutes early, stationing myself in the best spot in the classroom on a yoga mat, raring to go with my notebook and a series of crumpled photocopied poems and monologues. While I wait for Marcus to arrive, I daydream about what a fabulous, fun job it would be to be an actor. I get teased for being a teacher's pet by the older girls, and for what they suspect is a schoolgirl crush on Marcus. (For the record, I actually didn't fancy Marcus and I think some of my accusers, the ones who teased him mercilessly, may have been trying to divert attentions from their own growing infatuation. We'll get to the object of my twelve-year-old affections later . . .) I am mortified by this, so one week I decide to casually forego class and make a concerted effort to tone down my zealousness. Moodily, I creep into a corner of the lounge with my bead box and keep my head down as I work on a beaded fairy design in quiet. But barely five minutes pass before the door to the lounge bursts open, and there stands Marcus, wide-eyed and frantically scanning the lounge for me.

'Evanna! Drama class is starting now! Did you forget?' he enthuses, beaming, not for a second imagining that I would skip class.

'Oh . . .' I say, doing my best acting work at appearing aloof and uninterested. 'Right. Yeah, I'm just not in the mood right now.'

'What do you mean?!' Marcus cries, his smile not faltering for a moment. 'We're doing *Midsummer Night's Dream*! We need you for Puck!'

'Oh, OK then,' I answer coolly, as my heart soars with joy, and I quickly abandon my bead box.

The *Midsummer Night's Dream* show is a stroke of genius on Marcus's part. He is always looking for interesting new outlets for our creativity. He is the only one to identify our restless anger, our drive and ambition as untapped brilliance, as misdirected creative energy, and to try and channel our self-destructive impulses into self-expression. He's noticed, too, how heavily the reality of institution-alised oppression weighs on our spirits. Thus, one week he charges into the classroom just in time for drama class, his eyes shining, pos-sessed by the idea of taking all our rage, pain and sense of injustice towards Peaceful Pastures and channelling it into a show. He decides that we should challenge ourselves by putting together a series of sketches interspersed with monologues from *A Midsummer Night's Dream* and perform it in front of the whole ward at the weekly unit meeting, which happens every Wednesday in the classroom. The inspiration for the show came from the Shakespearean tradition of critiquing society through drama and using theatre to covertly lampoon the upper classes. 'We will use this play to speak truth to power!' he declares triumphantly to the classroom. 'People have been doing this for centuries! Ben Jonson in England in the 1600's! Aristophanes' *Lysistrata* in 411BC! Aristotle! The court jester poking fun at the king through satire!' he enthuses, excitement radiating from his pores, as we all sit around in a circle, blinking back at him. The staff agree to it, as they do most of Marcus's wild ideas. He is the only person in the building who seems genuinely pleased to be here, who shows up of his own volition to teach on certain evenings, even when he hasn't been asked to, so generally, whenever Marcus proposes an eyebrow-raising new scheme or show, the staff just shrug and leave him to it. As a result, no other staff members are present at our drama sessions on Thursday evenings, as we lie on the floor of the classroom and plot our revenge on the nurses. They have no idea that this is an act of political resistance. Marcus encourages us to write what we know, to say whatever we are burning to say, to take the repressed urges towards violence and resistance that flare up at mealtimes, and to put those raw feelings into characters and sketches.

'But won't we get told off and put on supervision for this?' asks Ruby, a sceptical expression on her face, a pen clutched in her hand over a sheet of paper. She is not a regular attendee of Marcus's classes but has been lured into joining the show by the tantalising prospect of taking artistic vengeance on the staff.

'Absolutely not!' beams Marcus, thrilled by the enthusiastic uptake of this latest creative endeavour. 'That's the beauty of art: we can do what we like. We have artistic licence! Even if they were to recognise themselves, there's nothing they can do. As long as we change the names, they can only speculate, and we can claim it's fiction.'

The following Wednesday morning, as usual, the staff and patients fold up the desks and form a large circle around the edges of the classroom for the Wednesday unit meeting. The other patients and the staff – the teachers, nurses, therapists, even the Farm's unit director, a terrifying, tyrannical, shadowy presence who we rarely see – take their seats in one half of the circle with expressions of mild interest, as our drama troupe squabble in the hallway over costume pieces and the running order of the scenes. A few students have lost their nerve, opting out of the show last minute despite Marcus's pleas, taking their seats in the circle and glowering sullenly at the floor, and this has sent the rest of us into spirals of panic. But Marcus, a consummate professional and true thespian, insists that the show must go on, whether it makes narrative sense or not. I have been cast as Puck, tasked with learning several excerpts from his monologues to add a vague framework to the show, so I step into the middle of the circle. My heart hammers in my ears as I stand before my arch-nemesis,

Sue, and the judgemental gaze of my more cynical peers at the Farm to deliver my opening lines.

It's funny how the body takes the helm and guides you through the motions when stage fright seizes you and you're convinced you're either going to pass out or shit yourself. That's the magic of practice, though: that no matter how terrified you feel when you first step out on that stage, moments later the body will kick in, say the lines and walk to the marks without your realising, and before you know it, you're immersed in the story and you don't have space to contemplate your mortality anymore. I get through my opening monologue and breathe a sigh of relief as I retreat offstage to a polite smattering of applause. Marcus gives me a hearty thumbs up, and the show goes on.

It *doesn't* make narrative sense, incidentally, and it probably would have worked better as a loose interpretation of *Macbeth* rather than *A Midsummer Night's Dream*. Ruby and Hazel take the stage as two evil witches. They huddle around an imaginary cauldron, concocting a milkshake composed of a stomach-churning list of double cream, animal fat and human remains, emitting high-pitched cackles and crying out the nutritional content of each ingredient as they mime dropping them into their cauldron. It isn't terribly funny, but it is good to see them expressing their feelings aloud rather than scheming quietly in the corner for a change. Juliet, a shy, dark-haired new arrival, surprises everyone by opting to join the show, and performs a mesmerising silent interpretative dance that ends, rather disturbingly, with her flailing and thrashing on the ground, making stabbing motions towards her own midriff. She would have made a fine Lady Macbeth. Lauren does some sort of frenetic, angry martial-arts display that is very obviously an excuse to burn calories, and she is reprimanded by Jen, who calls for her to 'Take it down a notch, Lauren . . . too vigorous.' Lexi and Jess perform a very thinly disguised parody of the unit director and Dr Walsch having an illicit affair, with her portrayed as a cruel dominatrix intent on suffocating Dr Walsch with a can of whipped cream. Marcus abruptly cuts this short, striding on to the stage and declaring that piece a work in progress. Next, Grace defuses the tension with a sad but sweet love sonnet. Finally, I take to the stage once more to deliver my final monologue, a piece Marcus had explained to the class will subtly apologise for any offence caused without claiming responsibility and declare it a work of fiction, an act of our collective imagination rather than the vicious attack on the staff that it actually is.

'If we shadows have offended, think but this, and all is mended: that you have but slumber'd here,' I tell the room peaceably, as various audience members nod and smile vaguely at me, either enjoying the show or relieved that it's ending. '. . . Now to 'scape the serpent's tongue,' I say, adding some grit and venom to my voice, and rounding on Sue, who sits there blank and expressionless, glancing every now and then at her folder, probably plotting the week's calories. Oh, it is delicious to stand there, to have a voice and vent openly at them as they blink back, obliged to sit and endure our tirades, because this is the stage, and the stage is sacred. '. . . Give me your hands if we be friends,' I finish, opening my arms to the staff as though I can dissolve any residual animosity with words, 'And Robin shall restore amends.'

Marcus and the other performers jog into the centre of the circle to join me as we take our bows and prepare for a frosty reception, but to our great surprise the nurses are smiling and clapping good-naturedly, neither bowled over nor deeply wounded by our display. Nigel, the headteacher, clears his throat and congratulates us on 'a spirited performance' as we shed our costumes and file off the stage that is suddenly just a classroom again, and take our places in the circle. We are still buzzing from the adrenaline of performance as Nigel launches into the weekly meeting and recites a series of announcements in his usual dull monotone. Throughout the day, various nurses compliment us on an entertaining show and sincere commitment to our work, and it dawns on us that they either had not noticed or had not cared that it was them personally who we'd been parodying. Miraculously, they don't seek to punish us for it, dismissing the whole event as drama, just drama, Marcus being Marcus . . .

Yes, life would have been much bleaker at the Farm without Marcus. It was his classes and his seemingly boundless zest for creativity that reignited hope in my heart and helped me begin to see the first glimmers of colour for a vision of life beyond anorexia. It was much better therapy than the actual therapy. He wove the fragile shining thread of creativity back into life at the Farm and urged us to protect it, nurture it, weave vibrant new threads in and around it, and to follow its winding path by instinct alone.

My advice for anyone toughing it out with the latter stages of the physical part of eating disorder recovery is simple: get distracted. Your body will feel huge, hideous, repugnant. You'll get panic attacks. You'll think your life is over. You'll look at yourself and won't be able to see past the fat. I know recovery is often described as a battle, a fierce, gritty struggle, and it is that in many ways, but I don't know that that is the most helpful metaphor, because recovery often feels far more like surrendering. In my opinion, words like 'war' and 'warrior' are much more aligned with the energy of anorexia, which likes to hurt, likes to punish, likes gruelling hard work and, ultimately, likes to conquer. And how would you ever win a battle, how would you tough out the tears and the sweat and the sacrifice, when you don't really know what you're fighting for yet? Who would ever start a war with the objective of gaining weight? Who would fight for fat? And even if you do initially start out with a keen intention to 'fight' your disorder, to fight for your health and your life, it's not a decision you make once and for all, but thousands and thousands of smaller decisions throughout the day. And, inevitably the daily struggle to eat – which stops feeling like a fight and feels more like weakness to your disorder – will wear you down, and you'll fail to remember why you were compelled to put yourself through this 'battle' in the first place. To me, recovery felt much more like surrendering, like giving up the fight, like turning my back on a trusted friend, like lying down on the ground and finally conceding, 'Yes, I am worthless.' But that's not an empowering narrative either. To live, to succeed, to thrive in this meritocratic society, we are compelled to deny and disprove our own worthlessness. It's too terrifying to sit there and be with your worthlessness. You'll have time to deal with your worthlessness later – believe me, it'll be there waiting for you on the other side of recovery – but it's best not to confront it when you're still trying to find your way out of the darkness. So, to me, it's better not to try and fight your disorder or frame recovery as a battle; it's better to just get distracted from it with something wonderful, exciting and intoxicating. The distraction should ideally take a long time and consume your energy and thoughts in much the same way your eating disorder does. But it could be anything really: a dissertation, a towering bronze sculpture, an insanely intricate embroidered gown, a book. A boy.

There weren't many boys at the Farm, let alone straight, attractive, interesting ones. The ratio of girls to boys at the Farm was approximately ten to one. The boys slept in a separate bedroom, but separating the sexes didn't really matter at the Farm, as we were all too obsessed with ourselves and the prominence of our own hip bones to have much energy left over for pandering to male attention. Besides, stewing in self-hate generally kept the notion of romantic love far from one's imagination. But there were boys around, and though they felt different to us and lingered more on the outskirts of our social circles, they tended to be unanimously liked. They didn't evoke the same animosity or bitchiness as certain girls did among themselves. To me, the boys at the Farm always felt like lost boys, a terrible loneliness and fragility hanging about them. There was Conor, an impressively obese thirteen-year-old who generously and delightedly demonstrated his ability to 'clear the pool' for his new anorexic family with ceiling-shuddering belly flops for the weekly swim at the local community centre. He was sweet and huge, and we all warmed to him because he cared so little about the kind of aesthetic we longed for, and his very presence floated the vague notion of unconditional love, somewhere, out there. There was Adam, the Nirvana hoodie-wearing, sly-eyed, sexually precocious ten-year-old who had seen too much too young. There was Colin, a pale, mousy-haired boy who loved Liverpool FC such an alarming amount that it was actually a relief when he switched to talking about calorie-burning strategies.

And then there was Alfie. He didn't breeze in the door in a leather jacket and a cloud of smoke, with hungry brown eyes and fashionably hollowed out cheeks, either. We never got our Deppian, forlorn, emo poet at clinic, sadly. Sixteen-year-old Alfie shuffled bitterly into that yellow hallway with hunched shoulders, a downy moustache and familiar, mistrusting eyes. His waist circumference quietened all of us in reverence. He was knobbly all over, and fluffy where he should have been hairy, and so, so petite.

For a while, Alfie kept to himself. Head bent over his school-work, elbows on the table, hands framing his face, a box of isolation. I didn't talk to him at first, admiring his cardboard midriff from across the classroom and wondering how many weeks of surreptitious star jumps in the downstairs bathroom would pass before the programme broke his spirit too. A few of the older girls took to sniffing him out, curious, teasing him and asking questions about his family, and Ruby even snooped through his locker one day after class and found a letter he'd been writing to a friend in which he described his female co-habitants as 'quite fit', which we all fell about laughing over, but which secretly intrigued me. The thing that brought Alfie into my orbit was MTV, and more specifically the 'Cha-Cha Slide'. Remember the 'Cha-Cha Slide'?! Wasn't it great?! Or maybe it was actually kind of lame – I can't tell, and will remain forever biased. Either way, in the spring of 2004 in an eating disorder inpatient facility, a pop hit that shouted aloud exercise moves and thus obliged you to get up and burn calories was everyone's favourite song. No sooner would the first few beats have kicked off, with DJ Casper exclaiming 'this time, we're gonna get FUNKY!' than the upstairs lounge would come alive with motion as each one of us sprang to our feet, ready to dance. *Slide to the left!* We practically crashed through walls! *Slide to the right!* We slammed back again. *Criss-cross!* Vases juddered! *Everybody clap yo' hands!* It was so much fun!

To this day, the 'Cha-Cha Slide' fills me with that same rush of manic glee, the feeling that I'm doing something extremely rebellious, and the irrational hope that I can box-step my way out of deep, unending despair. God bless the 'Cha-Cha Slide' for those moments of stolen fun in a regime of systematic daily morale-crushing. Soon the nurses caught on to what we were doing, and the song was immediately banned from the house. Nobody told MTV, however, and the 'Cha-Cha Slide' kept on – *kept on* – playing. If there were fewer than four of us, we would spring lightly – oh, so lightly – to our feet and nimbly hop from side to side in silent ecstasy. Sometimes they still caught us, and we would fall back into armchairs, wiping our sweaty brows on cushions and fumbling with the remote control to quickly switch over to *The Simpsons* whenever we heard them stomping angrily up the last few stairs, but even when a sour-faced nurse burst in, surveyed us through narrowed eyes and told us they'd have to increase our calories if they caught us, the sense of euphoria endured.

This is when Alfie and I took to looking out for each other, seeking out the 'Cha-Cha Slide' at every opportunity, manifesting it into our reality as we channel-surfed. We'd take turns standing guard and tag each other back in for the next chorus. It didn't take long for me to develop a firm crush on him. It didn't take much, either. He was the first boy I'd known who actually paid attention to me, who laughed at my jokes and sought me out as company, and that, to me, made him exceptional, worthy of my undying affection. He was also a nice boy, and there was a real sweetness beneath his initial teenage edginess – and something about his fragility really fascinated me. As for him, I was definitely an asset in his early days at the Farm, an excellent accomplice to his anorexia, which he was stubbornly fighting to protect. Alfie was only starting his programme as I was nearing the end, and he was struggling desperately with his compulsive exercise habit so I, a Peaceful Pastures habitué by now, who knew the rhythms and routines of each and every nurse intimately – the different sounds of their footfalls, the minute intervals at which they did routine scans of the unit – volunteered my assistance as his lookout while he did secret workouts. I wouldn't have been able to offer the same services for my female friends on the unit without feeling intensely guilty and triggered, but this was coming from a place of pure love and I'm a Leo; we are generous lovers. I manned the empty hallway as he did burpees behind the bathroom door with gladness in my heart.

Oh, I was so into him! I liked his knobbly hands, I liked his cool, working-class accent, I liked his sweeping brown fringe and the way he tossed it back for the 'Cha-Cha Slide'. I liked his impressively fleshless midriff, which he too liked to flaunt, tucking his thumbs into the waistband of his tracksuit pants to reveal his pointy hip bones. In short, he was HAWT to twelve-year-old me. I tailed after him all over the ward, and he didn't try and shake me off at any point or give me the cold shoulder. He was definitely self-conscious about the fact that I was twelve, though, and made one too many passing references to it.

'My friends would slag me off so much if they knew I was hanging out with a twelve-year-old,' he told me one afternoon in the lounge, as we were waiting for the 'Cha-Cha Slide' to make its rounds again. 'But you're not like other twelve-year-olds,' he added. This was clearly meant more to reassure himself of his own coolness than as an observation of my maturity, because I was *absolutely* as silly as any other twelve-year-old. But I was dazzled by infatuation and chose to take it as a profound compliment.

'Thank you,' I breathed, beaming and batting my eyelashes at him.

This love story never gets steamy – sorry, I was no sexually precocious nymphet and had basically flattened any burgeoning hormones for a good while. All we did was talk – about calories, about the future, about star signs, about our families – but that was enough for me to be utterly convinced we were twin flames. I thought of my mum and how she would often despair about my eating habits at the height of my disorder, telling me if I continued like this into adulthood, I would never be able to go on dates to a fancy restaurant if I was just going to sit there 'miserably nibbling a plain Ryvita cracker'. How wrong she was, I would think, dreamily studying Alfie's determined profile, his frustration mounting as he channel-surfed in search of the increasingly elusive 'Cha-Cha Slide', and I pictured our future together. We would both get out of here, lose all the weight and take on the world together. We would Cha-Cha Slide and star jump in ecstatic calorie-burning bliss! This would be our life, as anorexic lovers, with identical body shapes and an insatiable appetite for hunger! We would not conform, get fat or grow old together. We would never give in, never give up.

My distraction proved so effective that I hardly noticed the final few kilos creeping on to my body and, much sooner than I'd anticipated, my target weight and discharge date were upon me. And now that 10 May was finally here, I had very mixed feelings about being discharged. I missed my freedom and yearned for a day I didn't have to gain weight, but I was reluctant to go back into the real world. I had found a strange and dysfunctional family at Peaceful Pastures. I had made real friends, and though we were all different ages, with little in common with one another, we had one major thing in common that separated us from society, and that created a safe, sheltered sense of belonging, of being seen and liked for who we were. It was something I'd never found among other young people. I had no idea how to return to society with this new body, this pervasive sense of worthlessness that had been temporarily obscured by the warm feeling of acceptance amid my peers, but that was still very much a problem. Who would I be without my anorexia? With normal people who dieted and casually hated their own bodies and judged each other's worth off the most superficial aspects of their being?

'I don't think I want to go home,' I tell Ruby, sadly, as we watch Alfie and Grace play an energetic game of table tennis in the back garden, the sun beating down on our heads now that summer is here.

'Are you mad?' scoffs Ruby, turning to me, but then she sees that my eyes are brimming with tears and takes a gentler tone. 'You have to get out of here and get your life back. Besides, we'll all be gone in a few months too, you won't miss much. And if you leave now, you won't have to see me get to target weight,' she adds, darkly, and I laugh and grimace at the same time, pained by the unspoken fact that now I am at target, I am officially 'fat' in the eyes of my closest friends.

The weekend before my discharge date, my whole family flies to London. Patients are supposed to spend the last weekend before discharge at home in the family environment as a final test, but as my discharge date falls on a Monday, my parents have decided to book a few hotel rooms and treat the family to a little celebratory trip to London. My siblings, who I've not had much contact with throughout my time at the Farm, are cautious, slightly formal, and very, very nice to me, careful not to make any comments about my appearance, and giving me my way easily in arguments in a manner that feels oddly alienating. My mum, too, is going out of her way to make me feel good, and announces that 'the boys' will go off sight-seeing around Westminster while 'the girls' will spend the afternoon shopping. We wander around Zara, H&M and Topshop, and she tells me to pick out whatever I like. I can tell she is trying hard to reframe my vast weight gain as a glorious transformation, and though I can't see it that way, I am totally down with the shopping. I feel distinctly cheered up as we pick out a pink floral dress and a chiffon yellow skirt – bright, wild, happy items – and feel myself soothed by the wonderful adrenaline rush of a shopping spree, thinking maybe my future isn't so bleak after all. After we pay, I sit down in the changing room area, clutching my shopping bag happily, waiting for Mairéad to finish trying on some T-shirts. And then my gaze lands on a girl around my age who is trying on clothes with her friends, and I feel a sharp pang of envy. She is thin and lithe, wearing a fashionable crop top and short shorts, her belly practically concave, hip bones jutting out proudly. She has the aura of power that young, popular, beautiful people exude, knowing the shame and self-hate their presence evokes in their peers. It has been a long time since I've come face to face with this particular brand of playground nemesis in the real world. And as I look at her, I suddenly catch sight of someone else in the mirror behind her, a hapless, awkward-looking girl with a pink, puffy face and chubby upper arms. Humiliation sets in as I realise that I am this girl. I blink back, horrified, really seeing my new body for the first time. They have made me normal again, plain and flabby. A huge weight seems to settle on me as I realise that I am back to where I started: I've achieved nothing, done nothing to improve myself, to immunise myself from the sin of being so worthless. Why is this girl allowed to be so spectacularly skinny? Why can't I be special too? After everything I've put myself through to fix myself, they've simply swiped it off me in a matter of weeks, rubbed away my edges with mounds and mounds of food. I want to weep. I want to scream. I want to shout at this smug, beautiful girl that I used to be skinnier than her, that I was the best at being skinny. I want to yell out that impressive word 'anorexic' to the entire shop and claim it as mine, but looking back at this useless blob in the mirror, it is suddenly starkly clear that I do not deserve that word anymore: that it is gone, that nobody will look at me and see anorexia anymore, and there'll be nothing to distract them from seeing *me*.

'Ready to go, pet?' my mum asks cheerily, as Mairéad pays for her new loot, but then her face falls as she notices that I'm crying. She bends down beside me to investigate. 'What's wrong?'

'Nothing,' I tell her, my face burning with shame, as I try to hide it behind my hair. The cool, thin girls are now sniggering in their corner of the shop, and I'm certain they're laughing at me.

'Come on, pet,' my mum urges, putting a consoling arm around me and leaning in for me to whisper. 'What is it?'

'I'm just . . .' I tell her between sniffles, knowing she's not going to like my answer. 'I'm just . . . so fat.'

Her entire body stiffens and then wilts. She sighs heavily and looks at the floor.

'You're not fat,' she tells me predictably. 'You're lovely!' she

THE OPPOSITE OF BUTTERFLY HUNTING

tries, keeping her tone upbeat, but being called 'lovely' only makes me cry harder. 'Look, you're going to have to try to stay healthy. You're going to have to fight these thoughts,' she says finally, not acknowledging that she crushed the fighter in me fourteen weeks ago. I have no more fight left. 'We'd better go, the boys will be waiting. We can talk about it later,' she says, her voice stressed, and she gets up to leave. I wipe my face and follow her, clutching the purchases that had moments ago made me feel fabulous.

That's how long the shopping high lasts. I've done it again: I've popped the warm bubble of familial happiness, and now my mum is looking worn out, sad, and my sisters have scowls on their faces as we traipse out of the shop and on to the bustling London high street.

My final morning at the Farm passes in a blur. It's not like the last day of school, because everyone else is staying – I'm the only one for whom an era is coming to an end. Already, the separation and isolation I dread is happening. Lexi (who has bounced in and out of the Farm throughout my stay on her recurrent relapse visits) is the last one to sign my leaving book, handing it to me with a begrudging smile, hugging me fleetingly with just one arm, then trudging back up the corridor to the classroom. '*I fucking hated you when you arrived*,' her message reads, '*but you're actually alright. Good luck at home. Lexi.*' It is predictably blunt and unsentimental, but it still makes me smile. As expected, every single other person's leaving message is accompanied by pictures of tomatoes, and my now infamous line '*I haaaattteeee tomatooooooes*' is quoted over and over, along with other accounts of the adventures we've shared together. Ruby tells me how much fun she had as my roommate, and promises that she'll write to me. Hazel recalls the time I got in cahoots with Bridget, the friendly Irish cleaner, who managed to get me out of breakfast early by convincing the nurses that I absolutely had to attend the Mass at the church down the road to get my ashes for Ash Wednesday. Mona reminds me of how I somehow managed to convince the nurses that I *was* actually a very devout Catholic, and that I needed to be let out every Sunday morning for Mass, and she thanks me for insisting she tag along as 'chaperone'. Ava pastes lots of pictures of Westlife all over her message, and marvels at the time I vomited up my tuna pasta bake in the church courtyard one Sunday afternoon, and how I'd eventually confessed to the nurses and suffered my one and only milkshake. '*That's when I knew you were really crazy,*' she writes. Grace talks fondly about our 'Cha-Cha Slide' parties, and says it won't be the same anymore. And Alfie tells me again how I'm '*cool and mature for a twelve-year-old*', and I know I will read his message over and over for weeks. They all (except Alfie, noticeably) tell me I'm 'pretty' and 'look good at target' and I know they're lying, but it's still nice of them. After lunch, we sit in the sun outside and I try to take pictures of my friends with my disposable camera, but they all groan and shield their bodies, so I put it away and join in the gossip instead. They're all talking about a new girl who arrived three days ago, a dark-haired, dark-skinned girl from Armenia named Eva. They're debating whether her target weight will be proportionally lower according to the national average BMI in Armenia, which they've already discovered is lower than that of the UK. Eva is the narrowest person I've ever seen, and watching her across the garden, I'm reminded of the day Phoebe left and I took her place. I think about what a frightening sight my body must be to this new girl, a horrifying precursor of what lies in store for her.

After lunch, the others head back to class while I heave my suitcase downstairs and drift about the unit feeling deflated as I wait for my family to show up. I'm pacing up and down the hall when Marcus comes jogging towards me from the classroom and gives me a big hug. He then hands me a yellow form and explains to me that this is a form for 'Equity', an actors' union, and that I need to contact them and join. He's also written the website address and phone number for an extras acting company in Dublin for film and TV. He tells me I need to get headshots and sign up to this site.

'You must keep acting!,' he says, his glassy green eyes shining enthusiastically as he grips my shoulder and gently shakes it. 'You must pursue this passion!' He speaks with an insistence that indicates I have no choice but to agree.

'OK,' I tell him, nodding and scanning the Equity form. 'I will.' I smile at him and then he squeezes my shoulder once more and dashes back to the classroom, leaving me feeling slightly more hopeful.

Marcus was the very first person who singled me out for having any acting talent and conjured the idea that it was something I could do professionally. He stayed at the Farm for another year or so before it eventually wore him down too, and he had to retire from teaching there for his own mental health. 'I knew I had to leave,' he told me years later, shaking his head, a haunted look in his eyes, 'when I went to the pub one day after work and ordered a Guinness, and all I could see was a huge pile of calories.'

He moved to LA, continued acting, became a fully qualified yoga teacher and wrote several books. He was the victim of a near-fatal hit-and-run accident one day while walking home from synagogue and had to have two life-saving brain surgeries, but he bounced back within a year because literally nothing can stop Marcus and his undimmable passion for life. We are still good friends to this day, and he is still available for acting/singing/writing/yoga/business-coaching/life-mentoring/you fucking name it. Good old Marcus.

At 2.30pm, my family arrive, and I bid an unemotional farewell to the nursing staff as my parents help me drag my suitcase out of the hallway and down the driveway – finally, finally.

'Oh, look,' Dad says, as we reach the gate. 'Your friends . . .' He points back to the house, and I see Ruby, Hazel, Natalie, Grace and Alfie have been let out of class to see me off, and that's when I really start crying. Dad gets out his camera and they let him take pictures as I hug each of them tightly and say goodbye. And next thing, we have hoisted my suitcase into a large taxi, I'm squeezed in by the window next to my siblings, and we are on our way to Luton airport. My mum, hearing my sniffling, turns to look at me from the front.

'What a turnaround from all those weeks ago when you were desperate to get out,' she remarks, smiling vaguely, clearly confused as she thinks back to the suicide letters I'd pummelled her with. She looks alarmed as I continue to cry and searches my face, asking sincerely: 'What's wrong with you, pet? What's wrong?'

'I don't know,' I say, crying uncontrollably, as I watch the familiar landmarks of World's End flicker past the window and fade from view, feeling empty and rudderless and wishing my feelings made sense. 'I don't know.'

8

Mostly, when we talk about recovery, we talk about it being triumphant, glorious: all strength and power. You are a phoenix rising majestically from the ashes of your illness, a radiant, shimmering gold-and-scarlet-feathered mythical bird, a dazzling symbol of transformation and resilience! Would that it were like that, but if we are going to use the metaphor of being reborn, recovery feels much more like being a newborn baby spat from the womb-space into the sandy pit of a gladiator's arena, with eyes piercing you from every angle and the sun scorching your tender red flesh, the sudden sensory overload leaving you gasping for breath – oh, and there's a hungry lion pacing circles around you, and you're a baby with nothing to hide behind. This elemental, truly vulnerable, baby-state is the very thing you'd tried to protect yourself from, to *not* feel. Your eating disorder was the chosen armour you'd snatched up to protect the soft skin on your body that feels paper-thin. And now they've confiscated your armour and you're back in the arena of life, where people will judge you and criticise you, where they won't love you for you alone, where maybe some people preferred you when you were skinnier, and you agreed with them, and you

EVANNA LYNCH

have to quickly figure out another means of surviving the elements, even though, secretly, you have the sense the eating disorder armour was working quite well.

Recovering from physical recovery is about finding a new way to survive, and it is an intensely *awkward* process. Whenever journalists interview me and then proceed to publish an article under a boldly emblazoned title that declares 'How I Found the Strength to Beat Anorexia!', I cringe and look the other way, mortified by the self-congratulatory statement I definitely did not make, one that depicts my awkward and ungainly stumble towards recovery as a deeply heroic and inspiring tale. When I think back to this time in my life when I was just out of the Farm, ostensibly physically recovered but mentally still very much floundering, I think of the tantrums, the meltdowns, the humiliation, the embarrassment, the loss of control, the tears, the grief, the discomfort, and how much the reality of recovery jars with the emboldening narrative. I know that people like the fairy tales, and they can lend us a certain degree of strength, and I know that those are the simple, stark, uncomplicated narratives that gain clicks, but where recovery is concerned, I'm keen to dismantle this myth, because when other people are going through their own eating disorder recovery and it doesn't feel heroic or epic or mythical, I want to let you know that it shouldn't. Recovery is not a comfortable or straightforward process. All the gifts that people promised, to lure you from your dark enclosure into recovery – the freedom, the success, the love, the opportunities – are not here yet. It's just you and whatever you choose to do next. People usually assume the recovery journey ends somewhere around this point, but I really believe recovery from physical recovery is where the work to recover truly begins, and that it's a mistake to celebrate recovery at this juncture and to suppose it ended here. For me, recovery from recovery was probably the most confusing time – the most lonely, frustrating and psychologically challenging time. It did not feel heroic and it was also incredibly tedious. So, allow me to erase the captivating myth of my recovery journey and let's let it be what it was: awful.

Just as that summer previous, when I returned home from my first stint in hospital, everyone was oh-so-nice to me on my return: teachers let me get away with things, friends invited me places and relatives very tentatively asked how I was. Nobody really knows how to behave around you after recovery from an illness that had operated in secret, one that you had repeatedly insisted was in their imagination if they dared broach the subject at all, one that you probably never owned up to having. After recovery, anorexia becomes the sleeping dragon, and everyone around you is straining their hardest not to breathe too heavily or laugh too loudly in fear of awakening the beast. Everyone tentatively hopes it has slinked away and is not coming back this time, and they do everything conceivable not to evoke its interest. As for me, I didn't want to talk about my eating disorder either, because I wasn't sure if I even *had* an eating disorder anymore, and I didn't know how to cope with confronting the fact that I might not. My strategy now that I was back was to throw myself into my life, to keep moving, keep busy, and hurriedly move on from all that ugly business back there.

It was May when I got home, just over a month left of primary school, so I returned to class a few days after I got back from England. I wore the brightest, wildest knee-high socks on my return to school, figuring that maybe if I was loud and giggly and colourful, then nobody would notice that I had a new body. There was a strict uniform code at the school – navy jumpers, skirts and socks with a white shirt and red tie – and my colourful socks were certainly not de rigueur, but the teachers didn't say anything because they all knew about my issues. Soon, my school friends were wearing bright, colourful knee-high socks too, whether in solidarity or because they thought it looked cool, I don't know. Either way, it was nice and helped keep the focus off the thing I absolutely didn't want to discuss. The school made a fuss of my return, too, organising for me to make my Confirmation at a neighbouring school, and then staging a second Confirmation photo with the rest of my class, going out of their way to make me feel like I belonged here. There was plenty going on in those final weeks of school, with final exams and school outings and sports day, and endless discussions about secondary school and the future. And it felt OK to be back and in the real world as long as I made sure that I was busy, busy, busy.

Once home, I found I was relieved to be free of Peaceful Pastures. Now that I was back, I was determined to stay out of that place, and fear of going back, for a large part, kept me in line. I cooperated with the weight maintenance programme that the Farm had insisted all outpatients follow and that my mum duly adhered to, measuring out portions precisely on a scales with an expression of trepidation on her face that showed she wasn't entirely comfortable with this system of using metrics to decide how much I should eat. Almost as soon as I was home, the trauma of those early days at the Farm and of fourteen weeks on an enforced feeding regime reared its ugly head for processing, and I started having vivid, almost nightly nightmares of being back in Peaceful Pastures, pinioned to the ground by half a dozen nurses as they funnelled a stomach-churning vat of liquid fat directly into my mouth, telling me that I was sick, sick, sick! Other times in these nightmares, I was clinically obese, sitting at the table in the Brown Kitchen, my many chins wobbling as I cried over a bowl of sticky toffee pudding and tried to tell the nurses that I was already four times my target weight, that this was surely a human rights violation, and where in God's name was my mother, while they just stared back impassively, tapping their watches and taking notes.

I would wake from these nightmares in tears, hands pressed over my eyes, not ready to face the horrors of the Brown Kitchen, until tentative relief would creep through me as I dared to suspect it was nothing but a nightmare, and found myself, mercifully, in my own bed. I'd creep downstairs and eat my breakfast obediently, smiling vacantly at my parents and siblings, willing them all to buy into this act that everything was fine now, that everything was normal. Things were still tense with my siblings; they were polite and tolerant of me, but I don't think they'd forgiven me for the stress of the past two years and were wary that I might relapse like last time. As much as possible, we avoided talking about Peaceful Pastures. We didn't talk about that horrible first day, or the barrage of angry letters I'd sent, or why I'd ended up there, or what had changed while I'd been there, if anything had changed. And we didn't talk about my eating disorder either. Politely, lightly, we negotiated over portions of food and how much exercise I could do, but we weren't going to discuss it as a problem or say the 'a' word. So, even though my anorexia was still the thing I thought about all day, every day, and secretly suspected I always would, we didn't talk about it – and suddenly, I was just back home, living the life of a free thirteen-year-old rather than an anorexic convict. It was strange and surreal to wake up every day in my own bed with choices and privacy, and some mornings I lay there, numbly gazing at the ceiling in my bedroom wondering if the past two years had even happened.

But they *had* happened, and I was not ready to let go of my past. I made sure I stayed in close contact with my friends at Peaceful Pastures, the friends who knew and appreciated the real me. I hijacked Ruby's allotted phone call time and spoke to her, Grace, Hazel, Natalie and Alfie in rotation for a few minutes each. I was eager for all the latest news and gossip from the Farm: who was making their targets, who was back on supervision, and how the newbies were faring. They all chatted to me enthusiastically, passing the phone back and forth to affirm that they missed me and that the 'Cha-Cha Slide' wasn't as fun in my absence, and, for a while, I clung fiercely to the naive hope that we would stay this close forever. But, gradually, I noticed that life at the Farm was moving on without me, and I was no longer an intrinsic part of it. Suddenly, I was the one on the outside, the loved one showing up promptly at the end of the phone to speak to them for half an hour each week, and that just wasn't the same as sharing every minute of our lives together. I was missing out on every fresh new trauma, the battles we fought together that had bonded us so tightly. I started to suspect that I needed them more than they needed me, and soon fewer friends came to the phone, calling out hasty greetings in the background and saying they'd catch me next time before they dashed off to an aerobics class. Alfie, who I thought about every day, and for whom I still nursed a distinctly soft spot, became increasingly more distant with each phone call. One evening, as we were chatting – me working hard at conversation, asking all the questions and him fielding them with a series of shifty, non-committal responses – I heard Lexi singing in the background on Alfie's end, and it was impossible not to make out the words and the cruel intention she had in singing them aloud.

'*It's just a little crush!*' she trilled, '*not like I faint every time we touch!*' With a sinking feeling of horror, I realised that they were all on to me.

'Gotta go,' said Alfie hurriedly. 'I'll talk to you soon, yeah?' And then the dial tone filled my ears as he slammed down the phone before I could say a word. I sat there for a few minutes, my face burning in shame, wondering if all my friends were laughing at me behind my back. The next time I called, he didn't come to the phone, or any other time after that, and we never spoke again. *Coward*. A word of advice: next time you're looking for a suitable distraction from your eating disorder it's best that you choose something sturdy, inanimate and dependable, not an insecure teenage boy. I continued to call Ruby each week to catch up, but with less enthusiasm and with a growing feeling of sadness pressing on my insides. Then something unexpectedly terrible happened that drove a further wedge between me and my past.

'Oh!' said Ruby brightly one evening, interrupting our conversation with news of a new arrival. 'There's a new girl here! A new Irish girl! She sounds just like you!' Her name was Úna, and everyone liked her. Úna was fourteen and from Dublin. Úna was two weeks skinnier than I'd been, with a solidly respectable sixteen-week stay. Úna liked dance and drama too. Úna took my place easily in Marcus's class. Suddenly, all anyone could talk about was Úna. Úna this, Úna that. Within a matter of weeks, Úna had seemingly rendered my companionship in everyone's lives totally obsolete. There was only room for one anorexic Irish girl in people's hearts, and though I'd never spoken a word to her and everyone told me how much she

301

reminded them of me, I fucking hated Úna. Hazel informed me one evening that Alfie and Grace couldn't come to the phone because they were outside having a water fight with Úna, and then she decided to join them. I hung up the phone, enraged. And as I sat there quietly in the lonely shadows of our hallway, there was that familiar feeling of worthlessness, floating back to the surface of my consciousness again, reactivated by the very people who'd filled my life with friendship and had temporarily made that feeling melt away. But it had never actually gone away; it had only been momentarily obscured.

We'd already been drifting before my doppelgänger showed up in their lives, though: those friendships just weren't the same now I was home, and all of a sudden, we didn't have as much in common anymore. The thing about friendships founded on anorexia is that the only way those bonds can ever remain so tight is if you continue to court your eating disorder aggressively, and I wasn't sure I wanted to do that anymore. Being 'on the outside' instantly gave me back all the things my friends at the Farm yearned for and were being denied, the things that we'd previously dreamed about together – freedom, independence, privacy, self-autonomy, pockets at dinner time and the ability to eat food without every bite being mentally noted – and now that I had these privileges and wasn't using them to hide food, deceive my parents and lose weight, as they would the instant a nurse turned her back, I was suddenly, markedly different to them. My new freedoms haunted me with guilt, and I couldn't help but wonder what my friends would do if they were given my freedom. Would they have eaten that chocolate bar without protest? Would they be carefully tanking every night before the weekly home weight check? Would they pity me if they knew that, secretly, I was contemplating a faint idea that maybe I wanted to move on from anorexia, that maybe I wanted to pursue recovery? Would they all have relapsed by now if given the chance? Should I? While my mum kept a close eye on my weight, according to Peaceful Pastures's instructions, it would have been easy enough to trick her, to sneak portions of food out of the house and to snatch opportunities to burn more calories, but for the most part I chose not to take them – and I wasn't exactly sure why.

Summer came and school ended, and it became more difficult to stay busy. I resumed therapy with Natasha, but it was impossible to process all that had happened in one hour a week, and I found myself restless and moody that summer, quick to anger and frantically looking for hobbies to distract myself, frequently bursting into tears with the feeling of ineptitude every creative endeavour produced. The word anorexia, which we had previously delicately skirted and shied away from for the tension its presence evoked, now became completely taboo in our house, like the name of an ex-boyfriend whose existence everyone wants to forget, but can't. I forbade everyone from mentioning it aloud, not with words, but by devolving into tearful angry tantrums after someone brought it up, getting irrationally upset over the smallest things and blowing up at people for no apparent reason. The word itself just seemed to have this special, electrical charge surrounding it that made me jumpy and uncomfortable, as if saying it aloud was going to summon a spirit I was trying to run from. And above all things, the presiding feeling that struck me any time someone uttered the word 'anorexia' was one of an engulfing, all-consuming, insurmountable unworthiness. It's still the primary feeling I confront when I hear that word, though it doesn't trigger a catatonic meltdown anymore, and my reaction is more of a brief, irksome grimace. It's not a word I actively try to avoid (clearly, or I wouldn't be writing this book), but I think, no matter how many times I say it, the word will probably always conjure that feeling of worthlessness.

My theory on this is that you can't ever actually beat anorexia: you can only abandon it. If you're a fighter, a determined, wilful person, it's tempting to stay in its company and meet its constant goading and challenges. But in my opinion, anorexia is the ultimate fighter, the challenger, the energy that's always trembling with the need to dominate, to overcome, to beat out all the competition and be better than everyone else. I think that perhaps the only way to defeat anorexia is to defeat the feeling of worthlessness, but in order to do that, you would need to know the meaning of life, and, well, I'm just not that cocky, I suppose. I know that there'll be many moments in life where I confront the feeling of worthlessness, and that anorexia will still be there, positing an alternative, gently suggesting that this feeling would be more tolerable if I lost some weight. I know, too, that I'll often wonder if it has a point. But the way I see it now, the only way to win anorexia's game is to follow it to the very end, to sacrifice everything else to thinness and to die from it. Then you'll have won – you'll have proven to it that you did absolutely everything to not be worthless – but the price is your life. You either answer its beckons and embark on a lifelong struggle, or you lay down your weapons, you step away and you leave it behind to fester in the dark. I don't know that I'll ever stop glancing back at it occasionally and finding its challenge a tantalising one. I don't know if that word will ever just be a word, but I'll continue to speak it aloud to try and reduce its power and allure.

In the immediate aftermath of recovery, however, I think the word anorexia is too triggering, and it's best to try to avoid it. I think the strong emotional reaction it produced in me was because my anorexia was dying, and it was terrified of oblivion. I think every time someone spoke it aloud, it reminded me that I and anorexia were losing each other, and that sent me into paroxysms of fear, gave me this frantic compulsion to hang on to it, to claw it back and hold it tight. I think its presence in my life during this time *did* become something like that of a toxic ex-boyfriend, one who I loved and cherished, who I felt like I was betraying by living each new day without, who I was not quite sure I wanted to move on from, but who I suspected I could no longer go on living with.

There's not much point trying to avoid being triggered in the immediate aftermath of recovery because pretty much everything is triggering. Eating in front of people is triggering. Choosing what to eat. Watching other people eat. TV sitcoms where female characters casually joke about their eating disorders and claim not to have eaten bread in decades. Magazines, obviously. All models, all athletes, all dancers, especially ballet dancers. Naturally skinny people. Lanky children. Malnourished children in third-world countries on adverts appealing for charitable donations. Jesus on the cross with his enviable ribcage. Friends skipping dessert because they claim they're not hungry. Anyone leaving any scrap of food on their plate as you mentally calculate the calories they've omitted. Religious fasting. Animals in hibernation who don't eat for months on end and live off their fat reserves. Other people's hip bones, other people's belly buttons. Cartoon characters with waspish waists. Wasps. People who say, 'I was so busy I forgot to have lunch.' Every other person who has an eating disorder. The stories of other anorexics who died from their thinness. Boys with abs. People who run for fun. People who choose salad for lunch. The Olympics. Greyhounds. All of it, all of it, it's *all* so triggering, and there's no way around it, so you better be ready to cry in public and just generally be a human volcano who might blow and spill all your messy, uncomfortable feelings on the floor at any moment.

At this point, I felt completely, utterly out of control. I cried everywhere. I ate meals out with my family, and then ruined it by crying all the way home. I skipped friends' birthdays plans last minute because I hadn't showered in three days and I couldn't summon the emotional energy to face taking my clothes off and trying to cobble my appearance into a semblance of someone who had it together. Secondary school started, and it was a clean slate, a blank page, a chance to rewrite myself as someone normal, but I quickly generated rumours of being a lesbian pervert because I couldn't stop staring at all the other girls' legs. They all thought I fancied them, but I was really judging the fatness of their thighs, comparing and contrasting them to mine, trying to figure out where my body type fit in a line-up of my peers, and what the skinniest of them ate for lunch. It was just an intensely socially awkward time. I was struggling to define what normal was in a mind that still believed that any fat was a mistake and eating food, a sin.

In retrospect, I now see this period in the immediate aftermath of recovery as a time of grief. I see that I was grieving a huge part of me that I had not fully reconciled myself with letting go of. But it is tricky to name it as such, because you're not meant to feel sad over something that was so destructive to you and everyone in your life. It's taboo to grieve over something that everyone else is relieved to see the back of. You're meant to celebrate recovery and rejoice jubilantly at the wake of anorexia, and admitting 'I actually really miss my eating disorder' will only kill the vibe. But these are the people who don't understand that eating disorders are coping mechanisms, who portray recovery as all triumph and glory, who don't recognise that, for a long time, your eating disorder was your closest ally. They only see what it cost you, not the cherished moments of solace and steadiness that it lent you. It was always there for you in dark moments when others weren't. But you *are* grieving, even though you shouldn't, even though the thing you miss almost took you down: you're grieving the loss of this part of you that was integral to survival, that was, for a little while, your whole self. I think it's important to acknowledge that letting a part of yourself die is uncomfortable, and there'll be a substantial amount of resistance that comes with that. For so long, your ego has been inextricably linked to the image and feeling of being skinny. To lose that grasp on thinness is to suddenly have that perception and sense of self ripped away, and to not know what remains in its absence.

People think of anorexia as a killer, and fail to see that it starts as a fierce stab at staying alive, at having a purpose, at not being a human waste of space. So, in recovery, when you're losing your grip on thinness and it sometimes feels like you're dying, I think it's because part of you *is* dying. And there are many elements of having anorexia with which you have identified yourself, and losing each one of those feels like a small death. The obvious ones are the visible, tangible things, like a certain weight or dress size, prominent bones, the foods you eat or don't. But there are other, subtler things that fall away, like shopping for clothes in the children's section, or people telling you that you look pale and sick. Or not menstruating. Or being able to fit your hand around your upper arm. These things were markers of your virtuosity, and they fall away one by one in recovery, and, ready or not, with each loss, your identification with anorexia dies a little bit. These markers can be really obscure and personal to each person, private things like not licking stamps or a dress you were proud to fit into. Some losses you take on the chin – you saw them coming, and gritted your teeth in anticipation – but others take you by surprise, and you don't take them lying down. The anorexia is triggered and flares up angrily so as not to be dismantled. It's not ready to face oblivion, and you're not ready to face life without it so you scream and rage and fight back against recovery.

When you first recover physically, it's almost like you've just come up for air. You've been drowning for a long time, surrendering deeper and deeper to the downward pull, losing yourself in a vast ocean. Recovery brings you back to the surface and shows you the world you'd been part of before. Your newfound health keeps you afloat, but you only have a short time before you have to start fighting again to stay up. What do you like about life above the surface? Why not just give in and let yourself be pulled back under? I think in these early days, the impulse to sink is often stronger than the one to survive. But there must have been a reason you got back to the surface. Even if you were partially dragged there, even if you're regretting it now, there must have been something that intrigued you and called you out of the darkest depths. There must have been something in the world that captivated you, and, I think, it's at this point in recovery that you begin to lose your nerve: you're not sure that you want this anymore, and you feel so uncomfortable in your body, and it's just all too hard, and you're thinking it would be simpler to just let go and be submerged again. I think that's when you really need to remember that thing above the surface that called to your soul, and you have to hold on really tightly to that vision. I think something that is integral to the success of recovery is having people around you who hold on to that vision too, who can make it seem brighter and more real, who can call it to mind when you've forgotten, who will help you to build yourself anew. It can be really hard to hold on to it, especially when everyone is on edge and anxious about the eating disorder returning, but if you're only looking for the eating disorder, that's all you'll see. I think that everyone has to be daring in their thoughts at this point and work to see the person beyond their illness, to call that version of themselves forward. That's what friends and family of people in recovery need to do. You need to reimagine this person, because I've forgotten who she is. I'm not sure I believe in her yet; I'm not sure she's worth it.

I was lucky in this way; I had my parents and Natasha, and I think it was their collective efforts to support me and to nurture my dreams in the immediate aftermath of recovery that kept me afloat. We were still following the Peaceful Pastures outpatient programme for several weeks after my discharge, my mum cracking out our janky scale once a week on Monday morning to check my weight was not dropping, and then phoning the number into the office at the Farm. According to their programme, outpatients could not lose more than two kilograms without being readmitted, and the target weight had to be increased every few months to accommodate for an increase in age and height. They advised parents maintain tight control of their child's weight, insisting that if they followed these rules exactly, monitoring their child's weight hawkishly, the anorexia could be kept at bay. Very soon, this became a distressing routine. It just wasn't normal at twelve and then thirteen for my mother to be keeping a careful diary of my weekly weight fluctuations. It didn't feel fair for people to expect me to eat normal portions and socialise like a normal kid and attempt to build a normal life when my privacy was still being impinged on in very abnormal ways. I was embarrassed to step on the scale in front of her, to see the minor fluctuations from week to week, point two of a kilogram in either direction, and to try and read in her eyes what she thought of this whole charade. Was she surprised I was maintaining weight? Did she expect me to lose it? Was she as horrified by my new body as I was, but, as my mother, bound not to say it? Of course, I always believed my most paranoid thoughts, jumped right to them before they could catch me off guard from someone else's mouth.

Once again, there was no positive prognosis came from the weighing scales. I felt this immediate pressure to lose just under two kilograms – cutting it ever so close, but playing within the rules – and keep my weight precisely there. If I lost weight, my mum spent the day worrying, but if I gained, I devolved into panicked pacing around the house and demanding she tell me had she noticed me looking fatter. Once again, the only way to win the game and satisfy everyone was to stay precisely the same weight each week, down to the very gram, a maddeningly difficult feat that required total obsession. We were drifting back to that same place we'd been in before, in Deirdre's office once a week: the tug of war between the weighing scales and genuine efforts at recovery. It seemed that every time I tried to move on with my life, the weighing scales pulled me back, telling me there was something urgent and terrible to tend to in its digitised face. My mum could see this happening again, so one day after a weighing, where I had gained a pound and sat there crying, my face buried in my hands in shame on the bathroom chair, she made a decision.

'Look,' she said, taking my hands and squatting down to my eyeline. 'We're not going to weigh you anymore. I'm not going to call the Farm. This is just too stressful, and it isn't helping. We're just going to handle it between ourselves now, OK?'

'But won't they be cross with you?' I asked sceptically, knowing exactly what the nurses thought of parents who didn't follow the programme to the letter, and the kind of fearmongering they'd ambush her with. 'Won't they tell you off?'

'I'll deal with them,' she said bracingly. 'You just keep working with Natasha and focus on staying healthy, and I'll manage those wagons.'

I snort-laughed through my tears. 'Wagon' is perhaps my favourite Irish pejorative. It felt nice to have my mum on my side. She didn't call Peaceful Pastures that morning, and by afternoon they had called us. I heard her tell those wagons in the office, in a shaky voice, that she didn't agree with their approach and that we would be handling things among ourselves from now on. Peaceful Pastures did not approve, and reminded her that she was 'being manipulated by an anorexic', telling her she had given way to the anorexia far too easily. She told them she saw it differently and hung up the phone. They didn't bother us again after that. They'd got their pound of flesh – quite literally, in fact.

I know the weighing scales can be helpful in recovery to track progress, sort of a necessary evil, but I believe at a certain point you just have to throw them out. Human beings of flesh and blood are not meant to be evaluated via numbers and charts and measurements. Metrics are for robots and outer space. They're not a good assessment of a person. I let go of other things that were no longer helping me too. I quit reading fashion magazines, which had only ever made me feel bad about myself. I also quit ballet, which I'd done since I was a child, but no longer felt like a healthy environment for me, even though I was the first one to bring anorexia into the dance studio. I just didn't want to have to study my body in the mirror for several hours a week, or spend time around ballet dancers, notorious perfectionists. Finally, sometime in late June, I decided to stop calling my friends at the Farm. It was impossible to keep those friends close and let go of anorexia at the same time. Some of them were going home now anyway, we were all going our separate ways. I exchanged addresses with a few of them and wrote a handful of letters back and forth with Grace and Hazel, but soon those connections petered out. Ruby went home in July and we proceeded to write long, thoughtful letters to each other, remaining good friends, but at a more manageable distance. We are still friends to this day, and suffice to say I'm very proud of her.

I continued my strategy of staying busy that summer and decided to try and make something of my acting dream. I was speaking my dream aloud more and more now, my conviction and determination built up by Marcus's generous encouragement. My dream puzzled and bemused my parents, who would tentatively point out that I didn't even enjoy answering the phone to strangers, let alone delivering entire monologues to them. As teachers, my mum and dad regarded any vocation that didn't involve a nine-to-five daily grind that you consistently dreaded as a 'hobby'. I don't think they saw it leading anywhere serious, and they reacted much the same as they had when I'd told them I wanted to be a pony or a Pokémon trainer – with gentle smiles and a flicker of concern in their eyes. But they indulged me, and at least pretended to identify a glimmer of talent. Braving the phone myself, I contacted the extras agency that Marcus had passed on to me and asked to be included on their website for consideration for work as an extra on movies and TV productions in Ireland. They informed me the first thing I needed was to get some professional headshots taken and create my own profile with information of my training and 'special skills'. Headshots, special skill – it already sounded so fucking glamorous! I contacted the headshots photographer they recommended, who was doing sessions in Dublin in June, and promptly booked myself in. The day of the photo session, I got up early, straightened my hair and put on my pink-and-white floral dress, the one I'd worn for my discharge date from the Farm. My dad took me all the way to Dublin, a big deal for country bumpkins like ourselves, where you couldn't even access our house via public transport, and we made a whole day of it, getting there early and walking down O'Connell Street as he filled me in on who each statue was and their respective roles in the 1916 Easter Rising. I nodded along absently, my eyes hungrily scanning the shopfronts. I glimpsed my reflection in the panes of glass, noting my plain, pale face, my still-puffy cheeks, my straightened, dull blond hair, which now looked limp. I felt a sense of hopelessness ripple through me at the thought of being photographed. But I consoled myself with the knowledge that this man was a *professional* headshot photographer; he would make all those less comely details invisible.

We meandered down to Wicklow Street and followed the address instructions to a hotel, and a room where a dazzlingly bright photography studio had been erected for the day. It all happened so quickly. The sweat-drenched photographer was clearly stressed, barrelling through headshot hopefuls like inmates lining up for mugshots. I perched myself on the little black stool uneasily, ran my fingers through my hair in an attempt to create some volume my fine hair would never achieve, and hitched on a frozen smile. The light bulbs and camera popped in unison and I blinked back dazedly, wondering had he perhaps pressed the wrong button. It took several more goes for me to keep my eyes open during the flash, by which point the photographer was getting antsy. I slid off the stool and went to give my details and hand over a few crisp bank notes, courtesy of my dad – eighty euros a pop – and then we bumbled our way out of the glossy marble hotel lobby back into the Dublin sunshine, and I indulged part two of his history tour of statues, feeling hopeful and generous now that my dream was taking shape.

A few days later, my dad received an email with a link to my headshots. Eagerly, I bent over the computer and clicked the link with bated breath, ready to see the pictures that would launch my career as a movie star! The photo loaded jerkily from the top down, not terrible at first, but then revealing something so awful I actually gasped. To my utter horror, the straps of my pink-and-white floral dress, which sat cutely off the shoulder, stretching in a horizontal line across the décolletage, were not framed in the shot, giving the absolutely ghastly impression that I was totally *naked*. There was my gormless, gap-toothed smile, my chubby cheeks, my limp hair: me, with none of the myriad imperfections blurred out or smoothed over by this alleged professional. There I sat, exactly as I saw myself in the mirror, but apparently naked. Oh, it was obscene! I closed the link and never opened it again, quietly discarding all notion of my movie extras profile. Nobody was hiring me for onscreen work until I'd lost a significant amount of weight and put some clothes on. I dropped all mention of my burgeoning acting career to my parents, too embarrassed by the photos and knowing they didn't have another eighty euros to get them redone. They'd done their bit to help me: it was me who was unfit for my dream. Suddenly, it was abundantly clear, it was going to be a lot harder than everyone had let on to find something quite as satisfying as anorexia. So, you can see why, when I've told my story to journalists in the past and it's been relayed back to me as if I recovered and walked from an eating disorder clinic on to the set of *Harry Potter*, that it makes me want to cackle, or weep.

My eating habits got *weird* several months after recovery. It is naive to think that anyone who has struggled with an eating disorder for years could recover from it and then neatly fall into perfectly *ordered* eating habits, but that's what you hope for, not realising how fine the line is between restricting and bingeing. Nobody warns you about this, perhaps because it's so awkward, but after a few months, I completely lost control of my eating in a direction I wasn't prepared for: I started *over*eating. It happened out of nowhere. Suddenly, the meals and snacks that my mum prepared for me every day, a calorie count that had previously seemed to me a gross, insurmountable amount of food, were now not enough, and I found myself stealing to the kitchen while the family watched TV in the living room to sneak handfuls of raisins and fruit-and-nut muesli, which I'd eat in secret in my room. Soon, I was stealing whole 500g bags of raisins and not putting them back, just eating and eating them as I read books or did homework, and next thing I knew the packet was empty.

I think I picked things like dried fruit and cereal to binge on because they were ostensibly healthy, and that put my mind at ease, but it was hard to ignore the fact that I was eating hundreds of calories of sugar and far more fibre than the body knows what to do with. It was deeply embarrassing when my mum went to make scones and asked who'd taken the raisins, or when my digestive system made all sorts of incriminating noises, but my family dealt with it tactfully, my mum quickly realising where the raisin packets were being squirrelled away to and replacing them without comment. Privately, I was panicking about my binge-eating, entirely reluctant to even call it that, wondering would I ever get control of my eating again, or whether the next time I found myself in an eating disorder clinic would be for obesity. It was almost unfathomable to my ego that *I* could struggle with controlling my urges to indulge cravings when, just a few months ago I'd been known among all my friends and family for my iron willpower around food, notorious for never eating delicious foods and for a chronic problem with under-eating. *I* was the one who, until I had taken it too far, people had envied and admired for my ability to avoid the snack cupboard, the one whose parents' friends had complimented for my 'healthy habits' while my friends had asked for successful dieting tips. How could *I* have a problem with eating too much when so recently I'd been literally addicted to not eating enough?

Natasha was the only person I could bear to share these struggles with, and she assured me that it would pass, and that it was normal for the body to react this way after such a long period of starvation and repression of its natural functions. It was almost like my body was rebelling against what I'd put it through, claiming back her right to eat and taste and sense. It terrified me and I wondered when we'd ever be even, when these months of bingeing would finally have cancelled out my starving efforts. *I might as well never have had anorexia,* I would think darkly to myself after demolishing half a box of cornflakes in my bedroom. I couldn't stand it, and of course the greatest irony with the unpalatable feelings that eating disorders bring up is that the most efficient way that you can find to quell them is through food, be that eating lots of it or none at all. I think this is one of the most challenging and dangerous periods for people in anorexia recovery: it can so easily slip into bulimia, an even more vertiginously slippery slope with its own devastating set of physical consequences. Luckily for me, I had Natasha to confide these awkward new behaviours to, and the thing about sharing shameful, dark secrets out loud is that by exposing them to light, you can see them from all angles, objectively, for what they are, and the shame and discomfort you'd built up around them gradually dissolve. Natasha, who had life experience of both disorders, also warned me that bulimia was not the quick-fix solution I imagined it to be. Rather than helping me manage my weight, she explained, it would only bring me greater, messier, longer-term struggles, more problems that would obfuscate the root problem that we were finally trying to address. It was hard to trust her guidance, and even harder to trust that my body knew what it needed and would organically come to a place of equilibrium in its eating patterns, but it did eventually settle down, and after a couple months there was no more bingeing on breakfast cereal after midnight.

It is impossible to sum up or choose a neat anecdote to explain what my therapy sessions with Natasha in the aftermath of physical recovery comprised, because it's been years of therapy, hours and hours of work, one epic, continuous search for truth, meaning and answers, and I can't distinguish one session from another. There have been many 'a-ha' moments, but not one big one. I don't remember the day I figured out what the root cause of my eating disorder was, or discovered a final, resolute commitment to recover fully, for good. I don't think those revelations were contained in moments.

Therapy is not a simple, linear journey, and there's no quick fix to eating disorders. What I do know, hand on heart, is that without those therapy sessions and Natasha's expert, intuitive guidance, my recovery journey after Peaceful Pastures would have been a whole lot messier, and my eating disorder would probably either have flared up again or taken a new shape in the form of some other destructive coping mechanism. Because, as much as I had begun to envision a future for myself without anorexia, that future was still very much a fiction, mere images in my imagination – and when life becomes challenging, it's easy to give up on these fictions, to demote them to infantile fantasies, and to regress and cling to our tried-and-trusted methods of alleviating pain quickly. It's one thing to set your mind on recovery, to conjure the vision, but the journey towards it is beleaguered with obstacles, frightening encounters that might make you lose your nerve and turn back, and it will help immeasurably to find a guide to help you down that path, to bolster your spirit and give you courage when the terrain gets especially rough.

As with everything, though, there were good days and bad days in therapy. It wasn't simply a consistent series of profound spiritual breakthroughs, and it wasn't progress you could chart and visually interpret on a graph. Some days I left Natasha's house buzzing with positive energy, my heart resolutely set on recovery, my spirit reinvigorated and the notion of devoting my life to my skinny ideals having a comical absurdity to it. Sometimes we had deep, heady, mind-blowing conversations about the meaning of life, and I left her living room with armfuls of books – Eckhart Tolle's *A New Earth*, Victor Frankl's *Man's Search for Meaning* or Osho's *Book of*

Secrets – believing myself to be on the verge of true enlightenment. On other days, I found myself mired in grief for anorexia, triggered by something as simple as an oblivious uncle remarking that I looked 'healthy'. On those days, I simply bawled and seethed, swearing to Natasha that I could not give up my eating disorder and railing about how much I hated my parents for leaving me at Peaceful Pastures. Then there were the days I drifted out of therapy in something of a daze, speechless and befuddled, not really knowing who I was or what I felt anymore, responding quite truthfully to my mum's tentative enquiry about how the session went with: 'I really have no idea.'

From the most vapid, shallow aspects of anorexia to its uncharted, deepest depths, we worked through everything as it came up. Recovery is not a neat process. There is no formulaic, one-size-fits-all method to treating eating disorders, as much as hospitals and clinics would like there to be. They're not the ones who have to pick up the pieces and deal with the mess of recovery from their 'rinse-and-repeat' physical rehabilitation programmes.

'It's a very complex thing, as you know,' Natasha agreed as we discussed the complications of treating anorexia when I was interviewing her for this book. 'That's why psychiatrists don't like to touch it, and it's easier to medicate it than it is to sit with the raw pain of "why am I here?" Kids are getting younger with it; they're asking questions of "Why am I here? Who put me here to do what?", and those questions *must* be answered. If they can't find solutions to those questions, they're not going to bother buying into the three-dimensional currencies of food, sex, getting a job: all that stuff just feels rudimentary and pointless, so they don't bother. That's why these people tend to fall between the cracks, because they're not treated properly.'

That, in a nutshell was what we were working on in the aftermath of my disorder, and for several years after; the raw pain of 'why am I here?' It didn't and doesn't have a simple answer to it, but until we began to entertain that question, I really had no interest in recovery. I liked being thin and I liked not feeling worthless anymore, and recovery was an entirely abstract, unappealing concept until I began connecting with some firm reasons for why I wanted to *live* my life, and not simply survive it.

The thing about recovery, though, is that I never explicitly declared, 'Now I'm ready to recover.' For me, that moment never arrived. But Natasha and I had made some agreements once I was out of Peaceful Pastures, a focus point of mutual understanding for the work we were to do together. I agreed that I never wanted to let my anorexia get as bad as it had done before the Farm, and I agreed that I wanted to pursue my dreams. That was the common ground on which we worked together. I never agreed to relinquish my hold on anorexia, and Natasha didn't try and forcibly prise it from my grasp as every other doctor had been intent on doing. Her approach was gently, gently.

'I think initially you can't fully recover because that's too threatening to the host,' she mulled when I asked her about true recovery. Her words called to mind the panic attacks, the sense of oblivion, the heart palpitations triggered by sudden enforced weight gain, and how terrifying that was in the grip of anorexia, how it provoked an urge to fight back. She didn't pressure or bully me into eliminating all my disorderly habits at once, and she didn't punish me or take it personally when I stumbled, from one week to the next, on my road to recovery: she just stayed with me, held space for every feeling, all the fear, anxiety, regret and pain, and made sure, however unsteady I was on my feet, that I just kept going down the path.

Inevitably, one of the most devastating losses of recovery is gaining weight. After Peaceful Pastures, I made a pact with myself to never weigh anything heavier than my target weight on my discharge date at twelve years old. It was bad enough that I'd had to submit to that extent, that I'd let so much be taken from me. Cautiously and from time to time, my mum raised the matter of my target weight and the need to make sure it was increasing every few months to ensure my growth wasn't stunted, but I scoffed at these notions.

'I don't need to grow anymore,' I retorted one day over breakfast, dismissing her concerns promptly. 'I'm already taller than you, aren't I?'

She frowned and pursed her lips as she traced shapes in her toast crumbs with the tip of her index finger, but she dropped the subject and I refused to entertain it any time she tentatively brought it up again. As far as I was concerned, recovery was bearable as long as I ensured my weight stayed in the same place.

But approximately six months after my discharge from Peaceful Pastures, my mum comes to my room and nervously suggests she'd better weigh me, concerned that I am looking 'a bit pale'. I frown and grumble, telling her it is unnecessary, but finding myself flattered by her concern and morbidly curious about my weight, so I follow her downstairs. The worst possible outcome blinks back at me from the scale. I have actually gained one whole kilogram. My breathing shallows. I can't even think. I go back to bed and scream. Like, giving-birth screams. Guttural, anguished screams, muffled only by my duvet. It feels like my life is over, that something I need is being unceremoniously torn from my grasp with the irrevocability of dying. It is just so horribly painful and confusing.

My mums sits on the edge of my bed and tries to offer soothing words, but I just scream back at her that I hate being alive, that she doesn't understand, that I know she wants this, that she is secretly glad I am losing control of my body. Fuck everyone who said they believed in me and loved me and told me my life had intrinsic worth. I don't want their hollow promises or toxic positivity or sentimental twaddle: I just want anorexia back. Eventually, my mum gets to her feet, fed up, and tells me it's fine, I can lose all the weight again and starve to death and she will not interfere anymore.

'It's clearly the only thing in life that makes you happy!' she shouts, her voice trembling, and then she storms out, pulling my bedroom door firmly closed, leaving me alone, my own breathless sobs the only thing rupturing the silence. A moment later, I hear the front door slam and her car crunching down the driveway. She's gone to take my brother to hurling practice, because my siblings have dreams too. They have lives and problems as important and distinct as mine.

I stay in a heap in my bed, sobbing and sniffling, for a long time. The house grows quieter and darker, and I begin to get hungry. The feeling of hunger mocks and offends me. That lovely, empty feeling used to be a reminder of the good I was doing, how well I was correcting myself, an endorsement of my virtuosity, my iron willpower. Hunger used to remind me I was skinny and strong. How can my body dare to be hungry when I am so well fed? How can I be simultaneously hungry and fat? My body is so out of my control, out of sync with the balance I'd previously established, the routine I'd painstakingly created. And I don't know how to get control back over this new and unruly body. By now, I just want *out* of it.

My mum returns from town a couple hours later. I'm still lying in a heap under the covers. After a few minutes, I hear my door gently open.

'Look who came to see you,' my mum croons softly, and I know who it is.

My heart brightens despite myself, and I peek out from above the duvet cocoon and stretch my hands out for my familiar fur-and-whiskered friend, who is twisting energetically in my mum's hands. I sit quietly stroking my cat and admiring her intricately patterned tabby patches as I wipe my nose and sniffle quietly. My head pounds and my eyes itch with soreness from the hangover of crying too hard, but I feel the pain being soothed by this small, velvet bundle who turns around and nestles herself in a neat swirl on the bed, already purring contentedly. My mum and I don't say anything for several minutes as we both sit there, staring at this elegant feline, hypnotised by her purrs. Animals have a stilling power.

'Are you hungry?' my mum asks after some time.

I shake my head stubbornly, no.

'Do you not want some dinner?' she persists.

'No.'

'Well, would you like some cereal instead?'

I hesitate, deliberating. I am hungry and worn out, and breakfast cereal is a safe food. 'OK,' I answer, and I can't stop the tears cascading down my face again. My mum reaches out and hugs me and she holds me for a long time.

For me the post-physical recovery period was probably the loneliest point on the road to recovery, when the physical manifestation of anorexia had all but disappeared, but was still very much alive in my mind. For a long time, I felt confused and misunderstood, still mentally consumed by anorexia, but too ashamed by my physical wellness to keep talking about my recent past. Whenever people online and in the media write about recovery as a strong, brave or empowering experience, the image that comes to mind for me is being thirteen years old, curled like an overgrown baby on my bed, drenched in snot and tears and screaming at my mother that I'm a fat waste of space. It's tempting to believe fairy tales and imagine recovery is this meteoric rise from darkness, but I think it must be stated for the sake of honesty, integrity and solidarity with others going through it, that recovery doesn't feel at all like strength. It feels like giving up, like failing. It feels like lying in a useless lump all weekend, crying about the weight you gained. It feels like the deep shame you carry around all day because you actually can't stop yourself eating anymore. It feels like the maddening conflict of being hungry and healthy. You gaze back at your skinny pictures wondering what happened – was that really you? It was seemingly moments ago, but now you are asking yourself what happened to the girl who would have given her life to be thin. It feels like you're being weak and lazy and surrendering to your own worthlessness. It actually, on many days, feels like you've *lost* a battle.

One day, several months after Peaceful Pastures, I took to frantically rifling through photo stacks, searching for pictures of me at my skinniest. It was like I wanted to resurrect that girl, or check she'd been real. The skinny photos had been another anorexic phenomenon I'd picked up in Peaceful Pastures, where girls kept pictures of themselves at their worst tucked into the pages of diaries, like precious letters from deceased lovers, and took them out with careful fingers and wistful expressions to show to one another. It turned out my mum had hidden or destroyed most of the photos of me at my sickest, but there were a few left, which I dug out and pored over secretly in my room. There was one I was particularly obsessed with, showing me sitting on a wall in the south of France. I'm wearing a crop top, and my arms are like twigs, my face all teeth, my smile stretching the skin taut on my face. After a while, I propped the photo up on my windowsill as a reminder. I needed to remember who I'd been, the lengths I'd gone to for self-improvement, the sacrifices I'd made to fix myself. How *good* I'd once been. I'd look at the picture as time passed, feeling sadness, longing, jealousy, guilt, confusion, grief, wonder. The me in that photo was slipping further and further away. The picture got knocked and crumpled over time. Eventually, the sunlight destroyed it.

9

As the noted philosopher Britney Spears sang on her pop hit 'Circus': 'There's only two types of people in the world/ The ones that entertain and the ones that observe.' The older I get, the more depth and profundity this once fierce, fun, harmless pop-hit invocation acquires for me. By now, it has become a fundamental fact of life; we find our sense of identity either in loving or in being loved. We are the ravisher or the ravishee. If we don't find a place at the epicentre of the action under the dazzling warmth of the spotlight, we will take our seat ringside, in shadow and clutching snacks, to gaze, transfixed, at the story, because life is a series of stories, and whether we show up as entertainer or observer, we are still an integral part of it. So it was that between the ages of twelve and fourteen, when my dreams of edging my way into the centre of the ring weren't quite panning out, I was drawn instead to its peripheries: the silent, silhouetted enclave of the audience, the seat of the faceless voyeur. Or, in plainer, more modern terms: fandom.

After Peaceful Pastures, I found myself grasping for new ways to define myself. Essentially, I'd lost two years of self-development in every area of my life: I had kind friends, but not close ones; I had not bothered with schoolwork in months; I'd missed all the drama exams and was several grades behind my peers; I'd abandoned every other hobby; and the feeling of being determinedly fixated on any goal other than losing weight was a distant memory. I was a blank page, an unwritten script, mentally a child but technically now a teenager, the age when everyone develops interests in obscure genres of music, or when their childhood hobbies tip over into finely honed talents; people get interesting, or they get overlooked. I felt empty and lacking in all the skills and social currencies needed to connect with the people around me.

I tried my best, though. I went back to drama classes. I dyed my hair a screamingly bright shade of blonde and tried to convince everyone it was natural with baby pictures, to convince myself I could carry it off. I kept my weight in a carefully calculated place, eating the same bland and unappetising assortment of foods every day, but eating them nonetheless. I officially switched to vegetarianism, having read and seen too much to ever again regard strips of flesh as food, and now feeling a visceral empathy with the animals held captive on factory farms, whose sole, non-consensual objective in life is to end every day heavier than the last. Vegetarianism did lend me a degree of mental peace around food: I was soothed by the fact that if I couldn't control and curtail my own body, at least I wasn't eating someone else's. It also felt good to take a stance on something greater than myself, and to have developed what felt almost like an interesting personality trait. And yet, despite all my efforts, my desperate stabs at personhood, I was still keenly aware of all the gaps that anorexia had previously filled. Readjusting to society after anorexia felt something like being an alien, except that at least an alien would have been equipped with cool stories to share from their exotic planet. I couldn't talk about *my* exotic planet, because it triggered me and other people; it always came across as self-indulgent and attention-seeking. I also knew it would invite immediate scrutiny of my current size from people searching for verification of my unlikely tale. So, I didn't share what I was feeling or thinking with others, these thoughts that were consuming me, and I sat there, blank and wordless, whenever I met new people, as their conversations whirled around me.

Nature abhors a vacuum, however, and I quickly had to fill the void where there should have been a personality with something distracting. Though in many ways I was doing better now, my self-esteem was as low as it had ever been, and I did not know where to begin in trying to improve myself. I was worn out from the struggle of the past two years – with my parents, with the doctors, with my own warring impulses to recover one moment and starve the next – and I simply didn't have the will to find a new redeeming feature, something to love about myself. Self-love wasn't a real thing anyway. It was a marketing term: idealistic New Age garbage, as far as I was concerned. Self-acceptance was unlikely. My newest strategy for coping with being alive was all about disengaging from the self and putting my love and energy into others. Thus, a fangirl was born!

It's not that all fans are trying to fill a void; it's quite possible to be a fan of someone, to admire them and follow their work, while remaining an empowered, self-possessed, dignified individual. But when you are young, insecure and lack a distinct sense of self, I think that's when admiration for another – typically someone far away and who is mythically aspirational, someone who it is socially acceptable to worship – can quickly balloon into obsession. I think it's quite rare to meet an obsessive fan who doesn't have a deep-seated inferiority complex. I see this relationship as dysfunctional, but I don't see it as unacceptable. It has its place and purpose in life: loving someone else can keep you alive at times when it's impossible to love yourself. And sometimes, in loving someone else, you become a better version of yourself, someone who you still may not love, but might, to a certain extent, come to like. My shamanic teacher, a fabulous, wise, redheaded Irish lady named Catherine (who I work with nowadays and for whom I can think of no more accurate term to describe our relationship than 'spiritual fairy godmother'), has a theory on this: 'If you spot it, you've got it,' she continues to remind me in moments of too much jealousy or awe for another person. She means that when something or someone else captivates you to the point of distraction, it is because they are reflecting something within you that is longing to be expressed. There's something about them that is calling forth an undiscovered part of you. This can be hard to believe when you're a pale, shy, nondescript thirteen-year-old gazing adoringly at glamorous celebrities with gleaming skin and a charisma that suggests they were born better than everyone else. It is much more comfortable to just bow your head in shame and adulation and ascribe them an innate, God-given superiority. But there is more to the story if you see that the people you revere are mirroring hidden pieces of you.

The problem with fan culture is that people can get stuck in the place of always being a fan, of revering flawed human beings, and of never turning inwards to fix their own problems. Because even if (unlike Britney, our glorious, ephemeral princess of pop) you're not an entertainer by trade, there will be aspects of your life where you have to step out of the shadows, take centre stage and show up fully. You can't spend your entire life on the peripheries of the lives of others. At thirteen, however, I was not ready to address my problems, so I poured all my love and sense of self into those who were easy to love, people who were confident, beautiful, interesting, funny, charismatic and worthy of all the attention paid to them. And above all other celebrities, books and movies, I poured myself into the world of Harry Potter. Here was a space I saw myself belonging to, seamlessly. These were my people, these witches and wizards. They were smart, conscientious, weird kids, like me, the only significant difference being that they had magical powers. After a while, though, the *Harry Potter* books were not enough to fuel my appetite (these were the days where we had to wait years at a time for the next book instalment, and heated debates raged over whether Snape was good or evil). My obsession with the *Harry Potter* characters bled into their muggle counterparts, the actors who I hoped and imagined were just like the characters they portrayed, who would be my instant best friends if only we had the opportunity to meet. 'Weird *Harry Potter* girl' became a pejorative I got used to hearing muttered along school corridors or by the cool kids in drama class whenever I passed – and I didn't object. I was thrilled to be my community's go-to *Harry Potter* resource, and I took to the role with feverish enthusiasm. I papered my bedroom from floor to ceiling with posters of J. K. Rowling and the *Harry Potter* actors. I read the books over and over, frowning distastefully at the library books my mum would leave at the end of my bed, offended by the fact that people even bothered writing other books. I spent hours trawling the online fan forums for good fanfiction and interesting theories about Harry's fate. It's *very* lucky I was cast before I turned sixteen, or I might have had Daniel Radcliffe's autograph – which I possessed, obviously – tattooed on some intimate region of my body.

Still, Luna remained the character I loved most of all. I'd been captivated by her from the moment she'd appeared on the pages of *Order of the Phoenix*, and my love for her had only grown since. She was different to the other characters, who I was fascinated and enthralled by, but more distantly so. I was curiously challenged by Luna's presence each time she showed up, just as I had been on that first meeting in hospital. Somehow, I was simultaneously calmed by her and made distinctly conscious of myself. Her beautifully serene disposition always prodded at the edges of my consciousness. I longed to be like her, but could never allow myself to relax into the most core, fundamental aspect of her being: her capacity for self-acceptance, which stretched itself into an ability to let everyone and everything – nature itself – just *be*. She allowed people and things to be just as they were, regarding and appreciating them in precisely that moment, that place. Where Luna blossomed and leaned into her natural, unaltered oddness, never tempering or muting it for the comfort or approval of others, I worked furiously to cover myself up with whatever resources were at hand – thinness, *Harry Potter*, aggressive hair dye, even a regrettable fake tan phase. I just could not trust myself to be as I was, even as I watched Luna do it and be wonderful at it.

I continued to send letters to my kind friend Jo, who was also J. K. Rowling, and who consistently handwrote her incredible, wise letters after the relapse, throughout my time at Peaceful Pastures and every few months after that, offering me endless support, empathy and encouragement at every juncture. She never judged or expressed disappointment when I confessed to having doubts about recovery and struggling with anorexic thoughts, and she always urged me forwards on the path of my dreams. I'd told her by now that my dream was to be an actor, and specifically to play Luna Lovegood, and she encouraged me to write to the casting director, even providing a postal address, to which I sent letters and a tape of myself performing a few truncated Luna scenes from the books. These had been filmed with my dad's video camera, and two of my most long-suffering friends, Joanna and Amy, played Harry, Ron, Hermione, Neville and Ginny interchangeably, with the help of some heavy-handed editing. The *Philosopher's Stone* soundtrack played on a CD player in the background, jumping forward a few bars with every camera transition because I hadn't factored in how editing would butcher our live score. The casting directors wrote back a polite response, thanking me for my letters, but gently pointing out the fact that nationality played a significant part in casting, a rude reminder of my inescapable Irishness, an oddness I would never quite erase.

And then, in November 2005, I watched a live link to the premiere of the *Goblet of Fire* movie from my dad's small, windowless computer room via Mugglenet (my go-to *Harry Potter* website) as the actors – who seemed to get more glowy and attractive with each passing year – stepped out of shiny black cars to the cacophonous din of hordes of fans clamouring at the railings lining Leicester Square. I watched as an interviewer quizzed David Heyman, the producer, about pre-production for *Order of the Phoenix* and whether or not they'd found an actress for Luna, and I listened as he said, 'We've narrowed it down to a few, but we haven't yet cast her,' and later revealed that they had found five finalists, five final potential girls waiting in the wings to steal my dream. I watched until the end of the premiere coverage, after the last actor had trailed into the movie theatre, extinguishing all the glitz and glamour at once, leaving only rain and some drenched, discombobulated fans, and then I shut down the computer, not devastated by what I'd heard, but feeling glum, deflated. The dream was dead now. The part would go to someone else, one of those five girls, someone who was glowy and classically trained, who gave a very convincing impression of oddness, but inherently was not.

Then, out of nowhere, things got interesting.

One day after school in January 2006, I log on to my dad's computer and type 'Mugglenet.com' into the address bar, a ritual that by now has the routine familiarity of blessing oneself, to catch up on today's *Harry Potter* headlines. I know the bad news will be coming any day now – they are due to start filming in February – and I brace myself for her name. The name of the person who I will unequivocally hate. But her name never comes, and instead I blink, disbelieving, at a headline that reads 'Open Casting Call for Luna Lovegood'. Beneath it is a short article detailing the requirements for any young hopefuls wishing to audition for Luna. The auditions will be held on Saturday morning in Westminster. Girls between the ages of thirteen and sixteen can apply, and must have a valid passport. No acting experience is necessary, and they will see anyone fitting the age range from the UK, and – crucially – Ireland.

'MAAAAAAAMMM!' I screech, tearing from the computer room and through the kitchen, startling my mum as she enters the living room carrying several bags of groceries. 'Guesswhatguesswhatguesswhat!' I exclaim, my heart beating fast, and tell her the good news.

'Oh,' she replies, her eyes darkening, an expression of concern creasing her brow. She is considerably less excited by this glorious news than I am. For some reason, she doesn't seem to realise what a pivotal moment this is, doesn't seem to grasp that this is the precise opportunity we've been waiting for. 'Let's wait and see what Dad says when he's home.'

All evening, I debate with my parents. I'm fourteen, my mum points out, with lots of schoolwork and no professional acting experience. The flights are expensive at such short notice, my dad muses, sitting at the computer and clicking through Ryanair's options as he strokes his chin. The chances are very slim, my mum says. But I don't need multiple chances, I tell her, I just need one.

'I think we should go for it!' my dad declares, as he scans the Mugglenet casting notice once more and then turns to me, a jubilant glint in his eye. A sporting man and passionate Limerick hurling supporter, his spirits are always roused by an outlandish quest. A battle, a match, a chance to prove one's mettle, always brings a boyish glee to his features, and I can sense his excitement at the prospect of this reckless, brave and foolhardy mission. He loves an unlikely dream, a daring heart, the hopeful though ill-fated hero. He books two plane tickets – one for me and one for him – for Friday night, and a tiny room in a B&B with bunkbeds, and claps his hands together happily in anticipation of our bold adventure.

My mum had reservations though, as she tried to communicate to Dad in an anguished whisper. She was quoted in the paper shortly after my casting as having said I had 'a snowball's chance in hell, Donal,' a quote that pains her, but which she really did say. It was not, however (she has since been keen to clarify), because she thought her child was a useless waste of space, but simply out of concern for how I would handle it if I didn't get the part in my favourite movie series of all time. She was worried I was too fragile mentally, that I might not recover from that particular setback, and thought it would be preferable for me to stay at home, not get the part, and not face the unbearable reality of having my favourite thing, my one safe place, my heart, my home, look me in the eye and say, 'Thanks, but no thanks.' And she was right. *Harry Potter* would have been ruined for me. The magical world would have been irrevocably tainted by their rejection of me and the solid proof that it did not need me the way I needed it. Oh, it would have been awful! If I think about that possibility too long, I seriously start to believe that it would have been wiser to stay home on the couch, read my books, be sad but not crushed, and carry on safely on the sheltered side of the screen. The risk was terrifying, given the odds. But you have to put yourself out there for these things; you have to be foolish and idealistic and take risks. You have to try.

It was a curiously egoless mission for me. I'm not someone who lacks ego, clearly, given that my egoic obsession with thinness had almost consumed me, and I had been searching frantically for new methods of self-affirmation ever since, but this was different. I was strangely calm on the flight over to London and as we paced the streets of Westminster on Friday night to scope out the location for the morning. I was excited, sure, about the adventure we were on and about the prospect of manifesting my wildest dream, but I went to that audition in service of a character who I adored and was fiercely determined to protect. She was not just some role, an opportunity of a lifetime, a career boost or even a chance to go to Hogwarts – Luna was special. She was spiritual. She was joyful and colourful. She was a bright spot of light in the darkest night, for me, and undoubtedly for countless others. She had a legacy of kindness, curiosity and presence in every moment. She was not a costume you put on or a character you 'played' for accolades or financial retribution. She was someone you gave yourself up to, someone you stepped aside for so she could shine out. She was a human *being* and not a human *doing*, so hers wasn't a role you could *do* or act; you had to put yourself away and let her be. I felt sure that most actresses wouldn't understand this about Luna, however, wouldn't realise how special and important her spirit was, would try to 'do' the role – and might do so proficiently – but it wouldn't be enough. So, as we rolled up in a taxi to the Methodist hall where the audition was taking place, to throngs and throngs of excited, babbling young girls and their bleary-eyed parents already lining the surrounding streets, and made our way to the very back of the line, which was lengthening with each passing minute, I felt calm and untroubled, because I was there for Luna, to protect her legacy, her loveliness, and that was something so much bigger and more vital than just showing up for me.

We queue for four hours, slowly inching our way towards the entrance. The mood is chaotic and exuberant, with girls jostling for attention in front of TV crews, posing, dancing and recounting their lifelong dream to be in a *Harry Potter* movie. My dad is thrilled by it all, the professional slickness of the operation and the energetic hubbub, and he takes breaks from our spot in line to walk the length of the queue with his digital camera, documenting the whole experience. Meanwhile, I keep my head down, reading *Order of the Phoenix*, reconnecting with Luna's spirit and wondering which scenes they might choose.

Dad comes back and gets talking to the lady in front of us, Vanessa, and her daughter, Daisy, a shy blonde who confesses to being a *Harry Potter* mega fan. My dad and Vanessa pass the time trading stories of their daughters' *Harry Potter* mania, and then Dad presses her with a series of questions about her lineage until he finds an Irish great-grandparent, which satisfies him. ('If you ask a person enough questions, you'll always find an Irish connection,' is a theory of his that – amazingly – has yet to be disproven.) It's clear from the rowdy atmosphere in the queue that most of the girls lining up probably had no idea who Luna Lovegood was a week ago, or at least have not read the books very closely. The girls are mostly loud, confident, bolshy teens, breaking into songs and chants at random, much more suited to *The X Factor* than a *Harry Potter* film. But every few metres, my eyes land on a distinct oddball, dressed in rainbow hemp with long, loose braids, and I know my chances are largely riding on some shaky, whimsical good luck. I feel mildly threatened by shy, sweet Daisy in front of me, with her shoulder-length dirty blond hair and her calm disposition, but there is no need, for when we finally get to the front of the line, just before noon, and submit our passports, she is outed as being six months away from her thirteenth birthday and therefore ineligible to audition. Her mother begs for a little leeway as tears spring to Daisy's eyes, but the registrant is merciless, shaking his head firmly and asserting that the audition terms had been clear. He insists they step out of the queue. Lucky fourteen-year-old me waltzes through the large doors, waving cheerily to my dad, who is told to go to the exit on the other side of the building and wait for me there.

'Good luck!' he calls, his face bright and merry, as he fist-pumps in my direction. I reply with two determined thumbs up.

The audition process is ruthlessly efficient. Squealing teenage girls are shepherded in groups of thirty or forty into a large room with a stage and told to line up in front of it. Two women pace back and forth across the stage, scanning our faces with studious intent. They ask us to step forward, one at a time, and to say our name and where we came from, and this is when I get nervous. This part has nothing to do with talent or passion or *Harry Potter* trivia; this is the moment cold, hard snap decisions will be made based on the cruel inequalities of height, size and looks. My heart is hammering so loudly in my head I'm not sure if they can hear me speak, but they must do, because a moment later the two ladies whisper behind their hands and then point towards me precisely, along with three other girls, directing us through a doorway to our right. They politely thank the thirty or so other confused girls for their time, directing them through a separate door and wishing them a lovely day. Proud, loud would-be thespians with crystal-clear received pronunciation don't fare well in this process, shuffling away looking highly affronted. Neither do tall girls, who slope off sadly with their shoulders hunched. But their impediment today brings its own exclusive set of blessings – access to top shelves, excellent views at music concerts and modelling careers – so I don't feel too sorry for them. They don't need Luna like I do.

Our heights are recorded in the next room (my fangirl knowledge tells me I am shorter than Daniel Radcliffe – a fact I know because these are the kinds of details you research about your ideal future husband – and I also know this bodes well for me in the audition) and then we are each given a series of pages. These, I quickly realise, my heart leaping in disbelief, are actual scenes from the top-secret *Order of the Phoenix* film script, the scene where Harry happens upon Luna in the Forbidden Forest feeding thestrals. We are told to learn them to the best of our ability, and that we will be called one by one into the room to read the scene with the casting director. There are about a dozen girls sitting in a small room with chairs, clutching pages, chattering excitedly to each other about having made it this far, comparing notes on the scene, and discussing their acting experience – but I don't join in, because I am in Luna-mode, and that means I don't have to try. I don't have to impress anyone or prove my worth or earn their friendship; I just have to *be*. I sit quietly, taking in the scene, the words feeling as familiar as a child-hood nursery rhyme, and relax. Then I watch the other girls chat for a while, enjoying their excitement, appreciating their paisley skirts and spangly earrings, a multi-coloured tribe of Luna devotees. It is so easy to be Luna – so much easier than being me. All you have to do is breathe and surrender control, because no matter what you do as Luna, you will be OK.

'You're so like Luna,' one girl announces, calling me out of my daydreams in the Forbidden Forest. Her shrewd eyes search my face. 'I bet they'll like you.'

She has curly brown hair and a pretty smattering of freckles. She looks like Hermione in a polka-dot dress. I smile and thank her, accepting the compliment. That's something you can do as Luna: accept a compliment. You don't have to question its veracity or worry about whether you've earned it; and you don't have to fret about doling out a compliment in return, or what the person will think of you if you don't. It's just an observation, a simple gift, uncondition-ally given, more a symptom of the other person's generous nature than anything concerning you.

Fifteen minutes later, my name is called, and I follow a smiling, dark-haired lady into another large, empty room with huge arched windows. In the middle of it, two seats face each other, and there is a man with a video camera. The lady, Alice, asks me to read the scenes and to ignore the camera, staying 'out of the page' as much as possible. We read the scene. We read it again. Alice is smiling as she asks me what it is I like about Luna, and I tell her it's her open-mindedness, that she doesn't judge anyone and instead appreciates their differences. We read the scene again. Being Luna is as natural as breathing – and, more than that, it's a relief. I just have to relax, breathe, and there she is. Alice asks me to wait a couple of minutes as she goes to fetch 'Fiona' – a name I instantly recognise from the *Harry Potter* casting team. Fiona Weir is the casting director I've been sending letters to for several months, and I start to worry that she will recognise me from my dodgy tape and immediately dismiss me. Alice returns a few minutes later with one of the two ladies who'd picked me out from the stage. This is Fiona, a slim, attractive caramel-haired lady with a piercing green gaze. When she looks at me, it's like being X-rayed, but not in a way that feels like a violation. She stands back, clutching a mug to her chest with one hand and surveys me, head tilted, as I read the scene with Alice again. I feel myself getting nervous now. Under Fiona's watchful gaze, it feels like I have something to prove. Luna is slipping away, but I press on anyway. I read the scene twice for Fiona and then she thanks me, a pensive look on her face, and tells me they'll give me a call. I smile and thank them, then drift towards the door, unsure how to walk, but somehow I manage. I know that 'We'll call you' is something people say to actors when they don't intend to call them, but then what would she have said if she *was* going to call? At the exit, my dad takes me by surprise with an expression of wild panic, a very uncharacteristic state of being for him.

'You were in there ages!' he exclaims, momentarily grasping my shoulders as though to check all of me had made it out of the Methodist hall. 'Every other girl went in and came back out, and still no sign of you! I was about to go to the police!'

All sense of time had escaped me in the audition room, and I take Dad's account as a sign the audition has gone well. We step out into the sunlight, Dad declaring that he needs a large whiskey, and leave the Methodist hall behind, with hundreds of potential Lunas still filing into it.

As it turned out, they did call me – two days later, on Monday after school. The director and producers had loved my tape, Fiona told me, a smile in her voice, and they wanted to see me for a screen test on Friday. My parents watched me, wide-eyed, as I nodded along with Fiona's instructions and then called out my dad's email address for her to pass on to the transport coordinator. There would be no cheap-and-cheerful Ryanair flights this time: Warner Bros. were set to cover the entire trip, which felt absurd given that I would have quite happily donated a kidney to be able to merely visit the *Harry Potter* sets. Then Fiona asked me if it was OK for David Yates, the director, to give me a call. His was another name that, just one week before, I had been stalking on Mugglenet.

David called me that evening as I sat in my bedroom, feeling overwhelmed and dizzy. He was soft-spoken, his voice a hair above a friendly whisper, and reassuring. He reiterated Fiona's statement that he had loved my audition and was looking forward to meeting me on Friday. They would send me some audition materials to learn in advance, and we would spend the day working on scenes with 'Dan', as he called him, and I mentally noted that I would be in a setting with Daniel Radcliffe, where standing and screaming directly at him would probably scupper my chance of working with him, so it would be imperative to repress my inner fangirl. I had no idea how sincere they were about their interest in me, how many other girls would be there, or what had happened to the famous five who had got so close but not quite clinched the role. Would we all be there together, sitting in a green room locked in some surreal psychological experiment to out-Luna each other, staring into space and humming dreamily to ourselves as producers secretly watched behind screens? I dared not ask.

Dad and I take the day off on Friday, him confiding our expedition only to the principal of our school and the convent of nuns attached to it, asking them to pray on it. He insists that it's safe to divulge this news to the sisters; they are holy women, they are not about to alert the press. A smart black car rolls up the driveway at 6am in the near darkness, and an equally smart suited man steps out to greet us and to fit our shared suitcase into the boot. Mum waves us off from behind the door, trying to shield her pyjamas from the polished chauffeur, and Dad makes cheerful conversation with Brian, the driver, all the way to the airport as I sit quietly in the back reading my lines over and over, though by now I could easily recite them in my sleep. We have first-class seats on the British Airways flight, a completely novel experience for both of us. Dad hoots with laughter and loudly mocks the notion of a 'hot towel', but accepts every snack and drink on offer, stuffing the uneaten sandwich and salted pretzels I try to refuse into his black backpack 'for later'. He grumbles on the way out of the airport as shiny-haired, sharp-shouldered businessmen zip past us, their hard-shelled suitcases seeming to sprout wheels like an airplane landing on the tarmac as they glide along, loath to waste even one moment fumbling with a suitcase. 'Right yuppies,' Dad calls them, giggling away at their four-wheeled suitcases rolling neatly along beside them like show ponies, deeming them pretentious and silly.

He hoists our suitcase off the conveyor belt, a large, worn, cumbersome item that has two wheels – one of them broken – and does none of the work for you, and drags it proudly into the arrivals hall, where another suited man with a neat haircut and a sign that reads 'LYNCH' awaits us, statuesque. In this world, everyone is always clean, coiffed and prompt. The driver greets us perfunctorily and snatches the bag from my dad, his professionalism not slipping for a second as he smoothly readjusts his grip on the handle to accommodate the wonky wheel. He leaves us by the lift and instructs us to meet him on the fourth floor. By the time we have stepped out of the lift, he has already whizzed around in a shiny Mercedes to meet us, and is stepping out to open the car doors. London, baby! The London of film sets and cosmopolitan class, not of diabolical eating disorder incarceration centres, that is. Thank fuck.

My day at Leavesden Studios passes in a haze of names and faces that I know intimately, but who do not know me. Our first stop is the office belonging to the two producers, David Heyman and David Barron, who I instantly recognise from press junkets and DVD extras. David Heyman is tanned and ruggedly handsome, in a brown shearling coat, while David Barron has a round face and bright, protuberant eyes, and wears a white round-neck T-shirt under a navy-blue knitted jumper. They are as different as night and day, David Heyman leaning casually against the doorframe of his office as David Barron crosses his arms tightly across his chest and nods eagerly throughout the conversation. Immediately, they feel like uncles. They ask me about schoolwork and my love of *Harry Potter*, and I tell them about my hobbies, my favourite subjects at school, my affinity with Luna, my relationship with the *Harry Potter* books. I tell them everything except for one crucial detail: I don't mention my friendship with J. K. Rowling, because there is no way to explain to them our connection without also explaining the context of our correspondence and the fact that I have a terrible dark side, a snide, cruel voice in my head that overshadows everything and that betrays me as the absolute antithesis of Luna. No, I cannot tell them that. And luckily, there is no need – why would they ever suspect? Moments later, I am whisked off to the costume department to be outfitted in a Luna Lovegood-esque ensemble.

Jany, the costume designer, is French, elegant and disarmingly blunt. 'You are my *fav-ar-eet*,' she tells me with a wave of her hand, my first clue that I am one of several girls, as she adjusts the collar of a blue floral-patterned blouse on me. 'I told the Davids that you are 'er,' she tells me, and there is a finality to her tone that suggests her opinion is always the correct answer. She admires my handmade beaded earrings (two bright pink pigs with transparent wings, which I chose that morning as a symbol of impossible dreams being realised) and insists that I keep them on for the screen test, then she sends me off to hair and make-up in the dark blue patterned blouse, a purple skirt and midnight-blue tights.

In the hair and make-up department, I am at once accosted by a pair of enormous, startlingly blue eyes – Daniel Radcliffe, who introduces himself as Dan, warmly shaking my limp hand. Somehow, I manage not to pass out. The exchange only lasts a couple of minutes, pleasantries exchanged, and then my dad takes over the conversation, so I have a moment to just stand and admire Dan before I am wafted urgently into make-up and Dan tells me he'll see me down on set. A make-up artist dusts some powders on my face, saying Luna would be 'natural, natural', and then a hairdresser fluffs out my hair, winces at the feathery bleached ends, and decides to just pull it back off my face.

Next thing I know, I'm hurtling through Leavesden Studios on a golf cart. My dad sits up front next to a runner, and I am sitting beside Dan, who has gamely taken on the Trojan task of making me feel at ease. Suddenly I find myself in the unprecedented position of struggling to keep my attention on Daniel Radcliffe, because all around me pieces of the magical world are whizzing by my eyeline – a giant chess piece here, a Privet Drive sign there – but I really want this job, so I force myself to be still and focus on the individual around which this entire world orbits. It is so weird to see him talking back to me, neither a screen, a poster nor a neatly accessible figment of my imagination, but a real person with thoughts and reactions entirely his own, and it is hard not to gape and just let him talk, as he does in the films I've watched too many times. He has a nervous disposition, one foot jigging energetically (a habit I will always notice), and his hands tap a rhythm on his kneecaps as though his body is a percussive instrument. But he listens attentively and answers my questions. Questions are about all I can manage. An underlying terror of silence – and about what will happen if he asks me about *me* – keeps me talking – and luckily I have lots of questions. I ask him about his day, about the *Order of the Phoenix* script, about the studio, about his clean, cropped new haircut and the thinking behind the polarising shaggy mops all the boys sported in *Goblet of Fire*. I have the fangirl thirst for microscopic details that conveniently disguises the fact I can't make conversation. And today I am Luna,

I remind myself. It is OK for me to sit back, breathe and appreciate other people. There is no need to do, I need only be.

The screen test takes place in Dumbledore's office, a tall set composed of two circular rooms in the shape of a figure of eight, which has an atmosphere of otherworldly stillness, despite the hustle and bustle of a film crew preparing for action. The cupboards and bookcases lining the walls are filled with trinkets and dusty, jewel-toned books with gold lettering on the spines. These, David Barron proudly shows me, pulling down a hefty green tome and flicking through it, are real books. David Yates appears a moment later, greeting me enthusiastically and patting me lightly on the shoulder. He pulls out the scene for today, where Harry comes upon Luna with the thestrals in the forest, and we exchange ideas on what Luna might be doing in the forest by herself, her relationship with the thestrals, and what she makes of the famous Harry Potter. David calls me 'mate' a lot, which makes me feel less like a competition winner and more like a crew member, and gives me the confidence to voice the private thoughts and ideas about Luna that have lived in me for so long. He asks lots of questions and nods along thoughtfully to my answers. He is nothing like the image that comes to mind with the word 'director', which has always made me think of a loud, commanding, boorish presence foisting opinions and life experiences on to the hapless actors to obediently interpret. David is quiet, considerate and deeply curious, positing intriguing questions, prodding thoughts from me and triggering realisations that I hadn't quite articulated outside my own head. He beckons Dan over to join our sacred huddle and we talk a bit more about Luna's relationship with Harry and what it is they're really saying to each other in these scenes. Luna, I will later learn when playing less spiritually evolved characters, is easy to interpret thanks to her completely unique lack of subtext; she always speaks what she feels without a slyly disguised motive, so the work is simply to hold that truth in the face of others' plain discomfort.

We start filming, sitting on two chairs in Dumbledore's office, and the afternoon takes on that unusual timeless quality that I'd experienced in the first audition. We work through the scenes, moment by moment, pausing every now and then between takes to huddle again and mine for a deeper truth, the subtlest moments of understanding. *These huddles are where I want to spend my whole life*, I think, gathered together with other curious souls, unravelling stories and discussing the secret inner lives of beloved characters, like children in the playground inventing fantasy lands in whispers behind our hands while the adults work diligently around us, erecting the scaffolding and making the world safe to explore. Between scenes, I drift over to the producer-Davids, asking them how they intend to create thestrals, where they stand on the Snape is good/evil debate, and whether they've been told the ending to the final book. David Heyman speaks with captivating passion about the books, keenly cognisant of every minute detail of the magical world that I mention, and he gives compassionate explanations for why they had to cut precious moments from the books, like S. P. E. W. and Winky and Sir Cadogan. Silently, I vow to never again bitch about the filmmakers' editorial choices on the Mugglenet fan forums. At one point, David Barron wanders over to me, chuckling, and brings up a moment from my first audition last Saturday, where I told Alice that failing to cast me as Luna would be a mistake on their part, and he asks me to expand on that. I consider the question for a few moments, mulling silently as I gaze at a large bronze instrument depicting the solar system by Dumbledore's desk.

'I won't bear a grudge towards you,' I tell him, perhaps only half truthfully. 'But I will think you've made the wrong choice. I know who Luna is in my heart, and if you pick someone else, you'll be picking a different version of Luna, but it won't be the true Luna, as I know her.'

David smiles and nods, his eyes twinkling. It's a bold answer, one that could have landed badly, but it hasn't come from a place of temerity or cheek. It's just a feeling in my heart: that I have been called to show up and protect this character, that I know who Luna is, and I can offer them no more or less. And though I know that being rejected by them would be wholly devastating, and that I might never get through another *Harry Potter* book or film without dissolving into tears, I do also know that if they don't pick me, it actually won't be personal, or because of some inherent lack in me; it will simply be a difference of opinion. It's a choice I will respectfully disagree with. Perhaps this is how every fan feels about their favourite characters; perhaps there is no one true Luna or Harry or Hermione. Perhaps that is the private magic of books.

All too soon, we have completed the scenes, David giving one small, satisfied bunny hop on the spot (an idiosyncrasy of his I will come to look for after each scene), and Dan is released to make his way to other departments, who are jostling for a few minutes of his time. I am suddenly aware that I am just one of many appointments in his day, that he fully inhabits this world, has dozens of costumes to try on, rehearsals to attend, posters to sign – and probably several other Lunas to meet. He shakes my hand firmly again and tells me it was a pleasure to meet me, while my inner fangirl screams at me to ask him for a lock of his hair, or to simply reach out and yank it from his scalp. She has been so good all day, but I need her to behave a little longer, so, sternly, I tell her that she will have much greater access to stray locks of Daniel Radcliffe's hair if we manage to maintain this professional facade for the rest of the day and get the role. I thank him politely and tell him it was an honour to meet him, and he, his arctic blue eyes and all of his hair disappear around the corner of Dumbledore's office.

After that, David says he'd like to do an improv with me as Luna, an exercise I'm not prepared for, and I can feel Luna slipping away again as the urge to try very hard and manipulate the situation in my favour kicks in, because I know I have mere minutes left to realise this dream. In a few moments, the director and producers will tear their undivided focus away from me for the day, and maybe forever, and it is just impossible not to try under those circumstances. I decide to keep it simple, though, sitting on the steps and taking in some articles in a *Daily Prophet* prop they've handed to me, then wandering aimlessly around Dumbledore's office, tracing my fingers along his collection of brass and silver ornaments. Just as I am getting lost in a peculiar skipping game across the tiles of the office, David Yates says, 'Cut there,' and calls it a day. The improv didn't last very long, and I feel anxious and awkward suddenly, sure that I've ruined it now, having wasted precious and expensive minutes of these important people's lives playing a stupid skipping game. The lighting and camera tracks are already being dismantled with expert speed as I thank the Davids and say goodbye, once more firmly stifling the inner fangirl, who is weeping by now and pleading with me to latch on to David Yates's leg and implore him to keep me, to never send me home. In the wardrobe department, they give me back my weird muggle clothes, which I had bought especially for this occasion just two days ago, but now no longer want, and de-Luna me, stripping me of her every piece – her shoes, her clothes, her hairclips – everything except my winged pigs, which I keep on. And next thing I know, I am sitting beside my dad in another shiny black car, watching Leavesden Studios fade away in the rear-view mirror, feeling empty and clutching a new copy of *Order of the Phoenix* that the assistant director had handed to me on the way out as a gift from David Yates.

I open the front cover of the book and read the short inscription he has written to me: 'Dear Evanna, you did a great job today! Love, David.' I feel insulted by the assumption that I don't already own three copies of *Order of the Phoenix*, and devastated by his short message, which reads as unbearably patronising to me. And, quite unlike the Luna Lovegood scenes, these words seem heavily laced with subtext, which I comb through assiduously for the next couple of hours in the lavish hotel room that Warner Bros. has booked me for this evening. 'Have a nice life!' is one casually cutting interpretation of his words, whereas if you put the emphasis on 'today', he seems to be urging me to forget a career in the movies and never act again. A slightly crueller, though not entirely irrational reading of his message is: 'You are a nuisance who wasted my very valuable and precious time, but I don't want you to talk badly of me in the dungeon of fandom whence you came, so here is a meaningless gift with my signature that you can probably sell on eBay for a tidy little sum that you will inevitably splurge on more *Harry Potter* merchandise.' It ruins me for the evening, that humble, harmless message, and I hurl the book into my suitcase carelessly, because I know if I don't get the role, I will have no choice but to burn it.

The room is the largest and grandest hotel room I've ever been in, the bed big enough for the entire Dumbledore's office crew to climb aboard and have a picnic, if only I'd thought to invite them, but I am alone, so I curl up on the topmost corner of it and cry myself to sleep.

The next morning, Dad and I are ferried home by more pine-scented cars and impassive men in suits, and I embark on the longest weekend of my entire life. I spend most of it having increasingly unhinged private conversations with God, running through the list of things I would be willing to do in exchange for this part – six months in Peaceful Pastures, sacrifice a kitten, shave my head, become a nun – and promising the havoc I will wreak if it is denied me – convert to a pantheistic religion, egg a church, murder an up-and-coming young actress, starve.

By Monday, I am done, I am over it. I just want them to hit me with the bad news and let me get on with my miserable little life. I keep my phone on silent in my pocket during the school day, checking it discreetly behind piles of books at three-minute intervals to see if they've called me. After school, I insist, a note of terrifying hysteria in my voice, that we go straight home, because I am utterly convinced that if they call the house phone and nobody answers, they will think me quite uninterested in the role, shrug their shoulders and offer it to the next girl on the list, who will wisely be sitting with the phone nestled between her thighs like an egg about to hatch. On the way home, my mum tentatively says that she just needs to 'pop' into the shop – 'Just some bread and milk, please!' – so I tell her that *I* will go into the shop and get *only* bread and milk, lest she go in, meet half the village, get talking and lose me the part. Just as I am pacing the bakery section scanning for seeded brown bread, my phone rings.

It's Fiona Weir.

'Can you go somewhere where there are not a million people looking at you?' she asks, her voice warm and playful.

'Yep,' I answer, and I step out into the sunlight in front of Londis.

'We want you to be our Luna,' Fiona tells me, and I lock eyes with my mum and sister in the car, who are watching me, frozen and wide-eyed, and I give them a feeble thumbs up, and I honestly don't remember much after that, except that we forgot to get the bread and milk, and I went home and did my French homework because that was about all I could process that evening. It had happened. The role was mine. The thing that I had spotted, I had got.

Life changes dramatically after that moment. In less than ten days, I have quite literally gone from gazing adoringly at my cherished idols from my dad's computer to working with them in the flesh as a verified member of the cast. At the readthrough a week later, their faces loom at me in full 3D, complete with pores and imperfections rather than polished and deftly shaded smooth, shiny black posters that adorn my bedroom wall. I could even smell them if I wish, though I curtail that particular impulse.

I meet a cluster of them in the corridor that holds all the dressing rooms – Katie, Bonnie and Matt, who play Cho Chang, Ginny Weasley and Neville Longbottom respectively – and smile shyly at each of them, trying not to stare. The girls have such neat, symmetrical, pretty features, such thick and glossy hair, while Matt is already a towering, glowering teenager, wearing Ray-Bans indoors and clutching a coffee cup. Not ten days previous, if I had met any one of them in public, I would have bowed deeply and unironically, and asked them to sign my arm, and there would have been a protective metal barrier between us. They are all so nice to me, tentative in their approach, as though not to frighten me, nodding politely at my mum and I, and making friendly conversation about our journey from Ireland. I get the sense that someone has warned them I am a fangirl, that I'll practically be salivating in their presence, and that it would help if they could do their bit to welcome me into the fold. They ask me where in Ireland I'm from, and then mentally scan their respective family trees, claiming to have a distant relative from Wicklow, a third cousin maybe, or to have spent a long weekend in Cork in childhood, doing their best to relate to me – but they are not relatable, and I don't know how to talk to these people when they are not safely encased within screens.

In a bevy of shiny black cars, we make our way down to a small building near the entrance of Leavesden Studios, where the readthrough is taking place. The readthrough is notorious for being the most anxiety-inducing day on set, where you meet your new film family – an impressive array of colourful characters, vaguely or startlingly recognisable faces with booming voices and an easy gift for making people laugh or cry – and the immense pressure to make them laugh, or even just like you, almost renders you incapable of speech. My only way of coping with readthroughs nowadays is to commit to being deliberately shit, delivering my lines in a lifeless monotone and never making eye contact with the other actors, all while taking copious notes in the margins, pretending this is part of my 'process', that my acting instrument is too precious and nebulous – a spiritual channelling, if you will – to waste on a mere readthrough. This also serves to deliberately lower my co-stars' expectations of me, so that when it comes to the scenes and I am halfway decent, they can only be pleasantly surprised.

But in February 2006, on my first professional job, I don't know any of this and assume that Dan, Emma, Rupert and the entire Gryffindor common room, along with acting heavyweights Imelda Staunton, Helena Bonham Carter and Jason Isaacs, all assemble in a room at the start of each day to drink coffee, read scenes and regale each other with their heart-stopping talent. I am overawed by everything. It's too much, all of my wildest fantasies put together, a dream even I did not conceive of, as famous actor after famous actor glides through the doorway, exclaiming uproariously as they see one other – old friends from the stage – kiss each other on the cheek, and then step back in mock disbelief at how much the younger actors have grown. At this point, Dan, who is standing beside me, directs their gaze to me and introduces me by name, as though he is my personal assistant. Emma appears, with her beautiful brown eyes and her gorgeously groomed brows, and crouches slightly to greet me, a kind smile on her face, as though I am a tiny, featherless baby bird that has fallen from her nest, and says she's delighted to meet me. Then Rupert, in a casual hoodie, with his shock of silky ginger hair, says hello and nods sleepily at me. Then it's Devon, Alfie, James and Oliver (Seamus Finnegan, Dean Thomas, Fred and George Weasley, to all you normal, non-demented-fangirl people). I would have preferred if there *had* been a metal barrier between us; it would have made me more comfortable and given me somewhere to place my hands. I am relieved when they all start talking to each other, comparing Christmases and midterm exam results, and contentedly station myself in the corner to step back and admire them all.

Unfortunately, Dan has not given up on trying to get me to talk. He has seemingly assumed direct responsibility for the task of making me feel at home. Personally, I think he is the worst-suited candidate for this job, what with his *being* Harry Potter, but later I will observe that this is just his way. It is a role he embraces without being asked, walking straight up to trembling extras or children with terminal illnesses visiting Leavesden for the day, and insisting they address him as Dan, because he is a nice person, conscientious and determined to make everyone feel welcome on set.

'What kind of music do you like?' he asks, harmlessly, making another bold stab at conversation.

What he didn't realise is that he had just asked me one of my most dreaded questions and triggered my sense of mortal peril. Music is not a language I am proficient in. I like it. I enjoy listening to Britney Spears, Michael Jackson, a few obscure French indie-folk singers, the Disney soundtracks – and that's about it. I just don't have great taste in music, and there's nothing I can do about that.

The specific problem with *Daniel Radcliffe* asking this question was that I was well aware of every single one of his favourite bands, his penchant for eighties punk rock music, and, as a devoted fangirl, had saved up my pocket money for weeks to purchase CDs of The Sex Pistols, The Pixies and Nick Cave in an effort to understand him better. Rest assured that any album Dan had mentioned in any interview up to 2006, I had doggedly hunted down, listened to and learned the lyrics. My fangirl appetite for *Harry Potter* had compelled me to collect every magazine cover with his face, learn by heart every fact file comprising titbits of information about his birthday, his star sign, his likes and dislikes. His passions became my passions. Except they didn't, because I didn't actually like eighties punk rock music at all. I didn't relate to the songs or connect to the lyrics, with their lust for chaos, sex and drugs.

And I knew the moment I mentioned this precise list of bands that I could muster no genuine interest in, Dan would instantly discern that my alleged passion for this music was a thinly veiled passion for him, and that I had essentially borrowed his personality to cover up my own lack thereof. Standing there, struggling for words, desperately scanning my mind for any decent music not on Dan's playlist, I suddenly realised a vast mistake I'd made in trying to connect with my beloved idols: I had invested so much energy into trying to become someone they might like, only to realise that there was nothing original left of me. It had all been so straightforward up to this point; I'd been naturally guided by an inner compass. It was easy to be Luna – it didn't even feel like acting – and reading some scenes with Harry and then improvising a few quiet moments as Luna was just playtime for a regular frequenter of the fanfiction section of Mugglenet. But looking Daniel Radcliffe square in the face and being asked to clarify whether I was cool or not was a moment I had not prepared for.

'I like . . .' I say, still frantically searching for one solitary album that won't irredeemably alienate me from my once-imaginary best friend, '. . . the *Mulan* soundtrack.' I blurt it out before I can stop myself, and then look at him in terror, horrified – but compelled – to witness his reaction to this devastating admission.

'Oh . . .' he says, because what the fuck else could he say? 'Cool.' His voice trails off and his gaze wanders awkwardly to the other side of the room. He touches my elbow politely, electrifying the inner fangirl, and says, 'I'll chat to you later, I'm just going to go and say hello to Robbie.'

I die inside as he crosses the room to conduct what looks like a lovely and normal conversation with Robbie Coltrane.

Most conversations after that with my new castmates were to start and end thusly. It continued long after that readthrough and all throughout filming. I did not make it easy or comfortable for the other actors to be around me. I had trained myself in the language of fangirl, had followed their careers and personal lives out of a feeling of pious duty, of undying loyalty to know and love them better than anyone else. And up until now, this moment standing on set with them, doing a dreadful job at feigning insouciance, my social life had comprised whiling away hours on the fansites, locked in fierce battle with other anonymous users hiding under monikers that were always variations of '*siriusblacksbitch*228' or 'danradsgrrrrl87', vying for first place in a trivia quiz entitled 'How Well Do You Know Daniel Radcliffe?'

Mostly I remained silent, watching and listening, carefully repressing the crazily over-stimulated fangirl with her extensive knowledge of my new colleagues' private lives. Some days, it was a job to contain her, and all too often she bubbled to the surface, threatening to spill over. *How are Bubbles and Domino, your pet cats?!* my fangirl screeched in my head each morning upon seeing Emma. *Did you see* The Simpsons *last night?* she wanted to yell at Dan, *I only started watching because you do, and I don't really like it, but we can talk about any episode you like! Sing me the rap about Ron that you made up for your first audition, Rupert! Congratulations on your rumoured Chanel campaign! Is this the make-up artist you're reportedly dating? Ah, your parents, don't worry, I already know their names – Alan and Marcia! Oh, and did you ever get that Harry Potter doll I made out of felt and stockings and sent to your school address?*

You know how when you feel a kinship with a distant celebrity and you have all sorts of long, detailed, amazing conversations in your head with them, and you just wish you could meet them in person so that these conversations could play out for real and an epic, legendary relationship could blossom? Well, I had my shot at doing that every day on the *Harry Potter* set. In the car on the way to the studio, I would sit in silence, carefully outlining and plotting the arc of a conversation with Dan, Emma or Rupert. And every day, these conversations would peter out tragically a few awkward moments after they'd started. I was always over-rehearsed and under confident. I was a Professional Actor now, but I had no idea how to improvise a real-life conversation, and every night I would return home to the swanky furnished apartment in west London that Warner Bros. were paying for, feeling lonely and deflated. There, I'd resume my online stalking of my co-stars and mining for topics of conversation in the dark enclaves of the fan forums.

Some evenings, sweet, beautiful Katie Leung would drop by the apartment I lived in with my chaperone in a generous attempt at getting to know me. Katie, myself and a few of the other young actresses who were not from London, all resided with our parents or chaperones in the same building, a block of serviced, ludicrously expensive apartments, that were probably intended for millionaires on business trips and their mistresses. This arrangement would have been excellent fun if I hadn't had to scramble to close all the internet tabs of my co-stars' faces or hide all my fangirl memorabilia any time they rang my bell to suggest we go for dinner. How could I confess to them that I had just been whiling away the evening on Mugglenet, swooning over candid pictures of them all and taking copious notes on their outfits? They would have thought I was a serial killer.

I got away with it (mostly, I think) because I played the spaciest, dreamiest weirdo ever to attend a school of magical weirdos. 'She's not a million miles away from Luna Lovegood,' I watched Dan say in an interview posted online after the presenter asked him how the new girl on set was fitting in, and I remember feeling simultaneously sad and relieved that he really didn't know me at all. I continued to keep tight-lipped about my unease and discomfort, and to keep my secret fangirl hidden away. I let her out on occasion, though, to play wizard rock in the make-up chair in the morning, or to cheerily inform another actor that it was their character's birthday or that J. K. Rowling had released an important new titbit about their character on her website. I couldn't *stop* myself from interjecting loudly when I overheard anyone making errors when recalling details from the books. Thanks to this habit, I became known on set for being the person that people went to when they had a quick question about the logistics of a spell or about the Black family tree, and in that way, I sort of carved out a comfortable role for myself among the cast. But there was a huge distance between us that I couldn't allow myself to bridge. I was invited to dinners and birthday parties, and all of the cast made a concerted effort to include me in their social activities, but as badly as I wanted to be accepted and befriended – to belong – there was a huge part of me that did not want to get too close. I was not like them – they were born for the screen, while I had tricked my way on to it; they were attractive without make-up and skinny without having some messed up eating disorder. I didn't want them to know the real me. I knew that I had nothing to bring to this incredibly cool table besides an encyclopaedic knowledge of *Harry Potter* and the calorie content of postage stamps, and I was afraid of what they would ask me when I stepped out of Luna Lovegood's uniform and had to be me again: afraid that I wouldn't have the answers, afraid to discover that there was nothing there at all.

My saving grace amid all this social anxiety, this overwhelming sense of inferiority, was always Luna. She was my anchor to this world, as well as my sanctuary inside it. She allowed me to breathe and to be in a way I'd never had permission to before. I didn't know how to talk to other teenagers or how to behave, how to be cool or witty or interesting or famous, but I knew how to be Luna, and that was enough. Any time something odd I'd said provoked an awkward snigger or careful avoidance of each other's eyes amid crew members, and I got a sudden urge to slap myself or pull my jumper up over my head and cry, I reminded myself that I was Luna now, and it was OK to simply breathe, to be, to observe these behaviours without reacting to them. Luna did and said odd things every day of her life, and it didn't matter if people liked or ignored her, if they laughed at her or with her, avoided or befriended her, because she remained unaltered either way: always the same, always centred in who she was, true and wonderful. Always, somehow, despite her lack of trying hard, the most intriguing person on the page to me. And something special always happened when I focused on being Luna, when I let myself breathe as her. As Luna, my life was no longer about me. 'I' seemed to melt away, no longer my greatest obstacle.

Soon, it was just easier to hide behind her. It was just more comfortable being her. She gave me permission to look people in the eye, to accept their attention. I altered the pitch of my voice so that I always spoke in that dreamy, sing-song way. I got rid of all my edgy, frayed denim clothing and only dressed in bright floral patterns and zany tights. I started texting my friends using full words and thoughtful phrasing, abandoning abbreviated teenage text speak ('wot u up 2 bbz?') even though it meant the texts cost extra to send. It was method acting out of personal necessity rather than any lofty devotion to the craft. In a way, this was what I had always prayed for: to shrug off myself and trade her in for someone better. And, conveniently, people were paying me for it and someone brilliant was writing the script. This was my new life, I decided. This was who I was now. From now on, people would know me as Luna, accept me as her, expect me as her, and I was only too happy to play the part. My darkness need never be revealed. My parents had discreetly disclosed my previous struggles to the on-set doctor during the routine pre-filming medical assessment, though perhaps they had not underlined how serious my problem had gotten. The doctor had been satisfied with my progress and the account we gave of how I had maintained a stable weight for the past two years, and had declared me perfectly fit to work. Quietly, I fretted about what would happen when J. K. Rowling (bizarrely, both the queen of my new world and the only link connecting it with the dark one I'd left behind) found out about my casting, so I decided not to tell her, naively hoping she just wouldn't check the casting details, that she had far greater concerns than the names of actors. I planned to simply stop writing letters to her and hoped she'd forget me or assume I'd perished. It wasn't just that I was afraid she'd expose my shameful past; I feared that she'd be furious at the casting, devastated that one of her purest, sweetest characters was to be played by such an egotistical and selfish girl. I worried that she'd be too nice, too magnanimous to voice her disappointment, but that I'd always know. For the only time in my life, I tried to ignore J. K. Rowling. But of course, she did see the new cast list, which David Heyman always sent to her as a courtesy, and she immediately recognised my name and told the producers so. She wrote me the best letter I've ever received, full of excitement, hearty congratulations and multiple exclamation points, telling me how thrilled she was I'd got the part, and even calling me beautiful. Miraculously, also, she did not divulge the context of our friendship or let slip the secret of my disordered eating. It is a testament to her incredible class and profound sensitivity that she passed the nature of our correspondence off as a complete coincidence and never shared that just two years before, she'd been addressing my letters to an eating disorder clinic. It still makes me cry when I think of the depth of her kindness. She told the producers nothing about who I used to be. My secret history was safe.

No, it was not Jo who spilled my secret, but a shadowy figure from my past who was apparently feeling rather left out of all the excitement and publicity generated around me in the wake of my casting announcement. My casting in the films was announced on 2 February 2004, two years to the day since I'd been admitted as a patient at Peaceful Pastures clinic, a painful moment and place I wished never to return to, and memories I assumed were buried safely in the past. To this day, I can't quite fathom why this person did it; was it simply her cold, unbiased professional opinion that anorexia was an indefensible evil, its merest shadow needing to be brutishly trampled out of the public eye? Or was it, as I privately sensed, that she nursed a distinct dislike for me, a more personal, pointed loathing, had never relinquished the opinion that I was a sick person, and not a person, and therefore undeserving of all the fame and attention currently being paid to me? Whatever her motive, this person from my past made life very difficult for me when she wrote a public letter to a London newspaper addressing Warner Bros. and the *Harry Potter* films and criticising them for the irresponsible example they were setting by 'employing anorexic children'. I wasn't named, which would have been a breach of confidentiality, but she informed the paper that she had it on good authority that at least one of the young *Harry Potter* cast members was suffering from an eating disorder, and that by employing this person, Warner Bros. was brazenly colluding with an anorexic in promoting an unhealthy body image to impressionable young fans. She didn't stop at me, however, taking aim at the other female cast members, criticising their slim physiques and questioning if there wasn't something of an eating disorder pandemic spreading among the young actors. In allowing these slight young people to work, she said, Warner Bros. was directly responsible for exacerbating the mental health conditions of its vast international audience. Needless to say, her letter raised alarm bells at *Harry Potter* HQ. Putting two and two together, the producers called my parents, who were compelled to go into great detail of the extent of my disordered eating, and the next day my mum and I were summoned to David Barron's office for a meeting.

I kept my eyes downcast and my hands tightly clasped in my lap as my mum explained my situation, the programmes I'd completed, the efforts I'd made towards recovery, and how I'd succeeded in keeping my weight stable ever since Peaceful Pastures. She told how I'd been doing so much better for the past year and wanted to stay like that. David Barron, who had not been thrilled to be so blindsided by the letter to the paper, sat with his arms crossed, 'Mmm'-ing and 'aah'-ing thoughtfully as my mum spoke. He kept throwing glances over in my direction, but I couldn't meet his eyes – it was all I could do to keep from crying as I jigged a foot nervously and blinked repeatedly to clear the tears. It was still very triggering for me to talk about my eating disorder, to hear my name and 'anorexia' used in the same sentence, and I was deeply embarrassed for my kind, lovely new boss to know this ugly part of me. I was always afraid, after recovering physically, that nobody would believe I'd had an eating disorder, would think I was making it up in a bid for attention, would immediately scrutinise my healthy body and laugh at how fat I was. And I was convinced, now that my secret was out, that there would be serious discussions behind my back about recasting, that they would be furious to learn that I was not the carefree, dreamy girl they'd thought I was, and that my eating disorder was proof that they'd chosen the wrong person.

My mum finished speaking and David cleared his throat, thanking us for our honesty and saying he understood the delicacy of this situation, but that it was imperative that Warner Bros. understood the full picture. He said it would not do, if I were to get sick again, and Warner Bros. were accused of being negligent of my health, and that the big men in Burbank, California were very concerned about the situation and needed clear assurance of my health via ongoing medical assessments. It was agreed that I would have to start being weighed again on a weekly basis at the studio, and that I would attend therapy sessions at an outpatient eating disorder facility in London. He finished by saying that he wished he'd known about all this in advance, but that we were going to make it work. And then he looked at me, and I noted that his demeanour of warm fondness towards me had not changed one bit as he said, 'We love you here at Leavesden, and we want you to continue being our Luna, so we need you to stay well', and I couldn't help it then when a few tears fell out. He gave my mum and I each a hug and then we left his office, my mum breathing a heavy sigh of relief when we reached the corridor and saying the meeting had gone 'about as well as we could have hoped'.

I am always keen to dismantle the myth that someone offered me a part in *Harry Potter* in exchange for my commitment to recovery and that dutifully, easily, I obliged. It is not possible to simply incentivise recovery, and it is deeply disrespectful (not to mention irresponsible) towards people with eating disorders and their families to suggest that you can, when neither love, money, riches, nor a part in a *Harry Potter* will compel a person to recover from their eating disorder if they don't want to let it go. It is also completely naive to suggest that once the dream has been fulfilled, once the person has found the happiness, that their problems dissolve, the eating disorder melts away and there is no more struggle involved. Recovery is not a smooth, linear path, and though I was literally living my dreams, inhabiting this awe-inspiring world of storytelling, art and magic, I still woke up to myself every day: this person who I struggled to accept and had tried to undo. Beneath the costumes, hair extensions, make-up, editing, fame and fuss, she was still there, and she was not going anywhere. But I was lucky, because I had people around me who believed in me and who didn't measure my worth or health by the numbers on the scale. Warner Bros. were incredibly supportive of me and handled my situation in the most compassionate way possible, which is almost single-handedly due to the efforts of David Barron. He did not have an easy job fighting my corner and shielding me from scrutiny by the bigwigs in California. My insurance premium went way up after that infamous letter in the paper, which must have been a real headache for David as he fought to convince the higher-ups that this stray newcomer was worth the trouble and considerable expense. As a young, unknown actor I should have come at more of a bargain price: studios weren't accustomed to paying top dollar for the roughly hewn ingenue. He was also extremely protective of me, assuring me that not even the drivers who drove me to my weekly therapy session knew about my situation, and that he had only told the publicity department so they could ensure my story wasn't leaked in the press. The weekly weigh-ins were a source of continual stress to me, and I often tried to hide from them, disappearing to Hagrid's hut at lunchtime on Wednesdays when I knew my chaperone (who had taken over from my parents, as they were both full-time teachers back home in Ireland) would come looking for me to visit the medical cabin. But they always located me, and the doctor was friendly and kept up a light-hearted repartee as he squinted at the scales to record my weight. The weigh-ins and doctor's appointments caused several awkward moments among my new castmates, who knew me to eat quite well and had no idea about my previous problems.

'Come on, sweetie, we have to go,' my chaperone Tamara called cheerily one day, jerking her head towards the door of the canteen and trying to be discreet. I had just sat down to lunch with some other cast members, really hoping she'd forgotten what day it was.

'Uggghh, please can we leave it? It was fine last week,' I mumbled to her under my breath as Katie looked up at our exchange. She and I had started to become friends by this point. Katie is a sensitive, artistic soul, with a profound lack of tolerance for bullshit and pretentious-ness, which makes her a very grounding presence on a movie set or red carpet. Initially, we connected over our Celtic roots and shared experience of entering the world of the *Harry Potter* films through open auditions, and though I was still completely dazzled by her, I had managed to keep up a fairly credible facade of normality.

'Sorry, sweetie, you know you have to do this,' Tamara told me sympathetically.

'What's happening?' Katie asked, curious, and I tried for bare honesty.

'Have to get weighed,' I muttered angrily, in a vague attempt at intimating my problems. I was always grappling with wanting people to know who I was and then struggling to find the precise words to express it.

'Why?' she asked, looking baffled.

I was embarrassed to have mentioned anything, and tried to brush it off casually. 'Oh, just standard procedure,' I said. 'Don't they weigh you too?'

'No,' Katie answered, looking wildly perplexed, and as if I'd just told her I was being routinely molested.

'Huh.' I shrugged. 'Weird.' And then I scampered off after Tamara before Katie could see my reddening cheeks.

I ate consistently, and I was not unhealthy by any means during that time, but I was slightly underweight, several kilos below the optimal BMI, and the doctor was keen to keep a careful eye on my weight. I was weighed every week that I worked on *Order of the Phoenix*, and the weigh-ins definitely triggered a few setbacks. It was tempting to reach for old self-soothing mechanisms on days when I felt totally out of my depth and completely unworthy of my place among the cast, and I found myself, again, in that tricky, though all-too-familiar position of courting two contradictory objectives at once: of wanting to please the adults and honour their trust in me by maintaining a healthy weight, and of restoring my sense of equilibrium and inner peace by restricting my food intake and watching the numbers on the scales descend. There were a particularly tense few weeks where my weight kept dropping fractionally, and David called me into his office again to communicate to me the gravity of the situation. He explained that soon, if I did not play ball and commit to working with the weight targets the doctor set me, he would be unable to fight my corner against the men in California, who only knew me as numbers and as a serious financial risk. That was the moment, I think, where I realised that I'd been playing Russian roulette with my dream, that it could so easily be taken away, all the lights extinguished at once. I finally took his words at face value and realised I had to work purposefully to resist the voice of my eating disorder. David remained deeply invested in my situation, routinely checking on me, making sure I was settling into life in London and on set, even at one point offering to pay for a personal chef at home in the evenings, and calling my parents every couple of weeks to check that I was happy or to communicate an urgency to get me to gain some weight. At the same time, I made a concerted effort to balance my eating habits and to consciously check the impulses to restrict and hide food, and gradually my weight started to climb again. It wasn't fun and it didn't feel fair, but I gritted my teeth as the doctor recorded my weight and cheerfully congratulated me. I always tried not to look at the scales, but even when I did, it was considerably easier to deal with it now that I was living a glamorous, independent life in London and skipping off to the *Harry Potter* sets rather than the interior of the Brown Kitchen.

At the time, I don't think I appreciated quite how much David Barron stuck his neck out for me, or how sensitively Warner Bros. dealt with my situation. They could easily have fired me, could have decided it was too complicated and that I was not worth the trouble. They could have smoothly, seamlessly recast the role. The fandom did not know me as Luna Lovegood yet, and I would have been quickly forgotten, shrugged off, a small, uninteresting footnote in *Harry Potter* film history that only the most peculiar, hardcore fans would ever remember. But they stuck by me, they supported me, they did not immediately fire me, wrench my dreams from under my feet and let me fuck off back to my quiet dark cave of lists, numbers and rigid self-control – and this is how I think we can all help people recovering from eating disorders. We can love them, we can encourage them, we can meet them where they are on the road to recovery and coax them gently down the path of dreams. I count myself incredibly lucky that I had people who knew I needed my dreams far more than I needed food in order to be able to eat. I owe David Barron a huge debt of gratitude.

Filming for each *Harry Potter* film always lasted the best part of a year, but my scenes only required me to be there for a couple of weeks at a time and odd days here and there, so between bouts of filming I'd fly home to return to school in Ireland and focus on my studies. I found these sudden returns to reality dreadfully disappointing, my direct line to the magical world abruptly going dead, and even though I sat firmly convinced that I had the best role in all the *Harry Potter* films, I found myself envious of all the Gryffindor actors, who were called in far more often for background work and who seemed to while whole days away sitting in armchairs on the common room set bonding with one another. I would text my friend Ryan, a fellow Ravenclaw, who'd joined the cast of *Order of the Phoenix* as 'Slightly Creepy Boy', to check whether he'd been called in for any more Dumbledore's Army scenes, and to confer with him on scenes in the script where we might conceivably convince David Yates that some stray Ravenclaws in the background could add a touch of diversity. I found myself feeling isolated at school, where I'd never felt like I fit in, and now even less so, but neither were the cast of *Harry Potter* blowing up my phone – most of them had had the wherewithal not to give their personal mobile number to the rogue fangirl. These periods were lonely, but they gave me the opportunity to look back on filming and to self-reflect. I was sad to see how epic and awe-inspiring this dream made manifest was, how much it exceeded my wildest fantasies of it in every way – and how little I actually participated in it. I regretted how little I'd put myself out there to connect with my co-stars, how much I'd held back, and I realised that these days were rare and precious, and I had to shake off this debilitating inferiority complex while I still had time. At the end of the day, it didn't matter whether my low estimation of myself was true or not; the fact was, it was holding me back.

That summer, when filming went on hiatus I attended a summer camp for nerdy teens and worked hard to cultivate some basic social skills. I noticed, for the first time in my life, that people were intrigued by me. My connection to the upcoming *Harry Potter* movie didn't manage to make me cool, but it did make me interesting, and I watched, with a sort of detached interest, as heads swivelled towards me at the roll call, and as camera phone screens were tilted surreptitiously, they thought, in my direction before the perpetrator would catch me looking and fumble to take a picture of an innocuous flower. The attention didn't go to my head – I was too keenly aware of my own awkwardness and the fact that I would soon return to an environment where I was not special and was still, inescapably, the weird, quiet girl in the corner – but I observed how I suddenly had a considerable degree of social clout, and when I returned to set some weeks later for the second half of filming, I was determined to stop second-guessing every move I made, every word I uttered, and instead to accept where I was and try to enjoy it.

I turned my fangirl observational powers towards studying my castmates' behaviour for clues on how to be a convincing famous person, how to be worthy of all this, how not to stick out like a pale, overawed Irish person. I took note of the brand names on the containers lined up against the lighted mirrors of the make-up artists' tables, which contained luxurious face creams that they smoothed on to the main actors' faces at the end of each day, and I spent my weekends trawling Covent Garden looking for duplicates. I spent hours in the evenings by the mirror, pressing and dotting ridiculous little pots of eye cream into my face, thinking, *This is what worthiness smells like.* I observed the girls wore casual skinny jeans with layered strappy T-shirts, but then dramatically elevated the look with large, crumpled, leathery handbags with a tangle of straps, dozens of buckles and then a tiny, crucial gold plaque boasting the name of some Italian designer. So I made my way into Brown Thomas in Dublin one weekend, shuffled up to a polished and bemused sales assistant and pointed to a large tan satchel. A shiver of horror ran down my spine as she deducted over €900 from my glossy new debit card, but I left the shop hugging my bulky purchase and inhaling its fumes, (which I somehow only realised years later was actually the cruel smell of chemically treated dead cow skin). I carried my smart new satchel everywhere I went, attracting the attention of the other girls, who were forced to compliment it – not because it was nice, but because it was so clearly an embarrassingly blatant bid for approval, clashing hideously, as it did with my patterned tights and polka-dot skirts. I felt certain that though I would never belong to this ludicrous new reality of £100 eye creams and designer handbags, I could calculate a convincing assimilation into it.

I sought clues everywhere, asking the drivers who ferried me to and from set each day for anecdotes about my co-stars. What lofty tomes did they read in the car? Which ones only learned their lines in the morning on the way to work? Did any of the beautiful actresses secretly fart as they dozed? I learned from one of my favourite drivers, Jason, that I was known among the transport crew for leaving coils of long yellow-blond hair all over the back seat, and that they were all armed with lint rollers as a result to restore the luxe freshness of their film-star car interiors. Clémence Poésy, the stunning and intoxicatingly French actress who played Fleur Delacour, on the other hand, was spoken of by Jason in dreamy, reverent tones, and he confessed that all the drivers relished the task of taking her home. They traded opinions in the transport office, speculating on the name of that delightful floral scent she left lingering in the car that they all so enjoyed. I quickly discovered the perfume was Coco Mademoiselle and promptly bought some, spritzing myself liberally each morning before my pick-up time. I informed Jason that I was wearing it, asking him had he noticed, but he replied 'Hmm,' and said that it smelled different on me. I sighed heavily and looked out the window, calculating, calculating. There was that precise, intangible difference between me and all the other actors, the smell of being a plain, average and completely unworthy person that I couldn't seem to shake. I continued to wear the perfume to set, though. Maybe I would grow into it, glow into it.

There was a stark difference between the comportment of the adults and the younger actors at Leavesden: a giddiness and light-heartedness in them, where we were serious and self-conscious. Decades of hustling for auditions, slogging away for long hours on the stage and slowly, steadily establishing themselves as household names had lent them a greater appreciation for the scope of the production, and of the considerable resources we were so generously offered.

'Fill your boots, kids,' Mark Williams would tell a cluster of Hogwarts students waiting in line at the canteen with their blue lunch trays, a look of impish delight on his face as he shovelled one of each kind of chocolate bar into the pockets of Mr Weasley's tweed trousers. 'It's not like this on other films.'

The adults were always testing the limits of their privileges, sneaking empty Bertie Bott's Every Flavour Beans packages off set to take home to their kids, or turning up with a squadron of noisy nieces and nephews, when we'd been told by the runners that inviting throngs of visitors to work each day was frowned upon, and only permissible if you were Alan Rickman (and then only because everyone was too scared to ask him not to). The older actors were always encouraging us to enjoy this experience, to make the most of it, and warning that it might never be this good again, but I didn't really listen to them, preferring to believe that *Harry Potter* would go on forever.

The most profound lessons I learned from spending time with the older actors were always to be found in how they approached their work. While tapping into Luna before each day was a virtually effortless task for me, I found it impossible to shake the awareness that I was on a multimillion-pound film set, and worked towards the goal of 'nailing it' with each take. I aimed for perfection, not discovery, trying to play out each line and movement exactly as I'd planned it in microscopic detail in my head. I enjoyed the scenes, but felt gripped by fear each time the assistant director yelled 'Moving on!' and I realised that that was it, that was the scene that would be immortalised on film, which millions of people would watch and memorise and remember forever. Stressed, I would sidle up to David

Yates (himself notorious for insisting on 'one more, one more' and then filming eighteen more takes) and ask him was he *sure* he was happy, were we really done? So, it was something of a shock when I turned up early one day for a scene in the Department of Mysteries to witness Helena Bonham Carter and Jason Isaacs in the midst of an on-camera rehearsal for a dramatic battle scene, and acting like the biggest children on set. I watched in awe as they leapt and twirled about, cackling and swishing their robes flamboyantly in a wildly erratic display of . . . silliness. Or was it creativity? They weren't acting; they were playing. I stood in the shadows and gaped, as, each take, they did something different, bigger, wilder, more surprising, never stopping to analyse their work or second-guess their choices. Undoubtedly, those were challenging shoot days for the script supervisor, the onset pest responsible for continuity errors, who would tap your shoulder and remind you that you'd performed the spell in your left hand last take, and that your hair had actually been brushed behind your shoulder, and to please fix those things. But it was enthralling, exciting, *alive*. They were finding new things in each take, adding to and colouring their performances. And as I watched them, I felt something niggling at the edges of my subconscious, a feeling of unease or a small epiphany that perhaps artists are anti-perfectionists, and that creativity isn't about trying to nail it or impress David Yates or look good. Creativity in motion, from my vantage point watching these two joyful, experimental, mesmerising actors, looked messy, bold and playful. It didn't seem that there was any space for perfection in the face of this kind of feral, rampant creativity. And as fun and joyful as it looked, it was the hardest thing to do on a movie set, with hundreds of eyes scrutinising your performance. It was much more natural to be tense, calculated and controlling in that environment, but playfulness was how the colours came out. A disturbing thought occurred to me in that moment, that maybe the essence of creativity was not a careful, dogged fight for perfection, but simple, messy, ceaseless play. It was a thought that occurred to me, but that I was not ready for yet – perfection was still the security I sought, the sheltered corner I crawled to – so I filed it away to consider at a later date, some day when I was braver and older.

Perfection remained an alluring and soothing pursuit in other areas of life on a film set. Leavesden Studios was a joyous, exciting and unpredictable place to be every day that we were making *Harry Potter* films. Every day, that is, except photoshoot days. A heavy cloud of teenage angst would descend upon the dressing room corridor on the days the young cast were scheduled to have our promotional photos taken. It wouldn't start that way, however. It always started with excitement, confidence, aspiration, visions of our bright careers as promising young actors. We were movie stars now, after all! We were in the biggest fucking movie franchise of all time! But we were also normal fourteen-, fifteen- and sixteen-year-olds, who hadn't been born camera-ready and thirsty for the limelight. That is to say, we were mostly awkward, sensitive, thoughtful teenagers, trying to come to terms with our newfound stardom by wrestling with equal measures of narcissism and self-loathing.

Nevertheless, it is exciting, to be fourteen years old and called to a professional photographer's studio to take pictures that will end up on the sides of London buses. I practically skip in there, *I'm ready for my close-up,* a giddiness in my heart as someone hands me a wand and I step on set. Lights flash, cameras chirp, the photographer lays on the compliments. Everyone is smiling and nodding, pleased. But then I make the mistake of checking the playback on the laptop and my cheerful mood deflates in an instant. *Jesus Christ.* I can't believe how ugly I am. I can't believe that someone has chosen to employ me as an actress, has trussed me up in Hogwarts robes, that money is actually being paid to take photos of this hideous blond blob of a girl. The world tilts. Everyone is out of their minds – including me, for bullishly thrusting myself into this position in the first place. What am I *doing* here? Have I always been this ugly? Does nobody else realise? Why are we all standing around pretending that these pictures are OK, and that we should continue taking more of them?

'I look soooo awful,' I whisper to Tamara, keeping my eyes down and blinking away tears.

'Oh darling, no, you look lovely!'

I flinch at that odious word and scowl at Tamara, who is a pretty twenty-something-year-old blonde, and who, to the utter devastation of my tender fangirl heart, has been attracting admiring glances and flirtatious advances of late from a certain boy wizard. What the hell does she know about being the lumpy, ungainly resident oddbod?

'No, my face is fat and my nose is like a *Sesame Street* muppet,' I protest, hiding my face behind my hands and insisting that I can't take any more pictures.

'You're being far too self-critical,' Tamara coos. 'It's just a bad camera angle,' she ventures, but I continue to sniffle and hide my giant muppet nose from view. 'Do you want a minute outside?' Tamara enquires tentatively.

I take the minute, but I want a week. I want a month. I want the entire year to squirrel myself away in an underground dungeon where nobody will have to look at me and I can devote my life to self-starvation again, emerging neither beautiful nor camera-ready, but hopefully less of a catastrophic eyesore. I just want rid of my body, to live this fabulous dream as someone else entirely: someone better equipped and tailor-made for this wonderful, coveted movie-star life. But the minute passes, and all these grown adults are standing around, waiting for me to decide to be professional again, and I am wasting everyone's time, and it is going to take an *awfully* long time, longer than anyone has, to address my myriad imperfections, so I step back on set. When it's over, I sob for a long time in my dressing room. Tutoring is cancelled that day, by my decree! Vanity is the subject of the day. A couple of my castmates get wind of the drama and come to commiserate.

'What's going on?' another chaperone, Tina, enquires of Tamara as I bury my face in the couch cushions in a sniffling heap.

'She just had her promo shots today,' Tamara replies.

'Ahhhhh,' Tina, says knowingly, nodding sympathetically. 'Gotcha.'

Some days later, I am in the make-up chair when I overhear the make-up artists whispering about another young actress who has just been subject to her own set of promotional portraits.

'She won't come out of her room; she's upset about her pictures.'

It strikes me how everyone speaks about teenage self-hate in such reverent tones, but as I sit in that chair looking at my reflection, picking through a packet of dry, miserable, unsalted almonds, and thinking of a beautiful, talented actress down the hallway crying over her inadequate reflection, I am overcome with a wave of despair – and, I think, boredom. *God, it's all so mundane! We're all sick in the same ways!* In that moment, it is no longer glamorous and tragic: it is just pathetic. It has only been two days since I threw my own almighty hissy fit at the sight of my face and body on camera, but now I have to stop myself from rolling my eyes at the antics of my distressed co-star. Whereas as a twelve-year-old, my obsession with

377

perfection and devotion to self-flagellation had made me unique, different, admirable even, now, at fourteen, it seems it is practically the fashion to hate yourself.

Seeing my bright and interesting co-stars going through it too really gave me a new perspective on the whole thing. We were the young people to whom our peers looked for inspiration, for guidance. We got fan mail from people in India, Russia and Brazil, telling us our stories had inspired them to pursue acting, or that our portrayals of the characters they loved had given them permission to accept themselves. And here we all were, weeping over nothing greater than the circumference of our calves or the width of our noses. It was all so overwhelmingly boring, I thought, sitting in the make-up chair and feeling depressed. Wasn't there more to life than this?

People often ask me whether it was triggering to my disorder to be suddenly thrust (or to have thrust myself, more accurately) on to the world stage that was the *Harry Potter* set, and to be subject to the scrutiny of the international media, as well as the decidedly more malicious glare of bored, unhappy teenagers sitting behind computers. Oddly enough, I actually think being in the spotlight gave me a lot of distance from my eating disorder. One of the unlikely gifts of having an eating disorder is that nobody will ever be as mean as your disorder was. There is a profound sense of safety in being your own biggest bully, your own cruellest aggressor, which is why eating disorders are so addictive and so hard to let go of. There is something so comfortable and reassuring in getting to the edges of your darkest thought, in following it all the way to its fullest expression and burying yourself beneath it, where nobody can hurl it in your unsuspecting face.

So, it did not surprise me, after the announcement of my casting was published alongside a photo of me with my shockingly yellow hair, a timid smile barely masking profound discomfort and clutching a copy of *Order of the Phoenix* like it was a full body shield, to log on to my beloved Mugglenet and to see 285 comments by my brothers and sisters in fandom allyship ruthlessly tearing my image apart.

'Ugh, I'm sooooo disappointed,' grumbled one commenter, 'this is not how I imagined Luna Lovegood at all.'

'Ewww,' decried another particularly distressed fan. 'I can't stand her horrible bleached yellow hair and chubby chipmunk cheeks. Luna is supposed to look dreamy and carefree, not anxious and constipated.'

I nodded along with all of them.

'Her body confuses me,' insisted another commenter, giving a more detached, scientific assessment of my physical attributes. 'You can see she has thin legs but a very fat face. Anywayz, I hope she doesn't ruin Luna Lovegood.'

There were some kind comments, too, a few people saying I was exactly as they pictured Luna and admiring my eclectic outfit, appreciating the detail of my handmade parrot earrings, but I reflexively dismissed those people as mentally deficient. I scrolled and scrolled, rapidly scanning each comment and committing them to memory. I felt sad, as I recognised a few of the usernames of the mean commenters as people whose fanfiction I'd enjoyed, or whose incisive and unsparing criticisms of awkwardly directed moments in previous films I'd happily guffawed at. They were faceless people I'd connected with, and who I'd previously assumed wished me well. But I did not find their critique of my ungainly adolescent form shocking or excessively mean. These opinions were not news to me. Having an eating disorder had primed me to expect an avalanche of cruelty, to seek submersion in the deepest gutters of human consciousness, because I was certain the meanest thought was always the truest.

Scrolling to the very end of the comments, a faint feeling of dissatisfaction itching at me, a devilish idea occurred to me. These people were only playing a game at which I was a seasoned connoisseur. They were mere amateurs, while I was the irrefutable master of bullying myself. Above all things, I knew how to hit me where it really hurt. A thrill of perverse glee running through me, I logged in to my own profile on Mugglenet and added my own expert analysis.

'What an awkward, awful cretin of a girl!' I wrote, comfortably taking my place among the chorus of angry assailants. 'Did she have to skin a hundred Barbies for that fake blonde wig?! How dare she put her stubby little grease-stained fingers all over my favourite book!! She looks like she bathes in the grease of McDonald's chips. Is she storing up her next Big Mac meal in the folds of her flabby cheeks? Ugly inbred little troll!'

I exhaled calmly as I hit post, a beautiful feeling of serenity descending as I spewed my inner toxicity out into the world, and saw within a few minutes that many commenters were responding favourably to my contribution.

'Omg ur hilarious,' replied the commenter who had interpreted my shy smile as a constipated grimace. 'You totally nailed it!!'

'A bit cruel,' reasoned the poster who'd first drawn attention to my rounded cheeks. 'But I agree the hair is a mess.'

It was a curiously addictive hobby, secretly making my way to the comments section on fansites, hunting down my most passionately scathing detractors and joining in their conversations to verbally abuse me with increasingly more creative put-downs. Sometimes my comments were so mean that they got flagged by other users and then hidden by the moderators, and my username became known for my vicious commentary on all news items involving the Luna Lovegood actress and my unparalleled loathing for – they did not realise – myself. I knew these people were not my friends, but I had a compulsive itch to talk to them, and found an odd sense of companionship in participating in message boards designed to pick apart my every flaw in microscopic detail. Finally, I had some allies in targeted self-abuse! There was a feeling of security that came with seeing every mean thing said about me, a sense that if I could read every comment, I could get beneath the meanness, identify my cruellest persecutor and then lock her safely in my own head.

But the thing about meanness is that you will never actually get to the end of it, and the more you look for it, the more you will see its dark, murky residue tainting every surface. You will spend your life trying to get underneath the hate, and later discover that it has entirely robbed you of joy, of pleasure, of many precious moments where you could have chosen instead to look for something beautiful. The hours I whiled away self-flagellating in fan forums began to wear on me. The incessant stream of vile comments about my physical appearance played in my head each morning as I looked in the mirror and wondered how anyone could be so deluded as to cast me in a movie, or why my parents had fought so hard to keep me alive. And, much like self-starvation, the addiction to cruel comments could only ever be sated for a very short time, and I always found myself going back for more, searching deeper, uglier places on the internet. Sometimes, I finished reading my own threads and curiosity tipped me over into comment boards about the other young actors, and I was shocked to read a similar cadence of cruelty directed at the co-stars I revered and adored, who I regarded as virtually flawless, totally beyond reproach.

Going back to set after weeks spent corrupting my mind in venomous corners of the internet was always a distinct wake-up call to me. I wandered the studio departments between scenes when I wasn't needed on set and looked on as talented, passionate professionals pored over epic architectural drawings of the Hogwarts battlements, or toiled patiently for weeks on end with oil paints at vast scenic art screens depicting sun-dappled, snow-capped photorealistic mountains, or delicately brought a vibrant model phoenix to life, feather by smooth, scarlet-tipped feather. I watched a scene on playback, a warm glow in my heart, as David beckoned the trio – Dan, Emma and Rupert – over to him for a tight-knit huddle to discuss the emotional beats of the scene, their faces thoughtful, engaged and bright. I watched all my co-stars as they worked hard and laughed loudly, as they showed up each day on set and did their best. Every day, I saw a team of hundreds of creatives pouring hours, days, weeks, months of their lives into creating something that would probably never be perfect, and that would inevitably be gleefully trashed by critics, viewers and territorial fangirls all over the world, but that would come alive, would eventually be a fully realised story: a beautiful, textured film containing pieces of each of these people that would outlive every one of them, connecting people all over the world for generations to come. And I knew, looking at all these sensitive, creative people, that none of them would get out of bed in the mornings if they read and believed the cruel things that people wrote about them in festering corners of the internet. No stories would be told if we believed the most poisonous perspectives conceived about us. No *Harry Potter* films would be made at all. I could see there was a stark delineation between the hopeful, hard-working people who turned up ready to create every day on set, and the bitter, faceless online users who spent their evenings bitching about them, and that somehow I sat firmly between them. But I knew which side of the fence I wanted to be on, had always wanted to be on: the one that might never bring me safety, but would bring me moments of profound happiness and connection.

❧

I log on to the fan forums one evening after filming and read the latest comment on a newly released interview with me. The comment comes from one of my most prolific critics, one who I've come to notice patrolling this forum almost as frequently as I do, and with whom I've exchanged much colourfully cruel banter as we bonded over our mutual loathing of my face. I've noticed that lately she is picking up some choice insults of mine, getting cleverer and more imaginative in her diatribes.

'Ugh, I hate this little shrunken troll lady,' she spews. 'Why does her voice sound like she's on helium all the time?? Wish she would just tie her fake matted hair into a rope and hang herself.'

I've trained her well, I think, admiring the vitriolic bloodlust – a new touch – but then I type a reply.

'Maybe she's just nervous,' I tap out firmly on the keyboard, the Queen of Mean of the Evanna Lynch forum swerving unexpectedly, 'as you would be too if you were doing your first TV interview. And her hair actually has no matts at all. It is fashionably tousled, and, I think, looks quite nice.'

My blood pumping like I've just done something daringly illicit, I log out of the forum, erase the history and shut down the computer, reeling from the audacious kindness of my comment: my first wobbly but decisive step into the realm of self-love affirmations.

10

'Can I borrow a tampon?' a girl in my PE class asks me loudly, in case anyone passing in the corridor outside the changing rooms might not been privy to the fact that she has started her menses.

'Sorry,' I reply, louder still, making equally sure that any passers-by know that *I* haven't. 'I don't get periods. But if I did, I wouldn't let you *borrow* a tampon; I'd definitely let you keep it.'

'What?' she asks, frowning at me, slack-jawed. I can tell what she means is: *Why are you like this?*

'Nothing,' I say, commencing my carefully choreographed ritual of shimmying into my tracksuit bottoms beneath my school skirt and then mutter: 'Congratulations on your momentous initiation into womanhood.'

But she doesn't hear, because she's already circling the changing room canvassing for a tampon. The other girls are only too happy to oblige, diving eagerly into the depths of their schoolbags and emerging, victorious, triumphantly rattling the little yellow wrappers in her face as though they are priceless jewels.

I didn't get it, this obsession with growing up. All around me, my peers and classmates talked with excitement and smug knowingness about the beckons of womanhood. Proudly, they paraded their newly shapely bodies in just their underwear in the changing rooms and crinkled tampon wrappers deliberately as they rummaged in their schoolbags at breaktime, causing the buttoned-up young male teachers to cough. All of it was so repellent to me; so unseemly. The stretch marks, the acne, the bulging flesh, the sanitary products, the greasy-haired brooding boys their womanly scents draw to the peripheries of the school grounds every day after the bell rings. I was secretly appalled by the way these once-diminutive girls had suddenly blossomed, overflowing voluptuously and taking up so much space now. To me, a woman was a girl who had given up, an unmitigated tragedy, a feeble, pathetic, pitiable submission to nature, to our own innate weakness. I felt insulted any time anyone tried to foist the word 'woman' upon me, taking for granted that I had surrendered as they had. 'The young *girl*,' I would write back in emails to my publicist, firmly erasing the word 'woman' from articles she sent for approval describing me as such. I silently fumed at everyone around me for assuming womanhood was my destiny too. I had already surrendered too much. Now they wanted me to grow up and accept I was a woman. I was having none of it. Long ago, somewhere in my mind, I had crystallised the idea of menstruation as the fatal threshold into womanhood that, once crossed, could not be uncrossed. (Problematic, absolutely, but such were the rocky plains of my teenage psyche.) So, I made up my mind that as long as I evaded its curse, I could evade the altogether more devastating misfortune of being a fully formed, bleeding, messy, sinful, tainted woman.

My eating became more controlled again when I was around fifteen, focused as I was on repressing my body's natural functions. I was careful to avoid iron-rich foods, an easier feat as a vegetarian, and saw my consistent pallor as a positive omen. I had read that if girls didn't get their period by the age of eighteen, it was likely they never would (a condition known as amenorrhoea), and I watched, satisfied, as the years crawled by – fourteen, fifteen, sixteen – and still no period. Eighteen was not that far off. I was going to make it. My quest was not without its formidable villainess however, and just as she had faced off against my anorexia, my mother placed herself firmly between me and my goal to circumvent menstruation. She began consulting doctors again, and hijacking my diet, shoehorning spinach, lentils and kidney beans onto my plates of plain rice and Quorn. She stopped approving of my vegetarianism and came to regard it as an extremist puritanical sacrifice, as though I was paying for the animals' lives with my own fecund womb-space. She cooed less over the calves and lambs that populated the fields behind our house in the springtime, apparently holding them personally responsible for the grandchildren I would not bear her. She booked me an appointment for a blood test at the hospital, and was dismayed and unconvinced when the results came back declaring me in perfect health. She tried to bargain with me to eat meat, conjuring visions of a swarthy, virile husband whose undying love and devotion was to be easily secured by a pair of ripened ovaries.

'What will happen if you can't have children?' she probed, throwing an incriminating glare at my banana sandwich over lunch one afternoon.

'Then,' I tell her, affecting a tone of profound sorrow, 'I will lie down on the floor and die, because my life will have been rendered utterly meaningless.'

I snigger as she purses her lips in a look of silent reproach, knowing that she knew better than to challenge aloud that most sacrosanct emblem of feminist principles: a happy childless crone, even if she believed it to be a tragedy. Everywhere I went, people pitied me for my protracted sexual immaturity, which is how I got away with revelling in it.

'Oh,' a friend replied, sincere pity in her eyes, after I refused her a tampon on the basis of never having had to familiarise myself with them. 'Sorry.'

Don't worry about me, you silly bleeding woman! I thought, inwardly scoffing, *I am untouched, unspoiled and stronger than you!*

I felt otherworldly every time the girls around me would curl forwards, a grimace of pain contorting their features as they cradled their midriffs and complained of cramps. I felt like an alien or an AI configuration of a woman, possessed of all their superficial charms and none of their festering internal curses. My refusal to bleed was a secret I carried proudly. I felt like I had defied nature, outsmarted my own body, tiptoed stealthily past puberty. I knew that I would be a woman in other inescapable ways – in age, in haircuts, in theory – but I felt certain that if I could overcome sexual maturity in the same way I had once overcome hunger, I would be spared the worst, most unforgivable and disfiguring afflictions of womanhood. And I felt absolutely certain that I would never have a period.

But life, unlike idealistic teenage ultimatums, has an inherently capricious slant to it, and my carefully controlled routine was knocked askance when, one weekend after a week of filming in London, I made my way to a dance studio on a whim and promptly fell in love. There was something about dancing that just called to me at that moment in time. It might have been curiosity or mere boredom, but in retrospect, I look at it as the primal, unconscious reaction of a healthy body rebelling furiously against the years I'd spent trying to ignore its existence. My once agreeable, subservient little body was an unruly teenager now, and the only way it knew to get my attention and break out of the restraints I'd forced it into was to march me to a dance studio and insist, 'Bitch, I am here, and I am going to dance.' I became totally enamoured with dance: the movement, the focus, the freedom it lent, the way you could make such beautiful shapes with your body. The way a body, so useless, ungainly and extraneous in stillness could become a whirling storm of energy and dynamic movement in dance; could communicate passion, power and vulnerability in a way I could not. And even if you didn't get the move at first, and your body galumphed around gracelessly in the back making a spectacle of itself, you were always slightly better the next class, your body somehow miraculously assimilating the moves during sleep. There was something marvellous about that, as though a divine power was using the body as an instrument of its design. For the first time in my life, it felt like I was *working with* my body, not just its weary prisoner. With dance, my body felt vital. I danced for three hours a day after filming, flitting between whatever classes were scheduled, with bright red cheeks and sweat-drenched tank tops, right up until they closed the studio each night. I did the unthinkable and became one of those people pestering the assistant director for an approximate time I would finish filming that day, texting my driver the minute I'd wrapped to pull the car round so we might bolt across London to make my lyrical jazz class. In my early days of filming, I had been horrified by the crew members who tried to expedite lunchtime or complained aloud about working late, deeply offended by their apparent lack of willingness to devote their entire bodies and souls to Harry Potter's story. I was incensed when other cast members spoke of other films they were looking forward to filming after *Harry Potter*, or unashamedly admitted to not having finished reading *Deathly Hallows*, as though any story could ever be as worthy of telling as that of the Chosen One, but suddenly *I* was someone who had a life I couldn't wait to get back to in the evenings, a calling almost as pressing as my duty to Harry. Sometimes I'd turn up to classes with smudges of dirt and painted-on bloodied cuts from the battle scenes still peppered across my forehead, and other students would throw me funny looks as I rubbed them off in the mirror with my own glistening sweat.

The dance studio was where I fell in love in more ways than one. My interest was piqued by the tall, cool, confident teacher of a 'Locking and Popping' dance class one day as I passed by his class on the way to the changing rooms. The dance studios had glass panes that looked on to the corridors, allowing mothers, friends and a pair of lascivious teenage eyes a window through which to peer in at the dance classes taking place, and soon I took to stationing myself at the edge of the cluster of cooing mums and possessive boyfriends to ogle him before his class ended. I was far too intimidated by the energy of the class and the razor-sharp choreography my crush executed to perfection to join, so I pretended to be a regular at the breakdance class after his, spending one confusing hour per week flailing my arms about the floor in the manner of an upturned beetle, just for those ten precious minutes where I could drink in an unrestricted view of my tall, dark, dancing darling. Tragically, however, the windowpanes were equipped with blinds and sometimes, depending on his mood and the intensity of the onlookers' stares, he would stride over and whip them down abruptly, riling the watchful boyfriends and starving me of my weekly fix of his face. He began doing this more and more often, earlier and earlier in class, apparently irritated by his impromptu audience, an artiste proudly guarding his process. Even his anger thrilled me, but it was not enough to satiate my growing appetite for him. Unwittingly, he had nudged me towards that familiar pivotal moment of decision: to fling myself centre stage to be seen or shunned – you could never anticipate which – or to look on longingly from the audience.

I inhaled sharply as I turned the knob of the studio door on the first day I dared attend his class. The beat of Michael Jackson's 'Smooth Criminal' seemed to permeate my bones and intensify the pounding in my chest. It took him several weeks to notice me, though I think he had sensed my hungry gaze from all the way out in the corridor and was now warily conscious of my presence in the room. I was dreadful at both the 'locking' and the 'popping' in his class, but I was a fiendishly loyal and determined student, and they say genius is one per cent inspiration, ninety-nine per cent perspiration – and I did nothing if not perspire in that class. I was totally obsessed with my new teacher, whiling away my weekends stealing into dance shops to buy fancy new leotards, risking lower and lower-cut styles and then dashing home to continue careful surveillance of his Myspace activity. As it turned out, perseverance and presence were two qualities he appreciated in others, calling to the front his favourite students to flank him and demonstrate the moves to the graceless fools bumbling around in the back, and one Saturday afternoon towards the end of a class, my moment finally came.

'Little girl!' my dear one shouted, and with a jolt that seemed to ripple orgasmically through my entire body, I saw that his inscrutable brown eyes were fixed upon me. 'Come to the front,' he commanded, snapping his fingers, 'next to me!'

I skittered joyfully to the front row, ignoring the envious glares of the other girls, trying not to cartwheel in ecstasy, and spun and crotch-grabbed like my entire life depended on it. 'Little girl' was an undeniably condescending nickname, and though girlhood had always been the safe, sterile haven sheltering me from the horrors of womanhood, something about the word 'girl' now irked me as I stared back at this tall, striking man with his arresting gaze. It was an important development in the trajectory of our relationship, however – and my masterplan. He had seen me now, and could never unsee me. I stared intently at his curly black head as he 'pimp walked' (a locking term; you wouldn't understand . . .) back and forth across my vision, as he performed triple spins on the spot that sprayed the air around him, and my face and arms, with droplets of his sweat, stinging my bare skin, and I did not instantly wipe them away – nor for several hours afterwards. I set my gaze fixedly on the target. Within six months, I had made him my boyfriend.

Life was exciting and fast-paced and super *fun* all of a sudden! I had a *boyfriend*, a concept I enjoyed perhaps as much as I enjoyed the boyfriend. It had taken me seventeen years, but I had finally found someone who was verbally contracted to suffer me out of his own free will and – allegedly – love – and he was taller, cooler and older than everyone else's boyfriends! Quite a lot older, in fact. He was a towering twenty-six to my fresh-faced seventeen, a fact that you may balk at (as did my parents). But make no mistake: in that relationship, I was firmly the yellow-eyed predator, stalking him from the shadows and camouflaging myself to match his surroundings, while he was my unsuspecting prey. My seventeenth year was an exhilarating and dreadfully sophisticated time, as I embraced life in London away from any parental interference. Now cohabiting with my fabulous cousin Amy, I divided my time between filming, dancing, dating, and the occasional bit of schoolwork. I had (mostly) overcome my terror of and crippling sense of inferiority around my castmates by now, and spent many fun-filled weekends gallivanting around London with the other *Harry Potter* girls, living it up like wild college students, albeit ones with healthy bank balances. I was busy and excited by life, and I adapted my eating habits accordingly. Food was energy now, energy that I needed to keep up with all this dancing, all this excitement, all this love. I was so busy and distracted, I stopped measuring portions and analysing their nutritional content. I ate to fuel my movement. I ate without guilt and without the compulsion to subtract portions from future meals to compensate for all the extra food I was eating. And, miraculously, my weight stayed the same. Seventeen was the Roaring Twenties of my life: I was feasting and dancing to my heart's content with zero repercussions, too busy to stop and obsess over myself anymore, and too happy. I felt sure I had cracked life's complicated combination code. Finally.

We had some great times – fun, wild, heady experiences – but the relationship soured after a handful of months because we were both – surprise! – very dysfunctional people. The thing about a teacher/ student romantic relationship is that for it to be an equal and healthy partnership, the power dynamic has to shift radically, but the minute it does, the delectably taut sexual tension snaps, and dissipates. Better to engage in an elaborate roleplay with your mild-mannered colleague than to date your hot teacher. Leave him at the lectern in his thick woollen cardigan behind an intoxicating mist of knowledge and power. Most hot teachers don't like it when their fawning ingenue loses that misty-eyed glint and dares to look upon him as her equal. And you won't like discovering that most hot teachers are wounded little boys cowering behind a god complex. He punished me for prioritising my homework over him, and I punished him for daring to like my body, for paying it compliments, and then lapsed into tears when he exasperatedly tried to take them back. To quote Vladimir Nabokov: 'Let us skip sex.' It was a significant (and positive) experience to be touched by loving hands for the first time, but it is very difficult to love someone who loathes their own body, and too often my judgement of my own flesh seeped into my opinion of him; basically, it was hard to see anyone who attempted to love my body as anything other than quite pathetic, and at times his appreciation disgusted me, which wore his patience thin. He was always deleting me as a friend on Facebook and blocking my number, disappearing from my life for days at a time, giving absolutely no indication of when he would resurface, and I was always weaponising my eating disorder against him, threatening not to eat after a fight or foisting missed meals on to his conscience. My sisters found the whole saga terribly entertaining, Emily imagining scenarios in which in a violent fit of rage he had hurled his phone off a bridge. 'Did he fish it back out of the Thames?' she would ask, giggling hysterically after I'd received a not unexpected 'Hello, it's me' text from an unknown number three days later. My siblings all thought he was completely nuts, conveniently overlooking the fact that I was too. Filming ended and I moved back home, and though we stayed in touch and were on-and-off for the best part of a year, the relationship had mostly fizzled out by that point. Suddenly, I was back in Ireland, back to school, back to one dance class a week and no boyfriend. I was sad and bored and craving the sweet things in life, so I ate them. My lifestyle abruptly changed, while my new eating habits did not. And without even noticing it, my body changed too.

So it was, one afternoon in a grimy cubicle at school, that I gazed, horrified and transfixed, at the scarlet blood in the toilet bowl. Something was dying inside me, and I had not even noticed. Could it really happen so simply? Could womanhood arrive as suddenly as this, with such noiseless violence signalling the death of the pure, innocent girl whose blood now stained my fingertips? I sat with my head in my hands for a long time, trying not to hyperventilate, knowing that this was it forever and there was no going back, but clinging naively to the notion that if I never left this cubicle, then I need not accept defeat just yet. How had this happened? Why had my body betrayed me? I thought this day would never come, had quite forgotten about the looming danger, because I'd made a deal with my body: I would keep it on the edge of health if it would keep me ever the same. Only I had not kept strictly to this agreement, had strayed much further than the edge of health and into the full, blossoming richness of life, tasting and testing everything, losing my mind in its lusciousness, and I knew the inescapable rule of life and death from which I'd tried to hide and could no longer deny: you cannot freeze a body in time and fully live a life. I'd never hated myself so much as in that moment, as I paced the stall, my fists balled tensely and I rapped my knuckles against my midsection, as though to make sure my body knew I hated it too. There could be no escape from womanhood, now or ever again, and in momentarily indulging my lust for life, I had condemned myself to a lifetime of trying to repress the woman in me. There would be no turning eighteen, crossing a magical precipice and prancing, fairylike and unsullied by bloody fingerprints, into the sunset. I paced the bathroom stall for over an hour, ignoring the ruckus of other girls – nay, women – crashing in and out of the surrounding stalls, noisily obeying their bodies' demands. I waited until after the last bell of the day had gone and the crowds had abated, then crept quietly from the bathroom down the echoing corridors, feeling like a fallen warrior limping away from the site of my defeat.

It was another private tragedy, another period of mourning for a part of myself that was irredeemably lost, that I hadn't been prepared to say goodbye to. I was quiet and subdued in the weeks after, shell-shocked by who I was now, and furious at myself for losing control. I tried to ignore what was happening in my body, hoping vaguely that, with enough neglect, maybe my newly operational womb might wither and perish, like a forgotten Tamagotchi you left in your dad's car overnight. I tried to show my body as much discouragement for its inner machinations as possible, wearing organ crushing high-waisted jeans, restricting food and whispering a series of degrading affirmations to it like prayers every time I showered. Unfortunately, though, my body's will to thrive was far less tenuous than a Tamagotchi's health, and it pressed on like a totally independent entity, bleeding on the same day of each month with militaristic precision. Giving up on resistance, the only way I learned to cope with this relentless cycle was to feign supreme indifference to the whole issue, which ironically only ended up drawing much more attention to it. I cannot *tell* you the number of times I've almost bled through a designer dress I've borrowed for an interview or a press conference, all because I refused to acknowledge the process of menstruation, refused to keep track of my periods or travel equipped with the requisite apparatus. I was always the one hurtling back through hotel corridors to frantically rifle through the amenities, or grasping publicists by the elbow and communicating through wild eyes that I needed to get off the red carpet, *stat*. One time I found myself at a fancy dinner on a press tour in Italy that I discovered, too late, involved nine courses, so it was not entirely my fault when I bled through on to the chair, and left a tiny heart-shaped splodge on its plump upholstery. Back at the hotel, I begged my best friend to call the concierge and plead with them to send up tampons.

'TAMPONS,' she enunciated to the poor, befuddled Italian man. 'TAM – PON! Tam-poni?' she tried weakly, improvising an accent.

'We have . . . Kleenex?' he suggested nervously, after conferring with his equally confounded colleagues.

'Yeah, alright,' she answered, clenching her jaw anxiously as she watched me stuff fistfuls of toilet paper up my skirt. 'Just send everything.'

As somebody who's intimately familiar with the feminine hygiene offerings of most European cultures and almost every continent, I would caution you never to forget your personal stash when vacationing in Australia, where the complimentary tampons are gnarled and bullet-shaped, apparently designed by misogynists who loathe the female reproductive system almost as much as seventeen-year-old me did. Oh, I *hated* being a bleeding woman: hated, hated, *hated* it. I hated the smell. I hated the responsibility. I hated the crippling pain. I hated the repeated monthly reminders that my body was that of a mature, ripened woman ready to be fertilised at any given opportunity, as though I didn't have anything better to do each month than help proliferate this odious species. And I hated that the only way to stop it was to do something drastic, like remove an organ or medicate myself for the next forty-odd years. Most of all, though, I hated that this was my own fault. I had indulged myself, had enjoyed life far too much, and now I was paying the price. Love of life and of another had such a steep cost, and it had almost fooled me into thinking it was worth it. Love had made me take my eye off the ball and cede control of my body, and it had, for a moment, almost tricked me into looking at my own body through its soft-focused lens, into accepting it as it was. But love, I had so painfully discovered, did not last the way self-hate did. Boys would love your body for a short time and then leave you to love that discarded husk for the rest of your life. I resolved to remember that it was not safe to trust in love. But I would always find solace in my own self-hate.

I kept this hate inside me and carried on with my life, for it is quite socially acceptable to do so, but in therapy I had reached something of a stalemate. Natasha and I had navigated a lot in a decade: anorexia, recovery, relapse, recovery again, and then recovery from recovery; as well as school and social oblivion, fame and success, falling in love and falling out of love, growing up, growing out. I wondered was it possible that, at eighteen, I might already have experienced and survived every emotion I could ever feel – would the rest just be recycling? Had we, in fact, reached the end of therapy? And yet, even though the most stark and dangerous problems had evidently slunk away, and I had managed to move on and even begun to eke out a living for myself, even though all of the obvious, urgent problems had been placated and painted over, in many ways I felt as lost and empty as I'd ever done, so I continued going to Natasha, hoping she might take pity on me after all these years and just hand me the antidote to this pervasive feeling of worthlessness that nobody could say I hadn't valiantly tried to combat myself. Surely it was possible to pay psychotherapists for this.

'I think I might be asexual,' I tell her seriously, one evening in her new therapy hut in the countryside.

I'm pretty sure I'm not, but I want her to tell me I am so that I can seriously commit to not seeking attention from the male species, and my single status will look like a powerful statement of authenticity rather than a pitiable character deficit. Perhaps I can even have a coming-out party, and vouch for LGTBQIA+ rights with renewed vested passion, and just be done with the whole sorry, sordid business of awful, heterosexual men. That's all I want.

'Have you managed to make yourself orgasm yet?' she answers, just as seriously as my eardrums shrivel up in horror. Natasha is never one to shy from these brazen statements that cause a lapsed Catholic to cringe.

'You need to engage in the practice of self-love more. Otherwise, you will never know. There's no point us talking about asexuality until you've made love to yourself.'

Theoretically and politically, I heartily endorse the kind of sassy, liberated women who drink a tall glass of wine in the evenings and fiddle with themselves to completion, but physically the concept of putting my hands on my own body to derive a sense of pleasure is a suggestion bordering on the absurd. Masturbation seems an inherently contradictory concept to those for whom any sexual thrills will be abruptly flattened by accidentally grazing one's own meaty haunch. And surely, I reason, if I was sexually aroused by my own pink flesh, I would never have ended up on Natasha's couch in the first place.

I return home, choose a large, dense book on plant-based nutrition, shivering off her distinctly unappealing invitation. I wondered vaguely if it's possible to stir your own sexual appetite out of a visceral sense of disgust for your own lumpy body, in the same way you can use a surge of self-hate to motivate yourself to do things like get out of bed, go for a run and do your work, just as effectively (and often more quickly) as you could with self-love. Could one self-*dis*please themselves into convulsions of ecstasy? It strikes me as unfair that self-pleasure is strictly for the self-lovers when self-haters have a considerably more urgent need of the dopamine hit. I shake the notion of self-pleasure from my unenthused mind and carry on with my reading.

I decide to avoid therapy for the next four to six weeks, hoping that in that interim Natasha will have forgotten my 'homework' and I can try her again on the asexuality thing.

'I am so sad all the time. I want to run away from my life,' I whine in our next session. 'I want to tear down everything I've worked on so far. I want a new identity. I want to be a waitress in France and for all my friends to forget about me, and for an angry, sexist boss to tell me what to do every day. I want to join the circus. I want to be a brunette. I want to be a lowly servant in the old days living a simple life of chores and bread and water. I'd love to find a small and inconsequential crime that will put me in prison for three to six months and take me out of the world. I need to do something radical and dramatic that disrupts this monotony and restarts my entire life.' I exhale heavily and look at her expectantly. Surely, she will understand that this time it's desperate, that I'm out of ideas, that I've tried my very best and now she needs to hand me the answer. But she shakes her head, smiling wryly.

'This is nothing new, honey. You're always looking for an escape, when really you need to go deeper into yourself. You've been running from yourself for years, and you need to stop and give it up.

Here, let's do some breath work – and I'll send you the details of that ten-day silent retreat . . .'

That's it. That is the spiritual stalemate we have reached, and those are the only answers Natasha will offer me: meditation or masturbation. I ponder the notion that perhaps my own therapist has grown tired of me and is deliberately repeating her guidance so that I'll move on and she won't have to endure my solipsistic meanderings for another decade. I wouldn't blame her. Whatever her reasoning, she refuses to budge on this advice, or to qualify my pervasive sense of internal emptiness with an edgy psychological condition or an obscure sexual orientation, and instead repeatedly insists that I sit and breathe or grope myself. I have enormous resistance to both. I just can't make myself sit there and do either, because these are embodiment practices, and I've always survived by thinking my way through every problem. I don't trust the body, its unpredictability or imperfect design, and I'm afraid of what will happen if I sit there in that mysterious creature, if I stop denying that I live in a body and finally try to work with it, not against it.

So, I spend the next few years avoiding therapy. I audition for dance school at three different colleges, but I don't have the technique to back up my passion and receive three resounding 'no's, which crush me, so I immediately quit dancing – unrequited love is never fun. Filming ends, and I am devastated. For the past two years, we in the young cast have been fielding the same mind-numbingly inane question throughout the extensive series of interviews on film promotion tours: 'How are you going to feel when it all ends?' I've been asked this question so many times that it has lost all meaning.

I have no authentic feelings left to dredge up, and instead usually answer, through glaze-eyed numbness: 'It will be sad.' So when it actually does come to an abrupt end, one evening on the set of the Battle of Hogwarts, and the props guys quickly snatch away our wands, and the costume ladies cloak us in puffy North Face jackets for the last time, and frayed, bloodied Hogwarts students rise from the rubble and dust themselves down, and the entire cast of *Harry Potter* stumble about, clutching each other and looking teary and disorientated, I still don't really believe it's over. It's only late that evening, when I climb the stairs to the producer's office, where my journey had first begun, and my eyes rest on a cosy little bed nestled in the corner of David Barron's office for his cherished pug, Sam, that I realise I am neither their child nor their burden anymore. And that's when a cascade of grief and terror grips me, and it is all I can do to remain vertical, to not crumple on the floor of David's office, curl up in Sam's bed and beg him to adopt me as his pet.

School ends and I am relieved, but I haven't applied to any other colleges or planned for a future other than dance. For the first time in years, I find myself idle and unemployed, the outside world gone quiet, with no assertive, professional voice calling to tell me what to do or where to be. My agent recommends I be 'smart' and get qualified in something other than a career in the arts, cautioning that a life as an actor is a precarious vocation and that parlaying a period of childhood stardom into a stable career is a transition that few young actors successfully make, but I insist that I have no interest in anything other than the arts, in telling and enacting stories, and I find the suggestion to secure a sensible, alternative trade a bit insulting, frankly, coming from my agent, so we part ways. An American manager gets in touch, literally shimmying into my life at a concert of a client of his and emanating the exact opposite energy of my killjoy agent. He offers boundless enthusiasm and myriad creative ideas to bolster my career by immersing me in a series of auditions, meetings and photoshoots. I eagerly sign with him and hightail it to LA with hardly a second thought.

LA is a *trip*. What is not to love about LA for a bright-eyed, hopeful young actress? Life is sunny and upbeat and frothing at the mouth with opportunities. The absolutely undimmable positivity is the most infectious part, the sense of limitless potential truly dizzying, especially to a dazed Irish person. In Ireland, we're brought up to believe that some people are born special, gifted and destined for greatness, while the rest of us are inherently ordinary, about as unique as a mud-crusted sack of potatoes. Sacks of potatoes are earthbound, functional, hearty and versatile – all qualities that are highly regarded in Irish society – but they are decidedly unflashy, and it does not do to cultivate pretensions to stardom (or 'notions' as they are more commonly described at home) when you are a sack of potatoes. In LA, however, entire fortunes, careers and industries are built on the philosophy that even if you arrive as a potato, with enough hard work, passion, money and perseverance, you can evolve into something more exciting. In LA, everyone wakes up and zips to their gyms and yoga studios with a feeling of optimism, because they believe it is possible for anyone to manipulate their environment and contort themselves into a position of worthiness, success and international acclaim. Accordingly, there are gurus, experts and coaches corresponding to every part of your body and soul that needs cultivation, and who will buoy you on with hypnotic conviction as you slavishly seek to prove true the sacred Hollywood philosophy that relentless self-improvement will always lead to success. After a week in LA, I had my first audition, which I considered a largely successful enterprise due to the mere fact that I had narrowly avoided causing a multi-car pile up after following my sat-nav on to a freeway, an experience that I found to be reminiscent of the scene in *The Lion King* where young Simba is almost stampeded to death by a herd of wildebeests, moments before Scar murders his father. But the audition itself, apparently, had not gone well, and when I received the feedback that my interpretation of the character had been 'one-note', I collapsed on my sofa in despair, thinking it was all over, that I might as well pack my bags and ask our local supermarket back home about job openings. I called my parents in tears, only to find that they shared these sentiments, clucking sympathetically but gravely acknowledging that our collective gene pool did not naturally endow its offspring with the requisite charms for a life in front of the lens. *Remember you are a potato*, they seemed to be saying. They were already planning to call the admissions officers of all the universities in Ireland to see if a desperate latecomer might still be accepted for any of their courses before I recalled that this kind of soul-crushing modesty was the very reason I'd fled the country in the first place.

I hurriedly said goodbye and quickly called my manager to try and convince him to keep me as a client. His response stunned me: 'Forget about it – we'll just get you some acting lessons.' Apparently, in LA, the land of Disney princesses and starry-eyed dreamers, you did not even need to be a particularly good actor to make it as an actor! I was intoxicated by this new philosophy, and quickly adapted to never again calling my parents after dodgy auditions. I fully bought into the practice of being flanked by a bevy of pricey gurus in preparation for every meeting, every audition, every moment I dared open my mouth in the presence of a potential producer or director, and soon

I had collected one of each expert in LA. I had a trainer, an acting teacher, a dialect coach, a vocal coach, a life coach, an intuitive, a colourist, a manicurist, a stylist, an aesthetician, a publicist, and so on and so forth. If you had a fancy website, a celebrity testimonial and could easily point out some flaw that was surely going to hamper my prospects as an actor, and could tell me precisely how you would go about fixing it, I would pay you money. One time, an acting teacher told me that the reason I couldn't cry on cue was because my root chakra was blocked, and referred me to a tantric expert in Santa Monica. I paid $350 for this lady to lie me down on the floor of her meditation studio and hover her hands over my torso as she coaxed self-conscious sighs and moans out of me for an hour. In the next class, I eventually managed to cry over the fact that I couldn't cry, and also because Hollywood was bleeding me dry, spiritually and financially. The teacher made the class applaud, and told me there was 'some progress'. I didn't go back to that tantric lady again, though – even I am not that gullible.

All the work and effort and considerable expense eventually led to some success. I did a handful of movies and shorts, and made friends and lots of connections, and I found two acting classes where the teachers really cared about their students. I was quite happy in LA, but after a few years I decided to move back to London to try the UK industry again. I'd gone to LA on a cheerful whim, intending to stay for three months, and, in a blink, that had become five years – not because I had made any conscious decision to stay, but I think because of the allure of all that brimming potential, and of who you could meet and what might happen if you stuck around a little bit longer. I think it's quite possible to be happy and centred in LA if you find small, authentic communities, but I think a lot of people can spend their entire lives there daydreaming about the promise of tomorrow. So, after realising that I was on more intimate terms with the circle of gurus I paid to improve me than with my own family, I decided it was time to settle in London, something of a happy medium between dreamy, sunny LA and sober, rural Ireland. I worried that I might be making a mistake, throwing away all the foundations I'd laid and the work I'd done, and that I'd move to London and find I had zero career opportunities there. I shared these concerns with my wonderful acting teacher Julie in my last acting class in LA, and she promptly combatted them with some of the best advice I've ever received: 'Why don't you worry in the other direction?' she demanded, nailing me with her penetrating green gaze, which lovingly refused to ever let her students off the hook. 'Why don't you worry that it will *all* work out and you'll meet all your creative matches and you'll be *too* successful and *too* happy and *too* busy with how much work you have? Why must you always anticipate the absolute worst-case scenario, when you could worry that everything will just be too wonderful? Why do you do that? *Why?*'

Good point, I thought. *Why do I?*

London was a much more grounding place for me. People asked, with genuine interest, 'How are you?' before they asked 'What do you do?', and it was possible to cultivate other aspects of your life with the same care and detail as you applied to your career without spending sleepless nights worrying that you weren't 'hungry enough' for your dreams. I found that, while the acting industry in London was more tight-knit and exclusive, its inner circles harder to penetrate, the casting directors and producers didn't care so much about your celebrity profile or what you'd 'done' recently. They were much more interested in your presence in the room. Obviously, there were pros and cons to this: it was nice to be seen and evaluated based on who you were in that moment, but if you had a bad audition, you couldn't simply skip off to an acting masterclass and work through it – you just never got called back again. After several years of hustling in LA with the constant pressure to book a show or instantaneously 'make it', I was ready to work hard at my craft for little pay, and to slowly, methodically carve out a reputation as a committed actress.

I quickly fell in love with theatre: the warm embrace of a rehearsal room teeming with creative energy and the deep bonds actors formed within them; the heart-stopping adrenaline that gripped you every night you went onstage, convincing you that live theatre was a form of insanity before the nerves quickly dissipated and you suspected that the stage might be the only place where people were finally, totally honest. It only ever took a week for the cast of a play to feel like my artistic family, and theatre is where I've made lifelong friends. But acting is a lonely and unstable vocation, because eventually the show ends and the world you inhabited is dismantled, and everyone trundles sadly back to the train station with an overstuffed suitcase, back to their respective corners of the world, and it's just you again in your apartment, reciting lines to your cat and going slowly mad as you wonder if it's a coincidence that all the young actresses who book the top jobs get progressively smaller as their names get bigger, or is there something else you're missing? Acting is one of the best jobs in the world when you have work – it's fun, it's exhilarating, it's therapeutic – but there's no silence so deafening and devastating as the one that follows an audition you've poured your heart and soul into. In that silence, you realise the casting director was apparently so indifferent to your efforts that they won't even bother calling to tell you that you didn't book the role and can stop appealing to the heavens for that job. I've found that the most successful and happy actors are those who have other passions that feed their souls, and for whom a callback is not salvation from the brink of depression. Happy actors are also regenerative farmers, painters, wildlife photographers, playwrights.

Personally, I struggled with the constant anxiety and rejection that trying to be an actor brought, and I felt there was extra pressure surrounding my career because of the narrative built up around it ever since I'd spoken publicly about my eating disorder. By now, I'd been speaking to the press for several years about my previous struggles with anorexia. I think I wanted to get some distance from it and to reach out to other people lost amid that darkness. As it turned out, however, the mainstream media was not the best vehicle for having sensitive, in-depth discussions about mental health; nobody wanted to hear about the nuances of eating disorders and recovery, they just wanted you to tell them in a quavering voice that you'd been moments from death, and to prove it with a series of shocking photographs. I cringed and looked away every time tacky 'HARRY POTTER SAVED MY LIFE' pieces appeared in print. There was something so *off* about the idea that recovery had all been worth it because of my success, as though my entire worth was only realised by the fact that I'd achieved something in the eyes of society. These headlines always seemed disturbingly reminiscent of my inner thoughts as a sad, sick eleven-year-old, when I'd gazed at pictures of pop stars, actors and writers and thought hopelessly: *Lucky her, to not need an eating disorder to justify being alive.* Was recovery only worthwhile because

I'd gone and done something that piqued the public's interest? Was a life not worth redeeming simply because you'd been given it? A feeling of unease pervaded as I wondered about people who recovered from eating disorders who didn't go on to star in movies. What of those who recovered and worked quietly, diligently, in hospitals or classrooms and never received the public applause? What of other young girls whose spirits were being suffocated by their eating disorders, who read stories that told them that recovery would all be worth it once you manifested your dreams, but who gazed on sadly at the smiling faces and thought recovery was for the blessed, the beautiful, and for them it was not worth the risk? And what if Natasha had been right, that I still had deep healing to do, that my acting dream had not been the answer to all my problems, the fairy-tale ending not the end of the story? What if the fairy-tale ending – the idea that one could recover, manifest her wildest dream and secure eternal happiness – had turned into a trap? This all sort of caught up with me in late 2017 when life dealt me a series of blows in quick succession. A dear friend died unexpectedly. A dream role that I had been pursuing doggedly for several months – writing to the director, making him audition tapes and eventually convincing him to meet me for coffee – went to another actress. And it was at that precise moment in time that my beloved boyfriend, my sweet, adorable, kind-hearted boyfriend of two years, whom I worshipped and adored, and for whom I believed all the other ex-boyfriends had been worth enduring, promptly and abruptly decided to leave me – for a man.

I press on bitterly, because that's all I can do, now with a stubbornly nihilistic outlook on life. My broken heart has shattered my belief in happy endings. I no longer believe that things always work out in the end. I don't believe that if you work hard and stay humble and give to charity, you will get the happiness. I don't believe that if you love someone with your whole heart and offer them everything you have that it will ever be enough. I don't believe that anyone's life means anything. And I don't believe that life gets easier after recovery. I can see now that this is a bullshit ruse cited by parents and professionals so that you won't be such a problem to them anymore, and I envy other people with soul-sucking problems like anorexia, bulimia, and alcohol and drug addiction, because at least they've got a powerful numbing agent and don't have to feel how awful life is all of the time.

Life is not fun for the summer of 2018. I've had no acting jobs in months, I am living in a tiny apartment under an emotionally unstable young couple who frequently bellow their hatred for one another at a volume that makes the ceiling shudder, and I am still reeling from the shock of living a virtually fictitious romance for the past two years. Everywhere I go, I encounter reminders of my own pointlessness and useless bulk, from walking home in a blur of tears after an innocent lady in the post office enquires, 'Why don't we see you on screen anymore?' to the echoing silence from the person I've loved the most carrying on like I don't exist. I start writing hate letters to the universe, complaining that it is too hard, that I've done everything right and it still isn't enough. *Why have you put me here?* I demand. *What do you want? Why did you yank me back into this life fifteen years ago only to live it out as this hideous, meaningless lump of flesh?! Sometimes,* I continue, *I think the only reason I don't jump off a bridge is because I don't want to die fat.*

The vitriol of that statement takes me aback. I thought I had grown out of those thoughts. Forevermore, in my darkest moments, will it always come back to this? Will I always find myself reasoning with my hateful, fat-phobic eleven-year-old self once again? Bargaining for my happiness with this vicious, tireless bitch? I continue writing, begging the universe to send me something to remind me I still have something to offer the world, a reason to be alive. *You have to give me something*, I insist. *You can't just leave me hanging.*

The very next day, my agent calls to tell me I've been offered a spot on *Dancing with the Stars* in LA. It isn't exactly what I had in mind, a turn as a ballroom dancer on America's glitziest, tackiest reality TV show, but the universe works in mysterious ways, and I cannot deny that my letter has received a response. Leave grimy old London in winter for a glamorous sojourn in LA, where I'll be trussed up in satin and sequins, and where a ballroom dance world champion will be contractually obliged to make me look like a good dancer?

Fuck it, let's go.

Three days later, I am standing outside a rehearsal room in the *Dancing with the Stars* studio, a stone's throw away from Hollywood Boulevard. I'm about to meet my new dance partner, Keo, a tall, proud, chiselled South African. I had not previously watched the show and had no prior awareness of the hype and mystery surrounding the dance partnerships each season, but I quickly understood that although the famous participants were referred to as the 'stars' (and it would take me an embarrassingly short amount of time to identify myself under this nomenclature, quite unconsciously answering crew members' summons of 'Stars, come this way'), the professional dancers were the real celebrities on this show. I gathered, from a brief perusal of the comments sections on Instagram, that Keo was known as an underdog on the show, a striking dancer who had been disproportionately allocated the older, creakier star participants, who, though they were lovely and fun to watch, very rarely lasted long on the show. Fans passionately complained that Keo's chances at winning the coveted Mirrorball Trophy were being unfairly hampered by the rigidity of his partners' joints.

'Ugh, I bet this is just another old lady with a young-looking body,' huffs one fan in a comment under a promotional teaser picture depicting Keo beaming cheesily at the camera with one hand curled around my headless torso.

Keo overplays his enthusiasm by a lot when I walk into the rehearsal room to meet him, dropping to his knees before the camera and thanking the heavens, which makes me cringe inwardly, but I soon learn that this is an expertly judged performance, and that the 'real' you doesn't translate very favourably to reality TV, particularly if you're an introvert. You should always exaggerate your own character for these types of shows, aiming for a convincing impression of yourself after several tequilas. We exchange pleasantries and cover the basics, and then attempt some elementary dance steps, Keo exploding into paroxysms of delight over my merest shuffle.

Then he asks me a final question: 'What do you hope to get from this show?'

I ponder the question a moment, and am about to give a reflexively facetious answer like 'To get my teenage splits back', but instead decide to believe there must be a deeper reason I'm here and that the time has finally come to try and break a lifelong habit.

'I want to learn to think positively,' I tell him sincerely. 'I get into such negative thought patterns and then I ruin everything. I want to stop thinking such negative thoughts.' *I suspect they might be killing me*, I want to add, but don't. We'll save the melodrama for when we need the votes.

'OK,' answers Keo, nodding assertively. 'I can teach you that.'

Think what you will about the unapologetic gaudiness of *Dancing with the Stars*, it was one of the toughest and most rewarding jobs I've ever done – and I loved every minute. Days were jam-packed with five-hour rehearsals, costume fittings, media interviews and physio sessions, and there were barely five minutes in which to keep up with friends and family, save to pester them for votes every Monday. The professional dancers worked harder than I'd seen anyone do before, arriving promptly in the mornings to coach their panting celebrities through every precise detail of the minute-long routines that we spent an entire week refining, and then dashing off energetically in the evenings to rehearse dizzyingly complex opening numbers as their partners winced and limped to our cars to hurry home and submerge our throbbing feet in ice. The rehearsals were a stark shock to the system; I'd never trained my body so rigorously, and in the first few days had to take frequent breaks, collapsing into corners of the room and pressing my head between my knees so as not to vomit, while Keo stood there, glistening and waiting. All vanity and formalities between us were quickly abandoned when we'd catch each other pulling long sleeves over fingers to avoid palmfuls of the other's sweat.

But despite the omnipresent aches and the oily coating of perspiration, I couldn't help but appreciate how well my body worked. Every morning I hauled it to rehearsals, and though it had been ten years since I'd attempted any kind of dance, I watched in the mirror as it diligently worked to copy the shapes and spins and movements that Keo demonstrated, noticing how each day the moves got a little smoother, sharper and less laborious. Moves that seemed to knot electrical wires in my head on Tuesdays were always somehow miraculously understood and assimilated by my body on Thursdays, and every Monday evening on show night, when the intensity of the lights and the cheers and the stares of the American public set the pitch of my thoughts at that of a shrill scream, and I couldn't imagine standing still on stage and speaking, let alone performing a frantic jive, my body always somehow kicked in and did the dance for me. I can't say that all of a sudden I learned to like my body, but day by day, and dance by dance, it started to earn my grudging respect. I felt excited each day to see how fast I could pick up the moves and how bold I could be in adding my own flourishes. Why had I abandoned dancing all those years ago, when it had been teaching me the beauty of a symbiotic relationship between body and mind?

I watched, with interest, the pride and confidence with which the professional dancers held themselves, how they paraded their bodies around like show ponies while I shuffled shyly after them as if mine was a banjaxed old camper van. They treated their bodies with reverence, too, nourishing them with nine-dollar organic juices, rewarding them with visits to luxury spas, and listening attentively to them when they'd pushed too hard in rehearsal and needed to rest. It was truly revelatory – and a little disconcerting – to observe how you could use an iron sense of discipline to care for your body rather than punish it. They took self-care to new extremes, scheduling biweekly massages and arranging to meet for 'B12 shots', where a swollen-lipped nurse would hook you up to an IV that siphoned a cocktail of age- and injury-defying vitamins directly into your bloodstream. And while you could argue that their bronzed, sculpted bodies and disarming good looks made it easy for them to love and cherish their own flesh vehicles, I began to wonder which came first: a strong, healthy, attractive body, or an appreciation for it? What if a foundation of self-love was responsible for that radiant glow they all possessed?

My negative thinking continued to trip me up in rehearsals, though – literally and figuratively. At first, I struggled to meet my own eyes in the mirror or to imagine myself getting the moves. After a few failed attempts trying to nail fiddly little steps like batucadas in samba or the rapid tempo of the jive, my reaction was to throw up my hands and say I would never get it, but Keo firmly insisted I would, so we just kept repeating the moves until I did. Keo was a strict disciplinarian when it came to positive thinking, flatly refusing to indulge my doubts and anxieties.

'What if I fall doing this spin?' I asked him, a look of terror in my eyes as I met his gaze in the mirror and implored him to join me in a dark corner of my mind. 'What if I fall on national TV?!'

'You won't fall,' he answered, expressionlessly, reflexively flicking the invitation away.

'How can you know that?!' I demanded, clapping my hands to my head. 'I could easily fall! We should practise how to come out of a fall. Let's practise falling!'

'You won't fall,' he insisted more firmly still.

He was right; I never did fall, and I'll never be entirely sure if that was a miracle or because we simply had not practised falling.

I get better and better at the dances each week. We shimmy our way through a foxtrot, samba, jive and Viennese waltz, our judges' scores creeping up, but in week five we find ourselves in the bottom two, narrowly avoiding elimination by the public vote. I start to hear whispers that people find me boring and too stuck in my own head, which only sends me deeper into it. But I am not ready for this glamorous stint as a ballroom dancer to come to an end yet! I can work harder and be better; I can *think* my way through this obstacle. The other contestants are flashier or have bigger personalities, I can see that, but they don't have my hunger, so I resolve to try harder and devote more time to perfecting each step. And, as it always has done, my quest for perfection gives my mind a focus point amid all the chaos and anxiety. I try and try.

Disney week comes around and we are given one of my favourite songs from *Tangled*. I am sure that this is my moment to break through, so I give it everything, keeping a rigid daily routine and enlisting my circle of Hollywood gurus, dashing between a Pilates instructor, stylist, manicurist and flexibility coach after rehearsals every day. But it is not enough. The judges are unimpressed by our efforts, insisting that my timing is off and that they are looking for something dazzling, something *more*.

More? I wonder, fixing a tight grin on my face and nodding robotically at the camera. *More?!*

Keo seems to sense I am at boiling point, and once we are off camera, he leads me to cool off in the fresh October breeze outside the soundstage – but instead I have a meltdown. I am furious and hopeless and utterly disgusted with myself, sitting on the steps of CBS dressed as an overgrown Rapunzel. Why do I even bother? What is the point? Why is my best never ever enough?

I rail at innocent Keo for twenty minutes. Every so often, an anxious runner scuttles up to us to try and nudge us back to set, but Keo just shakes his head firmly, warning them to retreat, while I continue spewing a stream of vicious, hateful bile. It just keeps coming,

I feel I will never eliminate all of this anger and sadness. I am done with everything. I am done with this show. I am done with positive thinking. I am done with myself. I am sick of trying so, so hard at life, and coming up short. Keo continues to stand there, princely and ever patient. Eventually, I run out of words, and I take a long, ragged breath as I glower hopelessly at my shoes.

'Great,' Keo says, with perky finality. 'Now we have a story for our video package next week.'

I look up wearily and see him pointing off to my left, where the production crew are crouched with a camera and boom and not a hint of subtlety, capturing my every word. Ahhh, Hollywood!

We are voted through to the following week despite our lack-lustre scores, but I am out of ideas for how to win the judges over. The next week is Halloween, and we are given a tango and costumed as black cats, which is excellent *fuck everything* energy, so that's what we work with. On show day, a make-up artist informs me that it is, in fact, National Cat Day, which seems to bode well for us, and I resolve to hang on to my cool, cat-like composure all day and dance in tribute to the feline population. But the noise and the mayhem and the constant touch-ups eventually whip my nerves into such a frenzy that instead of sitting back, sleek and poised in the shadows to lazily eye everyone running about, I am dashing back and forth to the wardrobe department, appealing for someone to untape my butt cheeks from my pleather leotard for emergency trips to the bathroom.

Keo and I are chivvied to the stage to take our positions for our tango, and it's too much: every nerve in my body screams at me to make a run for it. I want so much for this to go well. I want so much to be loved, to be worthy, to be enough, to be perfect, but I know

I never will be. I know I am going to be voted out that night, and there is nothing I can do to change people's minds. The pressure, as I take my place behind a row of slinky dancers dressed as cats, is too intense, and I feel myself give up.

Suddenly, a new thought comes to me, right before the three shrill beats to signal the start of the music sound. *Fuck it,* says a strong, clear, pissed-off voice in my head. *They won't like you anyway. Might as well go out there and do what you like.*

Something snaps in that moment. I am fired up, focused, and though I can feel myself making small errors here and there, my skirt getting caught on my heel momentarily or my head whipping around too quickly, I do not give a flying fuck.

We finally get those elusive ten points from two of the judges that night, and everyone raves and fawns over us backstage, and we are voted through for another week. The praise is thrilling and intoxicating, and where a moment ago I'd thought I'd expelled my final two fucks and didn't care what people thought anymore, now all of a sudden, I am enjoying this flurry of affection and I care very much what they think. Whatever had snapped in that magic moment has unsnapped just as quickly.

'Keo!' I call to my partner outside the studio after the show, as he stands with a cluster of friends receiving hugs and claps on the back. 'Keo, come over here a minute.' I wave him over and pat the stone steps beside me, indicating for him to sit.

'What's up, partner?' he says, beaming widely and patting me on the shoulder.

'There were so many mistakes,' I tell him gravely, shaking my head. '*So many*. Let's sit down and watch the dance and comb through the mistakes.' I gesture to the phone in my hand.

At my words, his shoulders sag dramatically. He looks like I have popped him.

'No, girl,' he answers, a note of exhaustion in his tone. 'That dance is over now. We're done for tonight. See you tomorrow for rumba.'

I watch him quietly for a moment as he trudges heavily away to his car, and I can see that it must be wearing, that this incessant compulsion of mine to forensically sift through every mistake and negative thought is hard on other people too. I can see that the energy I carry is exhausting and off-putting, and I know I'd want to peace-out on that attitude too. I watch his car pull out, and wonder what place I could drive to where the negative thought patterns might not follow.

As I watched Keo drive away that night, I realised something profound about the choice between positive or negative thinking, between indulging fears or dreams, the worst thing happening or the best thing, and it was that a negative thought abruptly brings things to a halt, whereas a positive one facilitates growth. Negativity always leads you to a dead end; you can crawl into the darkest, dankest corner, and though it is lonely and miserable, you know where the wall is, your back firmly pressed against it, and there is something wonderfully safe about that. When you choose positivity, on the other hand, you choose limitless potential, and whatever you look at with positivity grows and spreads and unfurls in a thousand different directions. The realisation was exciting and unpredictable, but terrifying, because limitless potential would go on and on forever. There would be no end, and it would be wild and out of control and so far from perfect. If I wanted to reach a safe place where nobody could touch me, I needed only follow a negative thought down to it. But if I wanted to grow and create and evolve, I needed to follow the golden thread of creativity that didn't seem to have an end. It was a choice I'd been unconsciously making my entire life.

There was no denying it was a choice.

11

'What advice would you give to any of our viewers who are trying to recover from an eating disorder?' This enquiry comes from a well-meaning TV presenter one afternoon in the summer of 2019, as I sit across from her on a plump yellow sofa answering questions. I'm there to promote a play, but as usual the conversation is quickly steered into eating disorder territory, and soon comes to resemble a badly handled therapy session rather than a light-hearted chat-show segment.

It's been fifteen years since I was discharged from inpatient treatment, and ten since I first spoke publicly about my past struggles – but, apparently, it is still the most interesting and noteworthy aspect of my life. This is a fact that leaves me feeling irked and dispirited, but I suppose I have only myself to blame. I'm tired of these questions, but I believe in the power of sharing our stories and sometimes, admittedly, I worry that it really *is* the most interesting thing about me – that me and my work are not enough to hold people's attention, that I lost all my edginess when I let go of my eating disorder, that my body was only acceptable when I spent every ounce of energy trying to fix it – and so, it is out of a murky combination of altruism and insecurity that I indulge this morbid curiosity. I take a breath, searching for words that are simple and honest and hopefully somewhat illuminating, to answer the presenter's question, but before I can say anything, a scathing voice in my mind provides its unfiltered thoughts on pursuing recovery:

Don't, she cautions, bitterly. *It's not worth it. You'll never find the same security and solace from your dreams as you do from your disorder. Every day you'll feel flawed and vulnerable and ordinary, and you'll find that life stings a thousand times more without your armour of skinniness. You'll know you're deeply, incurably flawed, and some days you won't be able to cope with that, and all you'll want is your comforting dysfunction back.*

I wager that this is not the answer the viewers are looking for, so I catch myself and instead offer something glibly upbeat like, 'Recovery is difficult, but things get better afterwards,' or 'Remember your imperfections are your most interesting features.' After the interview, I traipse home, feeling exhausted and violated, as though the presenter had reached inside me and scraped the bottom of my being, fingernails scrabbling at the very base of my soul, leaving only a cavernous emptiness. It's hard to know where the boundaries are with journalists, and it's hard to know what answer to give to a question I'm still grappling with myself. I don't really know what I feel about recovery, I admit to myself, confused and drained. I don't know where to locate myself on the recovery journey.

And I don't know what to say to the dozens of letters I receive each month from people seeking guidance and inspiration; fathers writing on behalf of daughters, aunts on behalf of nieces, or young people going out on a limb for themselves, asking for strength, asking for advice, asking for answers. Most often when these letters arrive, I put them aside, vaguely planning to reply at some point in the distant future, but then more time passes, and the piles of letters start to totter and fall over, so I buy a large plastic box and I stash the letters in that. Soon, I buy a second box and start to fill that up too. Soon again, these desperate missives will spill over into a third box, and then I will buy a nice embroidered tablecloth and turn the boxes into a sturdy coffee table. But, for now, these boxes continue to bother me, and I see fragments of the letters through their plastic sides when I look under my desk, like ghosts of my past. Maybe some of these letter-writers *are* ghosts now. One third of anorexia sufferers do not get better – that's a fact. '*How do you recover from an eating disorder?*' the ghosts plead. '*Where did you find the strength to pursue your dreams?*' And, most hauntingly of all: '*Why should I recover?*'

Time marches on and I distract myself with plays and books and classes and petitions and friends' birthdays, and I continue to dodge these letters, hoping the ghosts, with their hungry raccoon eyes and their sharp-edged shoulders, will drift on and ask someone else, someone with the conviction and clarity of a cool-voiced deity, someone who never looks out of airplane windows drearily contemplating the emptiness of their existence. Because if I *were* to answer them, I would have to confess my most shameful secrets: that I recovered partly by brute force and partly by accident; that I merely fell in love with the world at pivotal moments and lost myself in its vast, alluring wildness, only to look back when I once again found myself assaulted by its dangers to realise – too late! – that I had strayed too far from the lonely, lovely island of perfection. And I would have to admit that recovery felt much more like surrender than like strength; that it felt like the warrior finally falling to her knees in bone-deep exhaustion at the end of a futile, unwinnable war, curling on the ground and weeping in hateful defeat as she succumbs to rest, food and soft caresses. As to the last question, it remains unanswerable, as elusive as the meaning of life.

Why did I recover? It's a question I continue to contemplate. I think about it as I look down into the enormous yellow eyes of my little cat Puff, her tiny, trusting, upturned face, this creature who I cherish and protect, but to whom I feed the corpses of hundreds of other lovable animals. Or when I don't get the job. Or even when my gaze falls on a small, boastful sign in JKF airport that reads: 'In New York, one person is born every four minutes.' I stare at the sign for too long, thinking one new person born every four minutes in the whole *world* seems like a gross excess.

'Why are we even here?' I moan to Puff in the winter of 2020 when the world has shut up shop and I am integral to no one but this small domesticated feline. 'What is it all for?'

'Mew,' she answers simply, but not unreasonably, her shiny orbs fixed unblinkingly on the tin can of tightly compressed meat, her pink tongue winding its way greedily to either side of her furry face. 'Mew' is perhaps a satisfactory answer for a cat, but as I watch her tearing noisily into the strips of meat, each bite buying another day of health, another day of life, I can't help but wonder: why do we eat? I continue to wonder and to ignore the letters because I don't want to admit my guiltiest secret of all: that sometimes, when I hear a story, told in hushed tones, of a woman who followed anorexia to her end, I feel a twinge of jealousy; that I am never sure if anorexia beat her or she beat it; that I think about the thirty-three per cent who never recovered, and I wonder which of us is better off; that, sometimes, I envy the ghosts.

'Sometimes' is an important word here, however, and envying the dead is not the same as wanting to die. It only takes a couple of nights' sleep deprivation, or sitting through an infuriating jingle played for forty-five minutes while you're on the phone to your bank for any one of us to fantasise about the quiet oblivion of the dead. I vacillate, you see, between feeling awed by something as simple as a cerulean blue sky on a clear spring day and my luck at being alive to experience it, and weeping bitterly on my couch over how long and unfair life is. I've grown up and changed and recovered, and even when the sun is lost behind dense layers of clouds, I believe sunshine is the earth's default state and the clouds just its transient visitors rather than vice versa – and that's significant progress. But I can't deny that there are still times when I long for the thing that numbed all joy and pain, when I look back on those days as the only time I had my life all figured out, when I truly miss my eating disorder. I'm ashamed to share these thoughts aloud, though. I'm supposed to be some kind of role model. I allegedly worked this out years ago. I'm not allowed to look back and wonder, was the other path the right one? And yet I do, and I can't remember the moment I chose this one. I have so many unanswered questions about the line between self-destruction and self-creation, and I have to ask them.

'It's a safe problem,' Natasha says over Skype one evening after I've asked for her thoughts on why eating disorders are so hard to let go of. Natasha and I don't work together as often these days, since I've moved away from home and have come to a point where I can handle what life throws at me relatively well on my own, but she has always been there for me, as she is today, to answer my most pressing questions on the allure, the healing, and the heart of eating disorders. 'An eating disorder is always a safe problem that keeps us protected from a risky adventure,' Natasha continues, 'but you will ultimately make a decision to play a life full out or to live a smaller life that feels certain and safe. And, of course, the irony is that the safe problem becomes the riskiest of all. The safe problem – if you continue down that path – becomes the rock on which you perish.'

But the safe problem, Natasha goes on, can graduate to being 'the safe hands on the wheel'. In her opinion, *true* recovery is impossible in the early stages of recovery, and the best way to recover, rather than trying to wrench away the eating disorder in one swift motion, is to learn to channel its considerable energy into higher pursuits. In Natasha's opinion, the path to recovery involves graduating away from using the mediums of food and weight as self-soothing devices and on to higher problems.

'It has to become more like a governing body, the co-pilot,' she says. 'You remove the emphasis from food and weight, and it becomes what it always was: a psychological device that just wanted to say, "Safety first." It actually upgrades to being the safe hands on the wheel across life. I think of it as an engineering device, and I think you never outgrow it, because it's part of your psyche. How can you cut off a part of yourself? You don't pull your ear off because you don't like what you hear. You're not going to root out a part of your inner design because you don't like what it's designing. You shift the design, you change the prototype, and then it prints off a better outcome for you, because you've outgrown the eating dis-order – but, yes, you always need to outgrow the eating disorder. I mean, you do always have a choice,' she adds. 'You can use your free will to keep anorexia going, or you can use your free will to swap it out for a higher plane, a higher you. But we're always meant to upgrade our problems.'

I feel a prickle of emotion listening to her speak, because these words resonate in a way that is painful. I don't think the doctors or nurses I encountered in treatment ever recognised the aspect of my eating disorder that was protecting me from a deeper pain, or saw the fierce, determined, obsessive energy I possessed as something that could be channelled into healthier pursuits. All I was, to them, was 'sick'. The eating disorder was a demonic, evil force to be stomped out by the most ruthless, time-efficient methods possible. 'You're not going to root out a part of your inner design because you don't like what it's designing,' Natasha had said, but that is exactly how the medical system approached treating eating disorders. I think when they ripped away the thing I'd cultivated to give me a small measure of self-worth, they denied me tools to fight my pain, and there was something about the forced surrender of my body, of ceding control of the only thing that was truly mine, that created a huge rift within me.

There's no denying that I needed professional help with over-coming anorexia, that my self-soothing mechanisms were out of control, and that I was too focused, too fierce, too ruthless, too obsessed. But I think Natasha is right – there was a brilliance and creativity to that energy, and I can't help but think that, had it been channelled into other things, I might have recovered a more complete person. Had I been taught to listen to, cherish and respect my body, rather than being frightened out of it with overfeeding and forced compliance, I might now have a better relationship with it. When medical authorities seized the reins, and I no longer had control of my body, being fully present in it became intolerable, and I think that's where an important connection was severed. It's a connection I've been endeavouring to repair through dance and movement and therapy, but I do believe it needn't have been broken in the first place. Of course, all of this is in the past, and I'm not looking for pity. I have my freedom and my health, and those are all the resources I need to continue my healing journey. My life has been remarkably blessed, and I've been very lucky to have met Natasha and a number of very wise healers and teachers who've helped me to grow into the resilient and hopeful person I am today. I am only musing on the medical system's approach to treating eating disorders. I am wondering, might there be a better way?

Recently, while discussing some of the memories I shared in the early chapters of this book with my dad, he recalled a moment I was not privy to, when I was refusing to cooperate with the programme in the hospital and the doctors were insisting on harsher conditions to get me to comply.

'They wanted to take away all your privileges: no visits from us or your siblings and friends – they were going to cut off all contact with the outside world. They were threatening to take away your books and your possessions to pressure you into compliance. There was a case review,' he remembers, his tone solemn, 'and your mother was determined that you wouldn't be treated like that. So, she brought in all your little art projects – the dolls you made, the cards and I-don't-know-what-else – and she laid them all out on the table in front of the doctors and said, "This is who my daughter is." She was trying to tell them that you were a sensitive, creative soul and needed to be treated as such. Of course,' he adds, shrugging, 'they didn't take any notice of those things. They just frowned at them.'

Dad recalls also, the intense pressure he and my mum were under to commit me to a more aggressive programme, and how frustrated the medical team got when they refused. 'There was one doctor,' he tells me, 'who was brought on to the team for your second hospital stay to back up Dr Nolan, who himself was fed up with us. This new doctor was very angry that we wouldn't sign off on the stricter practices they proposed. He said to me: "There are far sicker, more vulnerable children in this hospital, but she's the one I'm losing sleep over."'

The medical team were exasperated, he says, that so many resources were being funnelled into a patient who was stubbornly undoing all their work. So, when a little while later, the option of sending me to a specialised treatment centre presented itself, and the pressure was mounting for them to commit me to a programme that would actually yield measurable results and take the burden off the hospital, my parents quickly agreed – and you know the rest. For years afterwards, I was angry with my parents for leaving me at the Farm and for not rescuing me from what was a very scary, lonely and at times traumatic experience. I felt utterly betrayed and dismissed by everyone I loved, and I truly don't believe the approach that programme took was ethical. I've forgiven my parents now, because I understand that they'd been boxed into a corner and felt like they had run out of options. I have compassion for the parents and families of any person suffering from an eating disorder, and can understand how clinics that force-feed patients and rapidly restore their physical health must seem like a godsend. I am, also, not too stubborn to admit to the fact that places like the Farm did and do save lives. I'll never truly be able to say what would have happened to me without that kind of intervention. But I am stubborn enough to insist that places like this can cause unseen psychological trauma that will take a lot of therapy to heal, and that there are kinder, more holistic ways to treat anorexia. I also understand that hospitals don't have unlimited resources to spend on slow, individualised treatment, and that that is part of a bigger conversation about mental health care. I do realise that everyone was doing their best, and the medical professionals weren't *actually* tyrannical, power-drunk sadists (apart from that one nurse at the Farm . . . *that* shit was personal). But we must acknowledge that people with eating disorders don't usually *want* to restore their health, because they're not sure their life is worth living, so the medical approach to getting people better and back into the world will not work. I know I've harshly criticised the medical approach to treating anorexia in this book, and I haven't given an answer for the right way to handle it. Truthfully, I don't think there is one way. I think it takes a team of people supporting the physical, psychological, emotional and spiritual recovery of the person. From my understanding, people seeking treatment for eating disorders today in the public health system would be offered a mix of psychotherapy, CBT and family therapy, any of which can benefit someone who commits to recovery. The difficult part is finding the desire and the will to recover within yourself, because it's hard to make progress without that crucial first step. Personally, I know I was lucky to find a therapist I liked, trusted and admired and who helped me find that will to recover buried deep inside and who helped me define and strengthen my commitment to recovery. But even with Natasha, two devoted parents and all the support in the world, my journey to health was messy and I think that each person's recovery will inevitably be a long, complicated and personal journey, beleaguered with setbacks. So I haven't given conclusive answers here because I don't have them either, but I wrote this book in the hope that people might gain a deeper understanding of eating disorders and the kind of sensitive people they consume, and also as a plea to the medical field to treat people in their grip with more compassion, respect and humanity, no matter how young or sick they are.

I am walking along a cliff edge with my mum. A literal cliff edge, that is, in County Clare, on a windy summer's day in August 2020, several days before my twenty-ninth birthday. A six-month dearth of social interaction has triggered an uncharacteristic tactility in me and lulled me into believing that joining my whole family in a remote cottage in the west of Ireland for ten days is a charming idea. I love them, it is nice to see them after a long absence living in London during the lockdowns, of course, but by day two, I am already retreating to my bedroom for hours at a time to bury my nose in a book and breathe deeply as I recharge my rather tiny social battery. My sisters have grown and changed a lot from where I left them in the earlier chapters of this book, having emerged from the terrifying portal of puberty as strong, attractive, empowered women. Emily blossomed into a confident, capable, discerning person, an editor and a devoted mother. She's one of those super-active Dublin mums now, who plays doubles tennis tournaments with her husband, volunteers for community projects and still manages to read bedtime stories to her son. Mairéad is a cool-headed and capable primary school teacher, but elsewhere has maintained her fiery, defiant spirit, which can be glimpsed in the giant blue and purple splotchy bruises battered across her shin bones from the clash of camogie sticks, and in her flame-coloured ringlets, befitting of a formidable Irish goddess. My brother, Patrick, is on the spiritual path, dabbling in shamanism, psychedelics and all manner of alternative therapies. Every psychic he's ever been to tells him he's on his last life, and I don't know what I'll do without him as my buddy in the next life, so will probably have to go ahead and follow him into the next dimension. And my parents are chugging along happily. My dad vanquished his great enemy, the wireworm, many moons ago, and is now churning over a veritable rainbow of healthy crops – potatoes being the linchpin – while my mum is still teaching children with learning difficulties, reading French literature at the weekends and feeding everyone. We all get on from day to day, but as you can imagine, cramming the six of us, plus Mairéad's boyfriend, plus Emily's husband and child, into a country cottage in the August heat can be intense, and the kitchen area is always noisy, chaotic and covered in biscuit crumbs.

I always feel like something of a spare part among my family. It's nobody's fault – I'm always included in activities and my parents make a fuss whenever I'm home, waiting eagerly for me at the airport and filling their fridge with expensive vegan cheeses, but we just have different interests and sensibilities. They like going to hurling matches on the weekends and socialising with the entire parish, volunteering to wash jerseys and host bake sales, while my ideal Saturday involves slathering my skin in luxurious oils and taking a stack of books to my bed to spend the day absorbing moisture and stories. I am also, I confess, very jealous of my one-year-old nephew, for whom monopolising the attention and praise of my parents is an absolutely effortless endeavour, and I find myself getting irrationally frustrated by them cooing over his every moist gurgle, or when an entire dinner conversation devolves into a horribly graphic discussion about his constipation and then a game to figure out what precise sequence of foods might most effectively unblock his Highness.

'I finally finished *Anna Karenina*!' I'd announced to the kitchen one morning, prompting a series of polite murmurs of approval,

but it was nothing compared to the whoops of delight and the celebratory mood that had erupted when, on day three, Charlie finally
offered up a mighty bowel movement. He is obsessed with my mum,
instinctively picking up on her quintessential mammy energy, curling
his pudgy forearms possessively around her neck and glowering
at me. *Enjoy it while you can*, I think, jealously, shooting him back
an angry glare when my mum looks away. *Any day now you'll be a
gangly teenager with spots and body odour, and you'll have to do much
greater feats than poo in a pot to wow them.*

By the weekend, I'd had enough of this usurper's tactics, so I
sweetly invited my mum out on this nice cliff walk, just the two of
us, to catch up, while his Highness is escorted to a farm for the day
to meet some baby chicks.

My mum is much more comfortable, however, in a warm, brightly
lit kitchen, packing mashed potato and carrot concoctions into chubby
little cheeks, than she is adventuring along a pathway on the edge
of a treacherous cliff with the Atlantic Ocean crashing majestically
against its rocky base. She digs her nails into my upper arm as we
walk, an expression of terror etched on her face, convinced I'm going
to fall sideways to my death. Astrology has been my lockdown hobby,
and I enjoy explaining to her that her anxious disposition is because
Leo is in her twelfth house, the house of fears and self-undoing,
and so flashy, daring feats of performance like skipping along cliff
edges are extra challenging for her. I try to get her to take some
cool pictures of me perched atop piles of rocks, but she refuses to
let me out of arm's length, clutching the hem of my jumper as she
leans back to take the picture, and eventually I give up and just take
a few selfies with her on boring, flat terrain, coaxing a smile from
her when I finally consent to resuming our walk several metres in

from the cliff edge. We talk a bit more about books and astrology before the conversation lulls, and I decide now is perhaps my best opportunity to ask her some burning questions about her personal experience with anorexia. I only know the bare facts of her brush with an eating disorder – that she was fourteen, spent several weeks in hospital and was officially diagnosed as having anorexia nervosa – but I don't know where it started and ended, or how such a kind, sweet, maternal woman could have been afflicted by such a viciously mean inner voice. We step carefully across a small stream via some stepping stones, and I ask her what she thinks triggered it for her.

'Well,' she muses, frowning slightly as she steps daintily back on to the pathway, 'I was kind of getting more and more uneasy about growing up and changing, and about the prospect of puberty looming. I was quite frightened of it, and for some reason it was tied up with my relationship with my dad, and my feeling that I would lose whatever "loveability" I had. My older brothers were doing all these amazing things at school, and were clever and funny, and I just felt like nothing I could do would ever be enough again. I felt that the further I grew away from childhood, the more unattractive and – yes – unlovable I'd be. What I knew about adolescence seemed so off-putting and I couldn't identify with it. I had this kind of a high ideal of childhood innocence and sweetness. So then –' she sighs '– I started controlling my weight and it made me feel safe in my body again, and it went from there.' She turns to look at me crossing behind her and gives me a small smile.

'Wow,' I say, momentarily speechless, as I leap over the last two stones and land beside her on the pathway. I am stunned by the symmetry of our stories, at how much her words echo the thoughts I'd harboured as an eleven-year-old, but I am not brave enough to ask if she, too, notices the parallels, so I ask her what recovery was like, and how she got better.

'Well, I spent some time in hospital,' she says, her eyes darting watchfully between the rolling waves and the path in front of us. 'Like you,' she adds. 'We didn't have programmes like Peaceful Pastures, nothing so intensive, and there wasn't as great an awareness about eating disorders back then, but they fed me up again and sent me home. And then I think it was my mam,' she says, looking up now and gazing into the distance. 'She was very determined to get the food in, and she just kept an eye on me and made sure I managed to keep eating. I think it was her efforts that kept me on the straight and narrow. She was very determined,' she repeats, a sad and faraway expression on her face. 'She wouldn't let me give up.'

We walk in silence for a couple minutes, her pondering something private and me thinking about mothers who don't give up on their troubled children, and then I ask her when she thinks she fully recovered, expecting her to say somewhere in the region of six months to two years after hospital treatment.

'Probably . . .' she says, squinting into the sunlight and wrinkling her brow in thought, 'probably somewhere around the age of twenty-nine.'

And that is when I almost do topple off the edge of the cliff in shock.

'Twenty-nine?' I ask, stopping in my tracks to stare at her. 'It took you until you were twenty-*nine*?'

'Yes,' she affirms, with certainty, stopping too. 'Yes, I think it took getting pregnant with Emily to finally give up my disordered eating. It was already manageable by that stage, it wasn't as bad as it had been, but up until then I always kept a very careful eye on my weight and my eating. But that was my big dream,' she says, 'to have a baby.' A happy, dreamy expression lights up her entire face. 'And I wanted to be well for her.'

'Wow,' I say, speechless again, and we lapse into another pensive silence as the waves crash against the rocks, and I think about how much my mum loves babies, and how Charlie will probably always have the edge on me for that reason. I think about how Natasha says we have to upgrade our problems, and about what a brilliant mother my mum became when she channelled the energy that was keeping ano-rexia alive and her small into something creative, brave and abundant.

Circus is my new thing. I have always loved the circus, but my love for going to the circus has equally been tinged with a maddening envy for the performers hurling their strong, painted bodies through the air, making beautiful, awe-inspiring shapes that cause onlookers to gasp. To me, no human on earth is as free as a circus artist; they have total mastery of their bodies without being at war with them; they experience the joys and highs of performance without the trap-pings of fame; they have a home among their fellow performers, but no need of a house or mortgage. Once, on an optimistic whim as a teenager, I downloaded an application form and tried to apply for circus college in London, but when it came to the box requiring a parent's signature, my mother put her foot down firmly.

'Ah, come on,' she said shaking her head, a look of dismay in her eyes as she scanned the form, 'I've let you do a lot of crazy things, but this is the limit.'

I protested for a bit, but I knew I probably wouldn't be accepted anyway due to a complete lack of circus skills on my part, so I folded up the form, glumly accepting circus was for lucky people with a natural glamour and superhuman strength. Later, as an adult, I dabbled every now and then, signing up for an aerial class here and there in LA or London, but it was so extremely, shockingly difficult to perform even the most basic, fundamental moves, like climbing on to the trapeze bar *without* looking like an inebriated sloth, that I always ended up quitting, instead spending my savings on Cirque du Soleil shows all over the world, looking up with painful longing at the dazzling artists performing splits fifteen feet in the air while hanging from flowing red silks, or twirling in a mesmerising, glittery blur beneath steel hoops. But since making it to third place on *Dancing with the Stars*, I've had this curiosity, this urge to find out what else my body might manage to do if only I put my mind to it. I feel sort of sad that everyone in the world can't have a *Dancing with the Stars*-esque experience, where a master teacher trains you in an unfamiliar discipline and believes in you to such an extent that you manage to break through your own limiting beliefs. Personally, I am not about to waste this powerful new outlook on life by sitting at home and counting my missed opportunities, so in early September 2019, I follow my lifelong niggles and nudges towards the circus, signing up to a silks class – and I become *obsessed*. Make no mistake, it is still nigh-on impossible to perform the most basic moves, and the sweat pours down my flaming cheeks as I strain every muscle in my upper body in my efforts to heave myself a mere foot off the ground on to the silks. My negative thoughts interrupt my practice rudely, telling me it's impossible, that I'd be wiser to give up now, go home and read a book, that it was pathetic to imagine my woefully ordinary body could ever manage such impressive feats, but I no longer indiscriminately believe this voice, because I have witnessed my body defy my mind, I've seen it do things my mind was convinced it could not, and I know something I didn't before: that secretly, though we may never discover them all, the body contains miracles. The temptation to follow the negative thought spirals down don't go away, though, and by the end of the first class, when I still have not managed to climb more than two feet off the ground, I appeal to the teacher to examine these doubts.

'Are you absolutely sure,' I plead, sweaty and frustrated, hopping on one foot as I try desperately to extricate the other from a bafflingly complicated series of knots, 'that I'll be able to climb this silk? Are you *sure* there's nothing wrong with me?'

'There's nothing *wrong* with you,' she says, frowning at me with a look of utter bewilderment. 'This is only your first class.' she adds, coming over to rescue me from my accidental tourniquet after I've collapsed on the crash mat, dangling from an ankle. 'You just need to practise, that's all.' She shrugs.

And that's all I need to hear nowadays. I need a circle of positive, radiant people to remind me I can do things whenever the negative thoughts creep back in wagering that I can't. So, I nod determinedly, clambering to my feet again, and grit my teeth as I face off against the silks. By the end of the second class, I manage three climbs of the silks, and I fall back on to the crash mat in stunned disbelief. Above my head, dozens of muscular bodies are doing far more impressive things – piking, splitting and back-bending up by the ceiling's rafters – but I don't care about them, and I just want to leap to my feet and exclaim *'Did you see? Did you see the miracle? Did you see what my useless, ungainly body just did? Perhaps it is not so useless and ungainly after all!'*

In the fourth class I manage to climb all the way up to the ceiling, twenty feet in the air, and I return to the ground, gobsmacked, and reeling with delight, expecting the room to erupt in applause, but they all just continue spinning and contorting with looks of fierce concentration. But no matter; in my head I can hear raucous applause. Soon, I am spending every evening in circus classes, and it is the same hungry, fierce, determined energy I used to use to burn fat from my bones that I'm now funnelling into my passion for circus, a passion that requires a mind-body-soul partnership, and that seemingly involves the perfect balance of strength, beauty, storytelling and pain to keep my inclination towards self-destruction in check. And my new love is too consuming, too exhausting, too fascinating to spare any will towards perfecting my body, which instead requires nourishment and tender care to keep pace with my passion. There are breath-taking mountains to climb now, and I am desperate to see their summits.

It is not just the physical disciplines of circus that soothe my soul, though. There is a community spirit that is warm, welcoming, artistic, idealistic and playful. There isn't the same ruthless competitiveness or focus on aesthetic perfection as I had experienced in the dance community. In circus classes, people arrive in all shapes and sizes, from all backgrounds and all levels of athleticism, but it doesn't matter how vastly the levels vary, because you can guarantee, whatever the experience or fitness of each student, you will be united by one inescapable, levelling factor: pain. Circus remains painful and staggeringly difficult, no matter how good you get. Your body adapts to each new move you practise – again, a miracle – allowing you to climb the silks without sending painful tremors through your shoulders, and forming thick crusts of calluses on your palms so that hanging from the trapeze doesn't feel like tightly gripping a heated curling iron anymore, but once you overcome those agonies, there are fancier ways to climb up on the apparatus, and longer sequences with which to torture your grip strength. And pain is humbling; pain makes you more compassionate. Seasoned students don't become smug or arrogant, sashaying to the front of class to show off, but instead cheer the new students on, showing them trade secrets and tips, sliding a hand here and transferring weight there, because they remember just how hard the first class was, harder than all the others in fact, and everyone is proud of each other for simply showing up.

I quickly become infatuated with the women leading the circus community. Circus women are something to behold. They wear bright eyeliner, tie-dye leggings, T-shirts with holes at the armpits, and have wild messy hair with the odd dread or stripe of pink. Their bodies are decorated with intricate, beautiful tattoos of flowers, vines and mermaids, snaking patterns across their muscular backs and arms and hips. They walk with their shoulders thrown back, their heads held high: graceful, strong, and very much at one with their bodies. There is just something about the circus women I can't look away from, and it isn't even the death-defying drops they spin out of on the silks, or the fearless abandon with which they hurl themselves off a beam at a swinging trapeze; it's that they are totally inhabiting their own bodies. They aren't walking around like dismembered heads, avoiding looking at their flesh in the mirror or controlling it with joyless, restrictive diets. The circus women are endlessly curious about exploring the full strength and capacity of their bodies. And I am utterly enthralled.

I join a hoop class in early 2020. My teacher, Kerrie-Ann, is a petite, beaming redhead sporting pink leopard-print, knee-high socks. The scales of a snake tattoo peek out above her waistband: instant girl-crush material. On closer examination, her hair may not be red at all, but a rainbow of russet, chestnut, bronze, brunette and blonde shades, and possibly some stray scraps of material woven in, but she spins and whips through the air on her hoop too quickly for me to discern the components that make up this sparkling creature. I quickly learn that to hoop is to hurt. You simply cannot know the intimate crevices of the body it's possible to bruise until you have taken an aerial hoop class. The backs of my knees and calves erupt in a meadow of purple and yellow bruises from hanging off the hoop by the knee. Muscles I didn't know were muscles scream across my upper back and shoulders as I focus on grinding my teeth to dust to distract from the effort of pulling with all my might to hoist my weight up to sit in the hoop. Kerrie-Ann shows us an elbow-hang, a neat little trick that, all the same, is not nearly flashy enough to warrant the extreme pain it costs. Screwing up my face and screeching as I pry my fingers off the bar and attempt to hang from the crook of one elbow, I decide that this is as much pain as you can possibly feel in your elbow – short only of amputating it.

At the end of class, we hobble to the centre of the room and wearily stretch out our wrists, forearms and triceps as Kerrie-Ann babbles on about at-home abs exercises that will improve our straddles and remedies for the myriad aches and pains.

'Hot baths, folks, and lots of Epsom salts this evening.' She beams around at the room, and then claps her hands together with finality. 'And now the most important part: give your bodies a BIG hug and thank them for doing all these amazing things you put them through.' And she closes her eyes, wraps her arms tightly around herself and breathes deeply as she takes what looks like a truly divine, lovely, private moment with her powerful body. I glance around, feeling silly and self-conscious, wondering if this is just her quirky little sign-off that we will all carefully ignore, or if all these fully-grown, self-financed adults are going to tenderly hold their bruised old flesh vehicles in a roomful of strangers too, only to see that they do, that everyone around me is lost in dreamy, loving repose with their bodies. A large bald man in the corner even starts to rock himself gently from side to side like a tiny sleeping baby, and it is so gentle, so sweet, that I turn away and start to clammily finger my own forearms. I have just tentatively started stroking my upper arm with an index finger when Kerrie-Ann sighs breathily and calls everyone out of their warm self-hugs, inclines her head and thanks us for showing up to class. Everyone glides towards the changing rooms, pulling on hoodies and wrapping themselves in scarves, but I stand there in the middle of the room, still vaguely stroking my upper arm, feeling bewildered and, for a moment, so, so lonely, because it has been almost three decades of just me and this body, and I am still completely mystified as to how to even thank it.

I climb the steep hill to my apartment with every muscle protesting painfully. *Ow, ow, ow,* my body seems to say with every single step, cranking along like a rusty old tinman, and I find myself answering it, whispering, *It's OK, it's OK, it's OK* under my breath. I notice that I am still stroking my arm, and have been doing so all the way home. I feel a tremendous inner sadness as I rummage through my bathroom cabinets for bandages and ointment to wrap up my blistered hands and slather my bruised knees and thighs with arnica. I collapse on to my couch in exhaustion, and then my eye is caught by the sight of my own hands, curled in my lap. My hands are small and stubby – 'Chubby little hobbit hands,' I huff angrily at anyone daring to call them 'cute' – and now, as I stare at them, they look so much like a child's hands, and I don't know whether

EVANNA LYNCH

it's just because I'm tired or because of the intense physical ache all throughout my body, but suddenly my own blistered, bandaged hands look so helpless, so lonely and unloved, that I start to cry. I stare at these little trowels of mine, that have only ever done their best, that have been doing their best for thirty-odd years, serving me faithfully, keeping me alive and diligently weaving my dreams with their crenulated fingertips, and I cry because even they have not escaped my contemptuous ire. I cry and cry, and it's like something has become unstoppered in me, and suddenly I can't bear how cruel I've been to my body. All these years, I've been treating her as my slave. She's been asking for food, rest, love, pleasure, grace – or, failing all that, plain, simple acceptance. I think of all the times I've denied her those things, and how she has carried on doing my bidding anyway. I think of how, instead of defending my brave and resilient body from the world's hatred, misogyny and criticism, I've instead turned away from her and joined in the chorus of slurs and taunts, easily taking my place as her loudest aggressor. I think of how she keeps going anyway. I think of how hard it is for her to face a world that will gawk at, objectify, deride and dismiss her, make her feel wrong for even existing, and I think of how there is no respite from that spite, even in the silence of her own home.

I have been no better than an abuser, really. Sneering at, heckling and punishing this body. I shuffle to a mirror, still sniffling, and I turn about as I examine the bruises and freckles and blotches and curves and hollows and forks of vibrant blue and purple veins that make up my body, and I don't find it beautiful – I don't know that I ever will – but there is no denying that my body is miraculous. It's eaten when I screamed at it to stop; it's danced when I've scoffed at it to cover up; it's trudged its way home and wrapped itself in a

442

blanket when men treated it like it was disposable; it's struggled on and endured and fought for each breath in a world that demanded it pay for the space it took up. As I look at my body, I think back to a moment, long ago, when I had looked in the mirror as a child and wondered would anyone ever want this odd, pale, freckly creature. And I decide, now, in this moment, that *I* want it; I want this body. I want to inhabit her, enjoy her, care for her, and defend her in this world. And I no longer want to be yet another voice telling her she's disgusting or embarrassing or inadequate or too much. I want to be one of those arresting voices of love and compassion, to offer her a space where she can go to restore, to feel safe, to grow. And I don't want to be another person spreading hatred towards women in a society that has already profited too much from the pain of the female body. One day, not too far in the distant future, this body will be a pile of decaying flesh and dust in the ground. But for now, she's alive and vibrant, and I want to stop hurting her. I want to be the adult in this relationship: to look out for her, to have her back, because, more than anyone else, she has always had mine.

'You'll save more energy –' a polite voice interrupts my silks practice during class '– and get to the top quicker if you use a Russian climb.'

I'm bent double, panting for breath, having struggled up the silks three times in a row, and I look up to see a beautiful young woman with large brown eyes and long, curly brown hair peering tentatively at me from behind a pair of black silks.

'You're doing great,' she encourages, 'but you won't get so tired with a Russian climb. Do you know it?'

'No,' I say, eager for the help. 'Is it hard?'

'No, it's easier,' she enthuses, grasping for her silks. 'Let me show you.' She proceeds to show me the neat little trick of passing the fabrics under one foot and stepping on it with the other to hoist yourself up the silks a couple feet at a time, rather than the French method of spiralling the silks around your shin to secure the foot. (Trust the French to insist on climbing with an unattainable elegance.) It takes me a couple goes to remember where to place my knee and how to pick up the fabric, but eventually I get the knack.

'This so much easier,' I call down to her in delight from the top of the silks. 'Thanks!'

'No problem!' She beams and commences climbing and straddling her own silks effortlessly.

Bruna is her name. We quickly become friends, without having to schedule coffee dates or make plans, because our mutual obsession with circus is such that we keep turning up to the same classes all across London. She is friendly, passionate and obsessive, and has an insatiable appetite for learning that I admire and recognise. She's skilled and strong on the silks, but keen to tell me that it wasn't always this way, and she empathises with me when I am on the verge of crying with frustration over my hopeless straddle climb, admitting she shed tears of joy when she finally managed it. At first, our friendship is based strictly on technical discussions about the muscles required for a straight-arm straddle and precise placements of the hips in performing 'scorpion' to get the most impressive photo of the pose, but soon we find we have an uncanny number of parallel interests. We gab over our favourite Cirque du Soleil shows, over *Avatar: The Last Airbender* and which elemental bending power we'd like to have, and we exchange details of our favourite vegan haunts around the city.

One evening, she sends me a long, loquacious text after listening to an episode of my podcast on the topic of going vegan after an eating disorder, telling me she has 'so many thoughts and feelings' about the episode. She confides that she suffered from anorexia and bulimia herself throughout her teenage years, and admits that she initially adopted a vegan diet, not for the animals, but as an attempt to bring about a sense of balance and order to her eating to replace 'the mad binge-restrict bulimia cycles' that she was stuck in. Soon after, she learned about ethical veganism, which switched the emphasis of her diet from being a device to control her body, to a practice that was mindful, purposeful and helped her to finally heal her relationship with food. Instantly, a lot of things about her make sense – her hypersensitivity, curiosity and obsessive nature typify the kind of character that can easily fall victim to an eating disorder – and it is as if I always sensed she had this creative fire in her that could, if left unchecked, burn her up inside. It's perhaps the least surprising thing I've learned about her, and yet I feel a complicated swell of emotion upon reading her words: a mixture of pride, awe, sadness and joy. Eagerly, I text her back to say that I relate to every word and that, like her, veganism had helped me stop regarding food as a sworn enemy, and instead given me a way to treat it with mindfulness, to see it as a way of nurturing the things I most wanted to protect.

I don't know if you've ever tried to make a new friend – a true friend – while living in the city in your late twenties, but let me assure you it is a *novel* experience, and I am filled with childlike excitement any time Bruna texts or I bump into her shivering in the cold outside an aerial studio. I am invigorated by her presence and inspired by her passion for circus. But there is something deeper to it, too. Watching her gracefully swing her body into stunning shapes on some striking red silks, or taking in her excitement about a new fantasy series she's just discovered, or hearing the passion in her voice as she argues for legal recognition of animal sentience, I find myself utterly gripped by her, because she is reflecting back to me all the things I love about being alive. Her very presence is an affirmation of consistently choosing the path of creativity – and she is vibrant with it.

Bruna and I make plans, outside of classes for the first time, to see the Cirque du Soleil show *Luzia* at the Royal Albert Hall, where we sit and gaze up in awe at the acrobats, aerialists and contortionists hurling and catching each other's bodies through the air with stunning grace and apparent ease. The seething jealousy I once had for circus performers has simmered down considerably ever since I started participating in the community, and now I'm able to watch and admire their work with a deeper appreciation for the pain and discipline it requires. If you spot it, you've got it, and all that – there is healing that happens when we reclaim lost parts of ourselves that we find reflected in others. After the show, Bruna and I make our way to a nearby bar, rhapsodising about the performers and both vowing to train harder at silks and to push our bodies to perform greater feats.

But we have much to talk about beyond circus, and it seems the more questions I ask Bruna, the more surprising and fascinating a person she becomes. I listen in quiet awe as she talks animatedly about the events of her working day. She works as a researcher testing the effects of psilocybin, or 'magic mushrooms' as they're more commonly known, in a series of clinical trials on people with conditions such as depression, anxiety, PTSD and eating disorders. She is describing, her eyes wide and shining with excitement, a session where she supported a patient through a six-hour trip, when the barman interrupts our conversation to point out the late hour and prod us in the direction of the door. We part ways, and I make my way to the tube station marvelling at this interesting, complex new friend of mine, whose depths I've only just begun to fathom. I feel as amazed by her as I do by the Cirque du Soleil acrobats. She has so many interests and passions, and she flings herself into them with the same wild abandon and determined focus as the acrobats in *Luzia* leaping between the Russian swings, but it strikes me that she almost chose a very different path, arguably the one of least resistance. She could have chosen to stay small and in control of her nature, rather than letting it unravel all around her in many different, dizzying unprecedented directions. I think of Bruna, working in a lab testing out psychedelic drugs on people with depression and anxiety by day, and pulling herself up sky-high silks by night. I think of Natasha, who similarly spent years numbing her immense talents with anorexia and bulimia, and now spends her days helping people heal generations of ancestral trauma and deal with every manner of existential grief. I think of my mum, who nurtured a quieter, softer, though no less galvanising dream of becoming a mother, and how she now spends her days patiently working in a small classroom where nobody will witness and applaud her Herculean efforts to teach children with learning difficulties to try their best and to believe in themselves. And I think of all the young girls and boys I met at the Farm with that same fire raging behind their eyes that they had no idea how to handle except to turn it inwards on themselves.

My thoughts wander all the way home. I recall one of my recent conversations with Natasha, where she reflected on a moment when she felt utterly sure of her place in the world and knew her purpose in life was to heal people.

'. . .That's why I started doing this work: because it was the very first time in my life where *I* disappeared. My ego totally dissolved when I was in front of a client. I remember my first client like anything. She was bulimic, and it was like a carbon copy of my eating disorder. And I was maybe just a *page* ahead of her on the journey, maybe just a chapter, so it was so simple. I literally saw her as me and it was where I disappeared in service to something greater, you know, and it was just beautiful – so that's what began it for me. And I think, in gratitude for that, something then connected to me. Now I know what that is: it's grace; it's presence.'

I think that state of grace and presence Natasha describes, of finding a connection to something greater, is what people with eating disorders need most. I think they have to find a burning, beautiful dream to inspire within them the courage to leave their small, safe, dark place. I struggle to maintain that connection. There are many things that light me up and cause my ego to melt away in moments. Cats. Nature. The stars, the moon. Laughing with friends. Dancing. The circus. But I find my greatest sense of connection and purpose and presence, as I always have, in stories. I feel most alive and in love with life when I am a part of a story, be it in reading it, in telling it or in sharing it with others, but I struggle, when the stories end, to feel connected to something greater – and I still struggle with this creative path. Some days, it does not feel worth it. Some days, I just miss the safety of getting as low as I could get, physically and emotionally. I miss the security of being my own biggest bully. To dream is to hope and to hope is to leave yourself vulnerable to being hurt in many ways.

I don't think it's fair to say that people who died of anorexia didn't fight their illness. I think they fought it for as long as they possibly could. There is something heroic about people who manage to get up every day and somehow stay alive with their most vicious, hateful bully living within them. I don't think it's fair to judge them or term their entire journey a defeat. But I don't think they took the right path. I think they took the path of numbness, certainty and safety, and I think it was the safe choice cost them their life. I think the safe path always leads to a dead end.

Bruna and I meet each other again, unexpectedly – but unsurprisingly – on the first day of a new circus term outside an acrobalance class.

'I tried to sign up to silks,' I explain to her, 'but it was all booked up, so I figured I'd give this a try.'

'Me too!' she says, and we beam at each other.

Acrobalance class is sweaty, stinky and thrilling. I quickly discover that clambering up the backs of men to stand atop their shoulders is a *wildly* erotic experience, and make plans with Bruna to rent out dance studios and do extra acro practice where we will take turns to step all over unwitting male participants. We challenge each other to try out riskier versions of the moves that the teacher demonstrates, and alternate between being the flyer (standing on top of a person) and the base (being stood upon). In general, in acro class, people of corresponding sizes pair up, but these pairings don't always work out perfectly, and the etiquette of circus dictates that it is impolite and cowardly to refuse to 'base' someone simply because you're afraid your shoulders can't take their weight. When the students loiter nervously on the edges of the group while the tall, stocky students are looking to 'fly', pixie-sized teachers pipe up that they've based burly men twice their size. So, when a man with legs like tree trunks sidles shyly up to Bruna and I and politely asks are we up for helping him fly, I shoot Bruna a nervous glance and she responds with a swift, determined nod. I stand in a wide, stable stance, foot to foot next to Bruna, and set my face in a warlike grimace. The stocky gentleman deliberates nervously a moment or two, evidently sizing us up and questioning the hidden power in women's soft bodies, but then I feel a clammy foot use my hip as a foothold, and the weight of a small building seems to press down upon me. The foot jams itself on my shoulder then, and I concentrate very hard on my breathing and chance a glance at Bruna, who is tomato-red, a vein pulsing terri-fyingly in her temple, her every muscle trembling with the effort of allowing this giant man the feeling of being a nimble fairy – and I *love* this! I love having a body that can do unprecedented things, and I love the duality of standing atop men and feeling like an all-pow-erful sea-witch *and* of being climbed on by big, hairy, lumbering giants and feeling in my bones that my body is a miracle. And, just as it feels like my feet are going to start sinking into the stone floor beneath us, our passenger steps daintily down using hips and thighs as stepping stones, and we all high five each other as Bruna and I try to conceal the heaviness of our breathing. When no one is looking, I turn away and give my shoulder a quick, secret kiss. I may never be the kind of person who shakes her butt on the internet and declares her love for every square inch of it, and after so many years of being my body's most passionate hater, it is difficult to reconcile myself as her lover. But I can be her friend.

Our teacher calls the class to the centre of the room and announces we're ready to move on to two-person towers, with just one person on the base and the other person standing on their shoulders: a considerably more precarious feat than a three-person tower. To demonstrate, the teacher asks for a volunteer to fly with him as the base, and most of us shrink back nervously – he is well over six foot in stature – but Bruna's hand shoots up instantly. The teacher instructs us to position ourselves all around him in a circle and raise our hands protectively in case she falls. A circle of the tallest people closes in around Bruna as she climbs with tentative grace up to our teacher's shoulders and slowly, carefully rises to standing. Her jaw is tensed and her eyes fixed dead ahead in absolute concentration as she wobbles slightly and then manages to balance with no hands. I step back a few paces, realising my arms are not needed here – Bruna doesn't fall – and I look at the circle of hands raised around her. It looks for a moment as though they are worshipping her. I look up at her, standing high above, and it strikes me then how her energy is very much the opposite to an eating disorder. How wild and dazzling she is. She, with her experimental psycadelic work, her silks classes, her boundless energy and insatiable appetite to experience the most thrilling, unusual and sensuous pleasures life has to offer. She could have played it safe and stayed small and never left home and not taken the wild, unpredictable, oft treacherous path of dreaming and daring, or she could be here, standing tall, proud and brave: this wild, free, curious, mysterious, miraculous woman.

Afterword

I've always admired butterflies. Even as a child, before I could articulate my desire for freedom, beauty and colour, I was captivated by these tiny silken creatures that visited my dad's vegetable garden every summer. They inspired me to look up at the sky and dream about the magical places whence they came. Soon, I discovered that they didn't originate, as I'd imagined, in a faraway land where glittering rainbow-coloured streams flowed through grassy riverbanks and fallen petals arranged themselves around small furry bodies, lifting them skywards, but that they seemingly popped into being one day, crawling as teeny caterpillars out of a neat cluster of shiny, dandelion-yellow eggs. Their capacity for transformation was even more awe-inspiring than the idea that they were actually magic: that these wriggling, wiry tubes could pack themselves into crusty little cocoons, dissolve their own bodies into an amorphous pile of mush and then re-emerge in an entirely new shape, pulsating with life as their blood was pumped through new vessels that animated a radiantly patterned, utterly splendid set of wings that would bear them dancing and floating away on a gust of wind. They shared their colours and beauty with me for only a few moments, fluttering across my vision as I surged forwards on a swing, and I'd whip my head around to catch another glimpse of their dance before the glare of sunlight made me clamp my eyes shut. When I opened them again, the vision of loveliness was already gone. But I was always grateful that they visited, and that they left me with a sense of wonder and hope.

As I grew up, I continued to love and look for butterflies. I bought books about them with intricate scientific drawings, and I stuck posters on my wall depicting arrays of species native to certain regions. I liked surrounding myself with images of butterflies everywhere I went, on journals, fridge magnets, even a small tattoo on my left forearm. For me, they were symbols of transformation, freedom and beauty. I needed only look at them to feel my spirits lift with an inexplicable sense of hope. One of my favourite authors, Vladimir Nabokov, is also famous for his legacy as a lepidopterist. Like any Nabokov fan, I was enamoured by the whimsical loveliness of the photos of this big, learned man lumbering with a net in the wake of tiny, delicate butterflies on the wing. His famous statement: 'Literature and butterflies are the two sweetest passions known to man' made me sigh with pleasure, and I started reading more about his contributions to the field of lepidopterology and admiring his drawings of his beloved Karner blues.

And then, one day, while poring over a dense, beautifully illustrated book about butterflies, taking in the stunning array of polychromatic wings and speckled bodies, I suddenly noticed, for the first time, the sharp pins piercing the insects' perfect forms. In each photo, I saw a butterfly impaled by a gleaming silver spear. Once I had seen the pins, I could never again unsee the hidden violence of butterfly hunting. How had I not noticed it before? I shut the book abruptly, feeling sure that this could not be how butterflies were collected, that something so beautiful and enchanting as preserving the bodies of these tiny, wonderful creatures could not require so brutal a sacrifice. It could not be that someone could claim to love these mystical creatures and confess to killing them in the same breath. I rifled through the pages of the books in front of me, scanning for descriptions of the process of mounting and preserving butterflies, or of the fatal moments right before – and then I found it in a letter Nabokov himself wrote to a magazine when coordinating the type of photos to accompany an article on his butterfly-collecting exploits.

There is a special professional twist of the wrist immediately after the butterfly has been netted which is quite fetching. Then you could show my finger and thumb delicately pinching the thorax through the gauze of the netbag. And of course, the successive stages of preparing the insect on a setting board have never yet been shown the way I would like them to be shown.

There it was, a delicate 'pinching' of the thorax, the butterfly's life squashed tidily out between a thumb and fingertip as though it were an accident. The pictures in the books of hundreds of insects impaled on pins did not look like tributes to their beauty any more, but fatalities of their perfection. Somehow, distracted by the enchanting images, gorgeous bodies and dizzying patterns, I had never noticed that preserving perfection demanded so high a price. Their delicate bodies are frozen in mid-air and in time by a pin, and their radiance will never dim, but there is something undeniably sinister about pinching out a life to steal its beautiful corpse. I think of butterflies gleaming tragically on their pins, and of women who waste their unfathomable depths and limitless creativity – and eventually whittle themselves away to nothing – hunting for perfection in their own bodies. And I think maybe I'm better off not spending my life pining and hankering for the transient and useless fantasy of feminine perfection. Maybe perfection isn't for women at all. Maybe it's just for butterflies on the wing. Or flowers. Or drawings of women, or photos of women, or maybe even the briefest, most fleeting *moments* of women. Maybe actual women are always, in their fullest expression, bodies, not ideas or images or dreams of them, and maybe every body changes when we choose to fully live our lives. And maybe I will live a happier, wilder, more colourful and unpredictable life if I can finally abandon the debilitating and brutal pursuit of perfection. If I can learn to love butterflies from afar, and watch them fly away.

Acknowledgements

In *Goddesses in Everywoman*, Jean Shinoda Bolen writes: 'To make a dream come true, one must have a dream, believe in it, and work toward it. Often it is essential that another significant person believe that the dream is possible: that person is a vision carrier, whose faith is often crucial.'

I've been very blessed to have encountered many people who have been vision carriers for *The Opposite of Butterfly Hunting*, and without whom there would be no book.

Catherine Maguire and Amy Kiberd carried the vision for this book years before I dared mention it to anyone else. It took a profound stretch of the imagination to believe in this project for long enough to help me overcome my monumental resistance to writing, but they refused to let me off the hook and their consistent faith has been life changing.

To Catherine – my wise and radiant fairy godmother: you said many moons ago that writing a book was like giving birth and then took it upon yourself to be this book's midwife. You probably thought nine months was a generous estimate for a book's gestation period and didn't expect to be trapped in the metaphorical labour

ward for such an abominably long time – for that, I am very sorry.
Thank you for your patience with me and your determination to see
this book to completion. Thank you for being the first person to insist
I could and should write when there was very little to go by. Thank
you for the unparalleled generosity with which you offer your time
and energy, and for tempering my meltdowns with your boundless
wisdom and wicked sense of humour. I truly don't know where I'd
be without you as a teacher, a friend, and an example of a woman
standing in her sovereignty, though suffice to say I'd be quite lost.
They say the second birth is easier.

To Amy – my most magical of friends. Thank you for sharing
your gift for conjuring bold dreams and beautiful visions, ever since
I was little, sitting by you on the hammock listening to your fairy
tales. I feel very lucky to be related to you because if I wasn't I'd
have had to stalk you until you became my friend. Thank you for
the hours and hours you generously gave towards outlining and
refining this story, and for your certainty that it could be turned
into a book. Thank you for your professional opinions on crafting
the proposal and for looking out for my best interests. Thanks for
being the ideal writing partner and for motivating me with your
commitment to your stories – I can't wait for the rest of the world
to get to read them. And thank you for being the Flo' to my Go'. He
is much more manageable thanks to your influence, and I do actually
quite enjoy baths now.

To Rory Scarfe – my amazing agent, for your endless positivity,
support and guidance through this process, and for not recoiling in
horror when I sent you a very graphically detailed chapter about a
smear test, and then for somehow managing to get a book deal out
of it. I'm still horrified I sent you that, and marvel at your agent

wizardry in convincing some very important people that a heap of chaotic rambling had potential to be a book. Thank you for being so kind and enthusiastic about my writing when my confidence was in short supply, for holding the vision of the book and for knowing when I needed a push.

To Sarah Emsley – I could not imagine a more wonderful editor, and you know I have a very active imagination. Thank you so much for being the person who officially made this lifelong dream come true and for having absolute belief in it from the very beginning. Your confidence in this book was exactly the burst of energy I needed to throw myself into writing it. Thank you also for your total willingness to delve deep into some dark issues, for your sensitivity and deftness in helping me manage that voice and for making sure I kept sight of the brighter vision for the end of the book. I've heard other writers express regret for launching their literary career with a memoir, that starting out with their most precious, private story was a mistake; I feel precisely the opposite, that this was the best way to get into writing and I would not change a thing. I'm so grateful and glad I got to take this journey with you. Thank you for your patience with my very loose understanding of the term 'deadline', for allowing me the time I needed to finish it and for somehow getting it over the finish line. Phew.

To Erin Kane – thank you so much for believing in my writing and for sharing your enthusiasm and encouragement so generously. The letter you wrote to me after our first conversation was like a compass through some of the hardest writing days that helped me believe my words would resonate with others and that it would all be worthwhile. Thank you also for the kindness and sensitivity you brought to the edit, and for softening the text in places without removing its teeth.

To Mum and Dad – first and foremost, for putting up with me. Thank you for your unconditional love, and for fighting for me even when I was fighting against you. Thank you for supporting this book and for your bravery in letting me share these most private memories. Thank you also for your feedback on the early drafts and for sharing your own memories and reflections which added some much needed context and perspective. Mostly, thanks for being the two kindest people in the world and for always being there.

To Emily and Mairéad – thank you for your incredible generosity in letting me keep in some very sensitive, personal anecdotes from childhood. I know you like a quieter life and I've asked a lot of you, so thank you so much for seeing the bigger picture of this book and for helping me to tell this story properly. Thank you for invaluable feedback and for being such excellent big sisters too.

To Patrick – my fellow seeker! Thank you for being one of the first to read the book and for helping me navigate preparing the rest of the family for it. Thanks for the deep chats and friendship, for being a weird child too and for making sure I'm not the only one Mum worries about.

To Natasha – I wonder do many people know there's a genuine goddess living deep in the Irish countryside. Anyway, I'm glad I found you and that you opened your arms to me all those years ago. There really aren't words to express the impact you've had on my life, how you've inspired and shaped me. I know how lucky I am to have been one of the thousands of people you helped, and to continue to learn from you. Thank you for giving your time to be interviewed for this book and for such an eye-opening conversation about the treatment of eating disorders which afforded valuable insights into the philosophy behind your approach, and helped me crystallise my own ideas on effective, ethical treatment.

To Georgie Polhill and Tara O'Sullivan – for your painstaking attention to detail and for working to some *very* tight deadlines at all hours of the day and night and for never once pressuring me to work faster. Thank you for your expert eyes, your sensitivity and tact in delivering notes, and for finding ingenious ways to make the text flow better. Thank you for noticing parallels and patterns I didn't see and for finding one perfect word in places where I tried to use twenty.

To Dr Gareth James – thank you for reading this book with both your heart and your head. Thank you for your astute comments and suggestions that helped craft the text into a more mindful and, hopefully, illuminating book about mental health. Thank you for validating some of my hunches on effective treatment and for your passion for improving the system for individuals struggling with their mental health. I hope that more doctors will follow your lead.

To Meryl Evans – thank you for your insightful and thorough legal advice, for protecting the book and me, whilst ensuring my truth and feelings still rang out clear – not an easy balance. Thank you for your diligence and ingenuity in getting there.

To Vicky Beddow and Jess Farrugia – thank you for how hard you work to bring books and their readers together and for bridging the gap between writing books and selling them. Thank you for being so patient with my fussiness, and for your creativity and sensitivity in finding the most articulate way to communicate the message of this book.

Thank you to everyone at Headline who works tirelessly to pull all the threads together to make such beautiful books, and for your legacy of storytelling. Thank you for the care and precision you put into every detail of creating my book.

To Amy Fitzgerald – thank you so much for very early conversations about the book and for helping to develop it in its seedling stage. I'm sorry it took me so long to get my act together, but I hope you know how much your encouragement and guidance helped.

To Siobhan Hooper and Patrick Insole – thank you for all your care and attention to detail, and for your intuition and patience in finding exactly the right look and feel for this project.

To Lucy Rose – thank you for sharing your stunning gift to create a cover that was more beautiful and haunting than anything I could have imagined. It's a picture I'll never tire of admiring and I'm so honoured to have it wrapped around my story.

To Derek – thank you for firmly insisting I write this book and for helping me get my shit together enough to start. Thanks for the tough love, and all the delicious food.

To Sheva, Ricky, Samira, Geri and Alice – thank you for being so supportive of this journey and for allowing me to fully commit to the writing process. That support has been invaluable.

Thank you to The ChickPeeps community for being so spangly! Thanks for supporting this book and for being such empowered, compassionate, thoughtful activists. Your idealism and energy for animals inspires me.

Lastly, thank you to all the fans who have cheered me on while working on this and who are somehow still paying attention to my endeavours a decade after all the noise and excitement died down. Thank you to every person I've met who shared stories of their personal struggles and who prompted me to think deeply about my own past. Thank you for reminding me I had wisdom of my own to bring to this conversation, and for asking difficult questions – this book was my attempt at answering them.